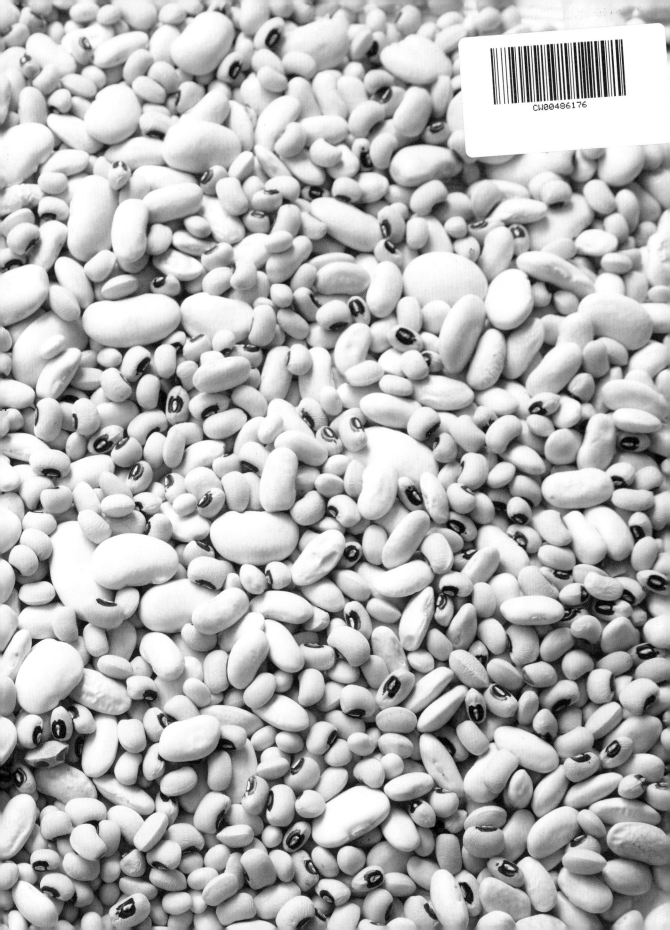

CW00486176

JENNY CHANDLER

PULSE

Truly modern recipes for beans, chickpeas and lentils
to tempt meat-eaters and vegetarians alike

Photography by Clare Winfield

PAVILION

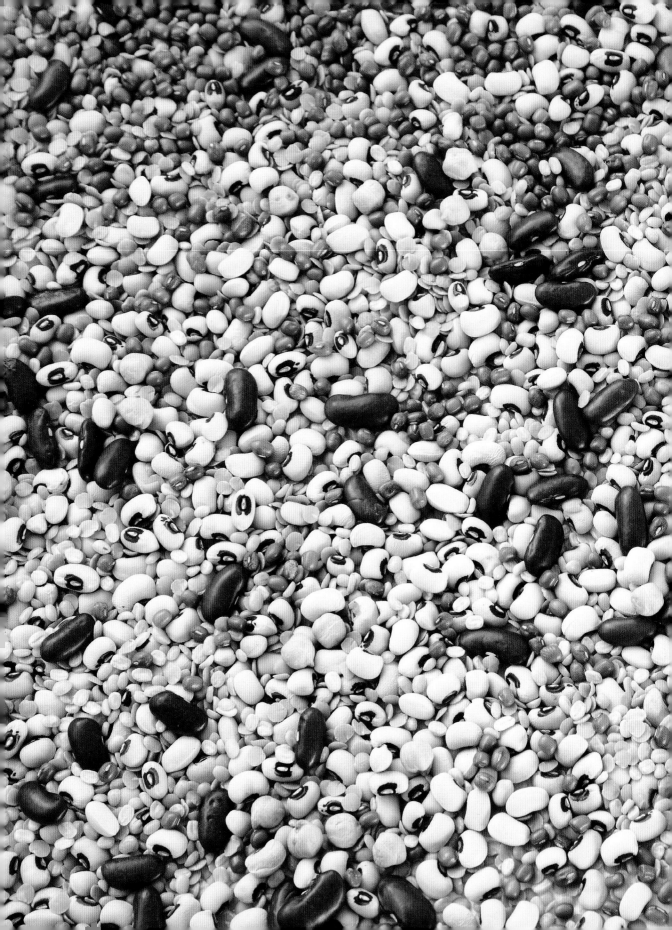

CONTENTS

INTRODUCTION

Pulses, or legumes, are some of my favourite things to eat, and that's after a year and a half of cooking and consuming them almost every day. Yes, you would hope that I'd be passionate about my subject, but my family had no choice in the matter as they became my guinea pigs. So you just can't imagine how thrilled I was when, after months of legume exposure, my six-year-old daughter opted for the Syrian lentils on a restaurant menu. The exciting thing is that beans, chickpeas and lentils offer such incredible scope, from the comforting creaminess of Italian chickpea soup to the zippy freshness of edamame, crab and noodle salad. You need never tire of them. Legumes are some of the most versatile, delicious and rewarding ingredients in the kitchen. I want to eat pulses firstly because they taste fabulous; all the other plus points, and there are so many of them, come as a bonus.

I discovered legumes in Spain as a teenager. My only previous experiences were tinned baked beans and the ubiquitous 1970s' kidney bean, green pepper and sweetcorn salad. Spanish dishes such as nutty brown lentils stewed with smoked chorizo and melt-in-the-mouth haricot beans with Catalan butifarra sausage were a revelation, a million miles away from the hemp-shirted hippy image that pulses still suffered back home. Where the British saw legumes as a vegetarian domain, the Europeans bathed them in pig or duck fat in celebrated meat fests such as Spain's fabada and France's cassoulet.

At last the pulse has emerged from its tie-dye teepee. Beans, chickpeas and lentils are still the mainstay of many vegan and vegetarian diets, but attitudes and styles have changed. Plant-based food has become so varied and exciting with all the Mediterranean, Middle Eastern and Asian influences we enjoy today, it's worlds apart from the wholemeal bean flan of old. Legumes can be stars in their own right and not just a meat substitute. Why stuff beans in a moussaka when you could be eating a classic Greek vegetarian dish, *gigantes plaki*?

Nowadays many great restaurants, such as London's Ottolenghi, Moro, Petersham Nurseries, Polpo, St John and Leon, serve up wonderful legumes. Who would have believed that the humble lentil could become trendy? But then camping has dumped its nylon-cagoule image and reinvented itself as glamping, and even that swirly kaftan of your mother's has become boho-chic. I believe our passion for pulses is much more than a fashion. The pulse is real food, it's here to stay, and here's why.

Most of us are reassessing what we eat for a number of reasons, the first being money. Reducing what you spend on food needn't mean buying cheap junk food, it just requires some planning and good recipes that you actually use. Pulses are remarkably cheap, especially if you buy them dried – but if you're short of time, even canned pulses are very economical. Gingery dal with a spiced tarka tipped over the top, served with some rice or flatbread, is one of my favourite suppers ever and it costs a matter of pence.

I'm not vegetarian but, like so many people I know, I am eating less meat. Instead of having cheap meat every day, I'd much rather eat more expensive but better-tasting meat once a week, or in smaller quantities alongside my pulses, knowing that the animal it came from was healthy and well-treated. Enjoying fabulous legume dishes, packed with plant-based protein, comes with no sense of deprivation and is quite simply more environmentally friendly. Fish is a treat, but there are sustainability issues too and it can be very pricey. However, you can savour a small but exquisite, carefully sourced bit of seafood with some filling legumes and feel perfectly satisfied. By cutting down on the meat and fish you eat, you are doing your bit for the planet too.

Pulses are, without a doubt, wonderfully good for you and, with cases of obesity reaching record levels, we really do need to rethink what we're consuming. I love food and I love cooking, so I quite naturally gravitate towards simple unadulterated ingredients. Legumes, whether dried, canned or frozen, are just that; you know what you are getting. It's up to you whether you prepare them as an indulgent feast or as a healthy salad.

Millions of legume dishes are cooked every day. Pulses are a staple in much of the developing world and they have played a vital role in the Western diet for centuries too, so every continent, country and region has its own classic ways. This book is not a collection of the most traditional or even the most famous recipes (I know that I will have offended many a bean enthusiast by omitting their local dish), but an eclectic mix of dishes using accessible ingredients that I love to cook, share and eat.

Many of my friends, and the students on my cooking courses, seem rather lost when it comes to pulses. They have only a few ideas up their sleeve when it comes to preparing them at home. This book should help you decide what to buy from the ever-increasing selection of pulses on offer in health food shops, delis and supermarkets. More and more households have mixed eating habits too, so it's useful to have dishes in your repertoire to keep the vegetarians and, with some minor tweaking, the carnivores happy too. I aim to demystify all the soaking and cooking conundrums – legumes really are a cinch to cook. Above all, I hope these recipes will inspire, get you cooking and leave you, quite literally, full of beans.

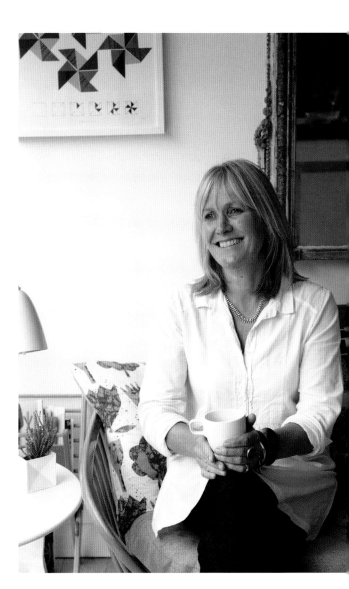

THE POWER OF THE PULSE

One of the great things about eating legumes is that you can feel good about yourself in body, mind and spirit. It's not just that these little wonder seeds are fantastically nutritious and packed with healthy fibre, they could help us save the planet too. While I'm determined not to leap on my soapbox, it is really important to realize just what valuable and under-exploited ingredients pulses are.

WHAT'S IN IT FOR ME?

Nutritionists are increasingly seeing pulses as one of the great weapons against obesity, diabetes, heart disease and cancer. Pulses have plenty of good complex carbohydrates loaded with fibre. They are relatively high in protein, low in fat and packed with nutrients, especially iron, calcium, zinc, potassium, and B vitamins.

Carbs and fibre

Starchy carbs (as opposed to the sugary ones) are the body's healthiest source of energy and should ideally supply about half of our daily calories.

Foods with high levels of fibre are not just filling at meal times but also make you feel full for much longer, so that you're unlikely to dive into the biscuit tin within a few hours of eating. This satiated feeling is closely linked to the speed at which our blood sugar levels rise and fall after eating certain foods, which are measured on the glycaemic index (GI). Pulses have a low GI, meaning that they produce a steady rise and equally steady fall of blood glucose levels instead of the peaks and troughs that have you snacking. So, eating plenty of pulses is incredibly helpful if you want to lose weight or simply maintain a healthy diet. Pulses can also be significant in preventing or managing type 2 diabetes.

While the fibre slows down the absorption of sugars, it also speeds up the passage of food through your body, accelerating the removal of toxins and excess cholesterol and keeping you regular, reducing the risk of colon and bowel cancer.

High protein

We all need protein in our diet: it's one of the building blocks of the human body, in our nerves, tissues and bones. It's necessary for growth and repair and the production of hormones, enzymes and even the antibodies that fight off viruses, bacteria and toxins. Pulses can provide the highest levels of protein in the plant world.

Proteins are made up of amino acids, some of which our bodies are able to make themselves and nine of which we need to absorb from our food. Whereas meat, fish, dairy and eggs can provide all nine of these amino acids, pulses lack one of them, methionine. Soya beans are the only exception: they are a source of 'complete' or 'high quality' protein. However, in one of those miracles of nature, grains, nuts and seeds can provide the last piece of the jigsaw. There's no need to consciously combine these ingredients within a meal, it's just a question of eating a varied diet with a good mix of these protein sources, particularly if you are vegan or vegetarian.

Low fat, no cholesterol

As most of us are aware, pulses can be a very important source of protein – but many of us eat plenty of protein anyway. However, increasingly, we're all being encouraged to substitute some of our meat and dairy intake with legumes. Dairy and meat products contain varying levels of saturated fat and cholesterol while most pulses are low in fat (and most of that's unsaturated) and are cholesterol free. Soya beans and peanuts are the exceptions, being higher in fat, but that's predominantly unsaturated 'good' fats. Our bodies need cholesterol but, to put it simply,

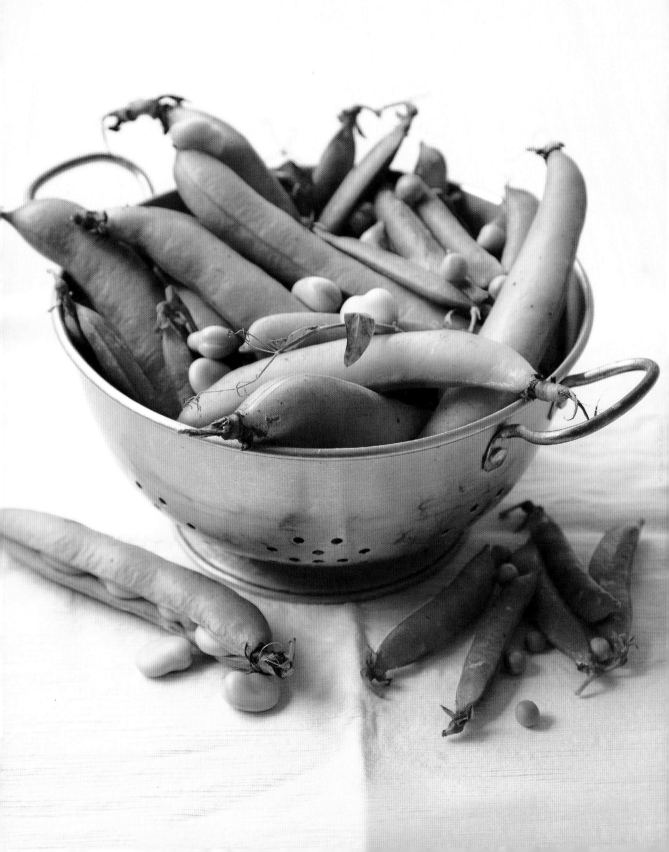

there's good and bad cholesterol; saturated fats are loaded with bad cholesterol that can clog up your blood vessels. By cutting back on saturated fats, you can reduce the risk of strokes, heart attacks and all the other forms of cardiovascular disease.

The other fats to avoid are the trans fats found in much processed, and commercially fried, food. These hydrogenated fats play havoc with cholesterol levels, so go for natural oils and fats with your beans and eliminate trans fats altogether.

The low-fat/high-fibre credentials of the legume make it a good contender for a weight-loss diet: filling and low fat, what could be better? Just remember to watch what you eat your pulses with and maybe halve the number of sausages in the casserole!

Minerals, vitamins and the rest of the good news

Legumes are good sources of calcium, magnesium and phosphorous, which are all vital in the formation and health of bones and teeth, especially critical during childhood and adolescence. These minerals are also required for muscle function, blood clotting, nerve reactions, normalizing blood sugar levels, lowering blood pressure and maintaining a healthy immune system.

Pulses have healthy levels of potassium, which is particularly helpful in lowering blood pressure, balancing out the negative effects of too much salt, and helping the kidneys work more efficiently.

Legumes are high in zinc, crucial for a healthy immune system and healing wounds; it's also said to improve fertility and libido. Many of us absorb a large proportion of our zinc from meat, so if you are vegetarian, do make sure that you eat plenty of pulses, nuts and seeds.

Pulses do contain plenty of iron, a particularly important consideration for vegetarians. However, unlike the more accessible iron found in meat, this 'non-haem' iron is more difficult for the body to assimilate, so you will need to combine your legumes with foods rich in vitamin C in order to absorb it

effectively. No problem, as long as you are eating some fresh vegetables or salad alongside your pulses – and don't underestimate the power of a good squeeze of lemon juice or a generous sprinkling of fresh parsley.

Pulses are good sources of many B vitamins, which help convert carbohydrates into energy. Folic acid, or folate as it is also known, is essential for healthy red blood cells; it is probably best known for reducing the risk of central nervous system defects (notably spina bifida) in unborn babies. Niacin is another important B vitamin that helps the body produce hormones and is also believed to lower bad cholesterol.

Fresh peas and beans are high in vitamin C, which protects the body against respiratory infections, skin diseases and cardiovascular problems.

Pulses are now recognized to have many other health benefits too. They contain antioxidants that help to neutralize free radicals (chemicals that damage cells in the body and lead to ageing and disease). The saponins found in pulses may reduce your risk of cancer and are also thought to prevent cancer cells from multiplying if you are already suffering from the disease. Saponins are also believed to stimulate the immune system and reduce high cholesterol levels.

So, in a nutshell (or pod)

Legumes are fabulously healthy things to eat. We are constantly being advised to eat more food from plant rather than animal sources. A helping of pulses counts as one of the recommended five-a-day fruits and vegetables we should all be consuming. They're filling, will stop you snacking, and can help to prevent obesity, diabetes, heart disease and cancer.

SAVING THE PLANET

Eating less meat

Pulses have an indispensable role to play in replacing meat as the primary protein source in the developed world. We simply can't continue, with a rapidly rising world population, to consume as much meat as we do. Meat and poultry production is having a devastating effect on the planet. This isn't some hairy-hippy theory: the facts were laid bare in a report named 'Livestock's Long Shadow' by the United Nations Food and Agriculture Organization (FAO) in 2006.

The FAO estimates that world livestock production is directly responsible for about 18% of the global greenhouse gas emissions contributing to global warming. World meat consumption quadrupled in the last 50 years and is set to soar with both the increased global population and China's newly awakened appetite for meat. Mark Bittman, a *New York Times* journalist, cites that 'it takes 2.2 calories of fossil fuel to grow 1 calorie of corn, but it takes 40 calories of fossil fuel – in the form of land use, chemical fertilizers (largely petroleum-based), pesticides, machinery, transport, drugs, water, and so on – to produce 1 calorie of beef'. It's just not sustainable.

There's the deforestation factor too, as vast swathes of rainforest are being cleared to make way for grazing land and crops to feed farmed animals. When do we stop? At current rates, there just won't be any forest left for future generations.

As animals are packed into factory farms to feed the growing demand for meat, the crowded conditions can propagate disease, which in turn leads to the greater use of antibiotics, vast amounts of which are excreted into our land and water. Not only the animals themselves but we too are developing increased antibiotic resistance. So, even ignoring the monstrous immorality of this type of farming, we have to recognize the negative impact.

As the Meat Free Monday Campaign set up by Paul McCartney and his daughters points out, each of us really can make a difference to the future of the planet by changing the way we eat, even if it's just cutting out meat for one day a week. So, although I'm not about to become a vegetarian, I am eating much less meat and more pulses. I'm not interested in meat analogues: they're highly processed, and why would I want a fake beef burger when I could be eating a fabulous homemade bean burger? Another area of research and a possible food of the future is '*in vitro*' meat, understandably described by some as 'Frankenfood'. This 'shmeat' is actually muscle flesh that's grown in a lab and has never been near a complete living animal. I'll stick to my beans, thanks!

Enriching the land

As well as being high in protein, pulses have yet another string to their bow. Our ancestors realized their miraculous powers. Not only can one little bean spring into life and provide you with a bountiful harvest, but the plant will actually enrich the soil – legumes have been used in crop rotation for thousands of years.

Leguminous plants are nitrogen fixers, which means that they can, with the help of soil bacteria called rhizobia, convert nitrogen gas from the atmosphere into the nitrogenous compounds required for their growth. So, no need for expensive or environmentally damaging fertilizers and, left to mulch back into the land as 'green manure', better nitrate-rich soil for next year's crop too.

THE WIND FACTOR

'*Gli amici sono come i fagioli. Parlano di dietro.*' 'Friends are like beans. They talk behind your back', goes the Italian proverb. I'm not sure about the 'friends', but as the saying shows it's widely accepted that pulses give you wind. Well, there had to be a downside and as far as I'm concerned a bit of flatulence is a small price to pay for all of legumes' plusses.

Legumes contain certain indigestible carbohydrates, the most troublesome being the oligosaccharides, that can't be dealt with by the digestive enzymes in the stomach. So these carbohydrates pass through the upper intestine largely unchanged and are finally fermented and broken down by harmless bacteria in the lower intestine. This rise in bacterial activity results in gas. There's also the high-fibre factor: if your normal diet is low in fibre then a sudden rise will cause gas too.

There are many ways of reducing the flatulent effects of pulses, the simplest being allowing your body to adapt gradually. The idea is to begin eating small quantities of legumes regularly rather than suddenly having a bean feast. I do feel a bit guilty about this, as we recently had a party when I decided to try out not one, but five bean dishes and even finished off with some black bean brownies. A great friend, who'll remain nameless, did call the next day and comment that the meal hadn't been an ideal precursor to a first date.

Some beans result in more gases than others, with soya beans, butter beans and haricots being the worst offenders (in that order). The Old World lentils, split peas and smaller beans such as mung, moth, adzuki, have the least repercussions, with chickpeas, favas and the rest somewhere in the middle. So maybe start off with the gentler pulses if wind is really a problem.

When I cook pulses from scratch, I throw away the soaking water but am not prepared to change the water during the cooking process as some cooks recommend. You do wash away some of the oligosaccharides but you also lose many nutrients, antioxidants and flavour. I'd rather have a bit of gas.

How to reduce the gas

There are a number of herbs and spices that are added to the pot with supposedly carminative properties, but the main thing is to make sure that your pulses are well cooked: intact, but soft and creamy within; undercooked pulses can unleash a whirlwind.

A piece of dried kombu seaweed (available among the Japanese ingredients in many supermarkets and health food shops) is placed with the beans as they soak and cook. The seaweed provides some seasoning too, and a packet will last for months.

A few leaves of fresh epazote or a teaspoon of dried (which I've found in my local Mexican shop and can be tracked down by mail order) are added to Mexican beans. Wind aside, the epazote adds a wonderful herbaceous flavour to the pot.

Asafoetida, also known rather ominously as devil's dung or stinking gum, is the Indian solution. Just don't stick your nose into a bag of the raw spice: flatulence will undoubtedly seem a better option. How anyone decided to put asafoetida near their food in the first place is baffling, but it miraculously transforms to a mellow garlicky flavour as it cooks.

Other herbs and spices that are said to reduce wind are turmeric, cumin, ginger, fennel and sage.

And if all else fails, there are certain over-the-counter remedies available from health food shops and pharmacists that can be taken with your beans. The most widely available is called (and it has nothing to do with Dennis the Menace) Beano.

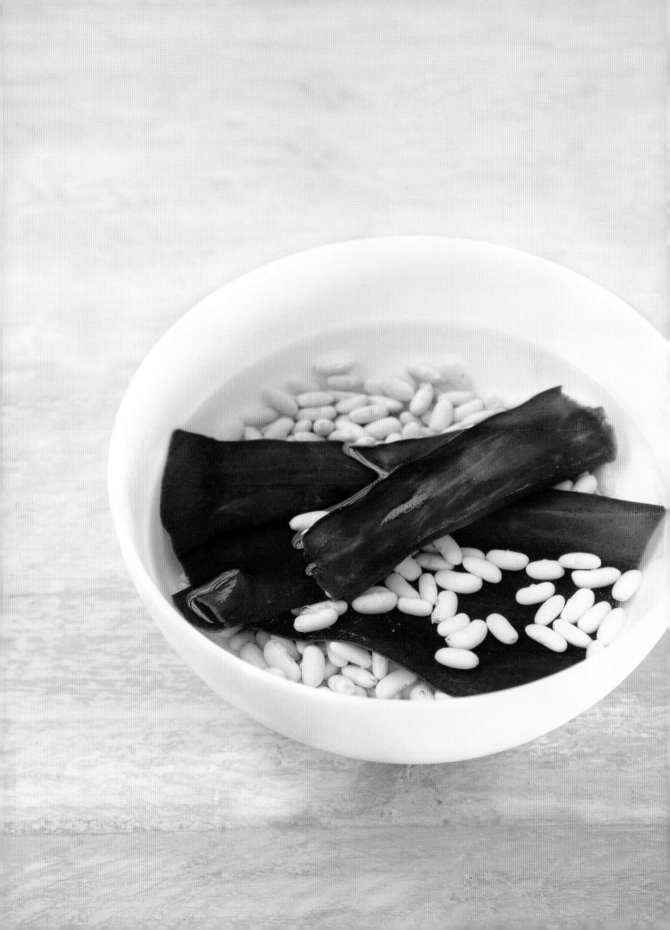

ALL YOU NEED TO KNOW

HOW TO BUY:
FRESH, CANNED OR DRIED?

The great thing with legumes is that you have a tremendous amount of choice, not just in the varieties available but also in the time and energy that you're prepared to spend on them. Fresh green peas and beans can mean a satisfying podding session while watching the tennis, or alternatively a quick dip into the freezer; dried pulses can entail hours of soaking and slow glub-glubbing over a low heat – or may be simply a matter of opening the can. Dried and canned pulses are fabulous storecupboard options as they keep for months and are among the most versatile ingredients in the kitchen.

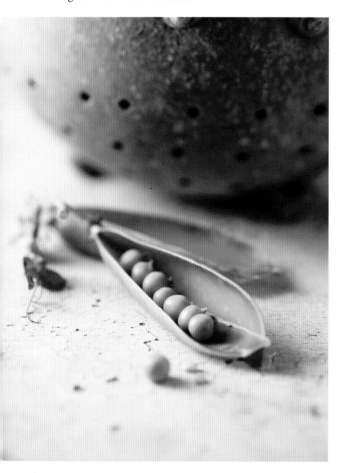

Fresh and semi-dried

Peas and beans fresh from the pod are best eaten within hours rather than days of picking; they're an absolute treat but are not available very often, so I'm happy to opt for frozen most of the time.

Meanwhile fresh mangetout and sugarsnap peas are available year round and add a bit of welcome green crunch to a salad or stir-fry. Edamame (soya beans) are increasingly popular; you can find the frozen, slightly larger beans in most supermarkets while you may have to go to an Asian store for the immature fresh, or frozen, pod-on beans.

Italian borlotti and cannellini beans are the most famous of the mature, semi-dried beans that are sold in their pods, but there are others too, such as the *pochas* of Spain's Rioja region and the *coco blanc* of France. Seek out firm, full-looking pods where the beans inside will be large and mature. Pod and cook them as soon as possible.

Canned

My cupboard is always stocked with a selection of canned beans and chickpeas. They really are the ultimate convenience food. We're not talking baked beans (although I do have a few of those too); I mean the unadulterated cooked pulses. Before you buy, check that there's no added salt or sugar; there really doesn't need to be anything but pulse and water. Some cans may contain antioxidants such as metabisulphite or firming agents like calcium chloride; avoid these if possible. You will need to rinse the beans thoroughly to get rid of the rather claggy water, which does smell rather unappetizing.

Canned pulses taste great, are highly nutritious and will undoubtedly save you time and energy. The downside is that a good-quality canned pulse will cost up to four times the equivalent home-cooked dried pulse by weight. But if you're catering for one, you could argue that all the power used during the prolonged cooking will offset the saving in any case.

While I'll happily buy canned chickpeas and beans, lentils are another story. Dried lentils require no soaking, cook in about half an hour, have a much better texture and flavour when home-cooked and cost half the price. Need I say more? For similar reasons, I rarely buy canned mung, adzuki or black-eyed peas, but they do take longer to cook than lentils, so I'll excuse you once in a while.

It's worth remembering that a 400 g/14 oz can of beans contains, on average, about 250 g/9 oz of drained beans.

Dried

There's something rather meditative about dipping your hand into a sack of dried beans and letting them cascade through your fingers. It's a common sight in markets in the traditional bean-eating nations, where discerning customers are literally weighing up the value and quality of the pulses before they buy. Pulses should feel relatively heavy (a light bean could be last year's or, worse still, a weevil-infested hollow shell). Uniform size and colour are sought out too. The skins should be taut with no sign of a wrinkle. When inspecting a bean, the hilum (in effect its little navel but often referred to as an eye) should be bright and never show any brown or yellow discoloration.

For most of us, this careful selection process is irrelevant; we simply pick up a bag from the local supermarket. Recently supermarkets have given much more thought, time and shelf space to legumes, in response to more widely recognized need for healthier eating, and I'm pleased to say that the quality and range of beans on offer has generally improved too. I no longer seem to come across beans that take a lifetime to cook (a sure sign of a 'has been' that's spent too long in a warehouse). The other advantage of supermarket pulses is that they have been well cleaned and sorted, so you're less likely to come across an unwelcome pebble. My local health food shop has a fabulous range of organic legumes and advice on sprouting, cooking and combining.

A trip to a specialist Spanish, Italian, Middle Eastern, Indian or other ethnic store is a great way to source exciting and very good-quality legumes. Once you've tasted a *blanco lechoso* chickpea from Spain or an Italian Castelluccio lentil, you'll realize that there are some real treats to be had, a little more extravagant than your average pulse but a snip compared to a good cheese, fillet of fish or meat.

Dried pulses can be incredibly good value: a bag of beans doubles in weight, at the very least, once cooked. But you do need a plan: legumes really only work for the budget-conscious cook if you prepare larger quantities. The idea is to get in the habit of boiling up a decent-sized pot of beans and using them over a few days in various different recipes or even bunging a few in the freezer.

Cleaning and sorting dried pulses used to be a time-consuming ritual, and still is in some countries. Nowadays most of the pulses we buy have been shaken and stirred, through a thorough cleaning process, to get rid of tiny bits of gravel, sticks and insect. I'm still slightly neurotic about checking through my legumes after a rather disastrous dal experience back in my yacht-cheffing days. A rogue 'rock', as the irate Aussie engineer put it, was responsible for some serious molar damage, which in the dentist-free waters of the Indian Ocean led to a rather tense atmosphere onboard. So I usually take the precaution of tipping out my beans onto a white tray and shuffling them, a few at a time, up to the opposite end of the tray. It's a good idea to give your pulses a good rinse before soaking or cooking to get rid of any dust or dirt: many are low-growing plants, so the odd bit of soil is often inevitable.

TO SOAK OR NOT TO SOAK?

It is entirely possible to cook pulses without any soaking at all. In Mexico, arguably the epicentre of world bean appreciation, there's no tradition of soaking the beans. Pulses just go in the pot with, or without, a few aromatics and perhaps a bit of fat and there they bubble away until tender and toothsome. So why not do the same?

Well, for one thing, dried pulses can take hours and hours to cook – depending on both their age and variety. The Mexican market does a brisk trade in beans, so while their beans are probably in their prime many of ours are likely to be distinctly older and will take an absolute age to cook if they're not soaked first.

While legumes require no attention at all during their overnight soak, a bubbling pot does demand a bit of hovering about. I want to keep the cooking to a minimum to save both energy and my time. A soaked bean cooks through more evenly, allowing the centre to become creamy and soft before the skin and outer flesh begin to collapse.

Finally, and most importantly, soaking is believed to improve our ability to absorb the wide range of nutrients found in beans. Washing away some of the phytic acid and the wind-induing oligosacharides makes the pulses more digestible whilst reducing any flatulent effects too (which we look into further on p.10).

There are two main ways to soak your beans:

The overnight soak

This is the way to get the most smooth-textured, evenly cooked beans. Place your beans in a large bowl, with about double their volume of water. Leave to soak overnight at room temperature (unless it's very warm, in which case they'll need to go into the fridge or another cool place, otherwise they can ferment and become rather whiffy). Drain before cooking.

The quick soak

I think of this as the 'resort to' option when you've forgotten to get ahead or you've just decided what to cook. It seems to me to require a bit more faff. Place the beans in a large pan and cover with plenty of water. Bring the water up to the boil and then remove from the heat and leave the beans soaking in the hot water for an hour. Drain the beans and start cooking.

Soaking and cooking times

The table below suggests the optimum soaking times and approximate cooking times. These may vary in individual recipes. Broadly speaking, the smaller the pulse, the less time it takes to soak and cook. I do give smaller beans a short soak as it cuts down the cooking time and seems to result in fewer split skins and more evenly cooked results.

No soak	Optional short soak: 2–3hrs	Recommended short soak: 2–3hrs	Long soak: at least 4hrs	Long soak: at least 8hrs or overnight
Lentils, split peas, split beans (often known as dal), moth beans, mung beans Usually cook in 30–45 minutes	Adzuki beans, black-eyed peas Usually cook in 30–45 minutes	Chana dal (split chickpeas), pigeon peas Usually cook in under 1 hour	All the New World beans: butter beans, lima beans, haricots, flageolets, kidney beans, black beans, borlotti, cannellini and pinto beans Usually cook in 1–2 hours	Peas, fava beans, chickpeas, soya beans Usually cook in 1½–3 hours A pressure cooker will cut the cooking time. Or perhaps add a pinch of bicarbonate of soda (see opposite)

COOKING FROM SCRATCH

Why bother cooking your own legumes rather than simply opening a can? It's not just about saving money, or being able to track down some of the more highly prized and elusive varieties. When you prepare your own pulses, you can ensure they reach the perfect creamy texture, as well as enhancing their flavour with herbs, vegetables, bones and fats. There's the added bonus of the cooking liquid, too; this wonderful stock provides the base of many soups and stews. So don't tip your bean water down the sink – it's full of nutrients and flavour.

Cooking dried pulses requires nothing more than a bit of patience and a large pan. There are a few very general rules to follow.

Cover the pulses (soaked if necessary, see opposite) by just a few centimetres (an inch) of water, otherwise you will leach away much of the goodness. Colour, flavour and valuable nutrients are lost if you use too much cooking water. You will need to keep an eye on the beans as they cook and add a splash more water from time to time as required (just enough to keep the beans covered). Spanish cooks swear by adding chilled water to 'shock' the beans, helping them retain their skins, while in Mexico scalding hot water is the answer. My advice is not to get caught up in all the bean dogma. Cooking beans really isn't rocket science.

Begin by boiling your beans for about 5 minutes. Red kidney beans require 10 minutes of boiling, to ensure that their high levels of toxins are deactivated (see p.263).

Reduce the heat to a very low simmer: too much turbulence and you'll lose the skins and end up with a mushy mess. Cover the pan and check occasionally that you have enough water. The simmer can take anything from 30 minutes to 3 hours or more, depending on the size, variety and age of your pulses. In general, the no-soakers take about half an hour, the quick-soakers under an hour and many of the long-soakers under two (see opposite). Your beans should, in true 007 style, be shaken but not stirred from time to time to ensure that they are not sticking (stirring will break them up).

Salt Adding salt to the water is reputed to toughen the skins and lengthen the cooking time, although nowadays many scientists are making the opposite claim. I stick with tradition as I find that early salting can give a mealy texture to the pulses. So, season the beans once cooked; it's easier to gauge how much salt to add at this stage. Pulses do cry out for seasoning otherwise they can seem bland, so I usually add at least 1 teaspoon of salt to 1 kg/about 2 lb of cooked beans.

Bicarbonate of soda Many cooks suggest adding bicarbonate of soda to the cooking water, especially if you live in an area with particularly hard water (with high concentrations of minerals). There's no doubt that the skins do soften more quickly and the whole cooking process is speeded up, but at what cost? You will reduce the nutritional value of the beans considerably and sometimes end up with a rather soapy flavour. I only resort to baking soda with marrowfat peas and fava beans, which can take a lifetime to cook otherwise.

Acids and sugars These will stop the beans softening quickly, so tomatoes, molasses, wine and other sweet or sharp ingredients should usually be added only after the beans have cooked. This can be used to your advantage when you want to add cooked beans to casseroles and bakes without them collapsing. Such is the case for Boston baked beans (p.224), which bake for 3–4 hours and still retain their shape and texture.

Are they cooked?

A cooked bean should remain intact but the flesh will collapse into a creamy pulp when you squash it in your fingers; if there is any slightly granular texture, it needs more cooking.

Split lentils will collapse to a velvety purée, larger lentils will become soft and lack definition, while smaller lentils will hold their shape but should squash between your fingers or they will be mealy.

Chickpeas will hold their shape even if they lose their skins, but do check that they are slightly creamy when squashed and have lost their starchy dry centre.

Pressure cookers

Pressure cookers can dramatically reduce cooking times, and I find them very useful for cooking chickpeas, whole fava beans and marrowfat peas.

However, with most pulses I'd only bother with the pressure cooker if I was really pressed for time. Beans do have the propensity to collapse if they are a little overcooked and it's impossible to gauge what's going on inside the pot. If I do use the pressure cooker for my precious beans, I reduce the recommended cooking time considerably, using the pressure cooker as a kick-start and finishing off the cooking with the lid off. Lentils and split peas are ready so quickly that they're better just simmered in a saucepan.

Timings will vary according to the model of your pressure cooker. Nowadays they come with extremely comprehensive instructions, but if yours is an ancient family hand-me-down that looks like something from the Ark, then you'll have to take some ancestral advice.

Only half-fill the pressure cooker, as beans do expand and froth up; adding a tablespoon of oil to the cooking water will reduce the foaming.

Slow cookers and crock-pots

Cooking your beans long and slow can give delicious results, but there are a couple of things to keep in mind before you begin. Smaller beans (short-soak varieties, see p.14), lentils and split peas are ready so quickly that you might as well cook them conventionally in a pot on the hob. Chickpeas, marrowfat peas and the bigger beans are better suited to the crock-pot.

It's wise to boil beans for a few minutes before putting them in the slow cooker. This is an absolutely vital step in the case of red kidney beans (see p.263) otherwise toxin levels can increase during the cooking.

Gauging cooking times is tricky – there is no way of telling how old your beans are. Check bigger beans after about 4 hours (even on the lowest heat setting) and then at 30-minute intervals thereafter.

This method is ideal for Aga owners too. Start your beans off on the top, cover the pan and place in a low oven. Begin checking after about 4 hours.

Things to add to the pot

Herbs It is often an idea to cook up a plain batch of pulses that can sit in the fridge and be used as a starting point for all sorts of different dishes. I can't resist adding a few herbs to the pot, though, and find that a small muslin bag, rather like a lavender bag that I've stitched up rather crudely, is ideal and can be used again and again. I slip in a few sprigs of thyme, rosemary, sage leaves, parsley or whatever takes my fancy, tie it up with some string and leave it in to simmer along with the beans. You could gather up a little Dick Whittington-style bundle out of some muslin if you don't own a needle and thread (Nigella suggests a pop sock, but I'm not sure I can face that). Once the beans are done, you hoick out the bag and don't have to faff about picking out little twigs or shards of rosemary. Empty, rinse and hang up your little bag (or pop sock!) and you're ready for next time.

Vegetables Many recipes call for a base of chopped, lightly cooked vegetables (known as a *mirepoix* in France or a *soffritto* in Italy) to set the beans on their way. Dice equal quantities of onion, carrot and celery and fry them in a little olive oil until beginning to soften before adding the beans and water. And you can never go wrong with a few peeled and bruised cloves of garlic thrown into the pot. I use this method for all sorts of beans, with the herb bag (see above) thrown in too, but do keep in mind that – because of the onion – they will sour after a couple of days, so not ideal if you're cooking the weekly pot.

Stocks, bones and fats Many bean dishes call for some pork fat or ham bones to be thrown in with the beans. You can fry off your vegetables with chopped bacon or good-quality lard (see p.162) to add flavour. In some recipes, you can use chicken stock to cook the pulses if you require more depth of flavour. I tend to prepare pulses this way only when I'm cooking a particular dish for a crowd. It gives the beans a distinctive character but they will not keep as long as plainly cooked beans and are not quite so versatile.

To reduce gas Pulses can cause flatulence, there's no doubt about it. In the big bean-eating cultures, certain herbs and spices that are meant to reduce wind are added to the pot (see p.10). It's rather a tricky thing to gauge but I like to think I'm doing some good.

MAKING YOUR PULSES SING

This book is packed with recipes from all over the world, from chefs and home kitchens. There are many combinations that I've put together over the years and I do hope that you will feel inspired to throw together your own creations too. There are a few general points to keep in mind.

Pulses are wonderfully versatile because they provide a subtle base where other flavours shine, so you must add plenty of seasoning. I add salt to legumes once they're cooked. Even if you're trying to reduce your salt intake, you'll be consuming considerably less salt in your diet if you're cooking your own food rather than eating processed food.

As well as salt, I like a bit of pizzazz, be it black pepper or chilli heat, the kick of mustard or wasabi or the zippy ting of ginger. Bring life to your beans.

Some bean dishes taste flat and flabby and they're just screaming for fresh acidity. Citrus juices – lemon, orange, lime – and vinegars (some, like balsamic, have sweetness too) to the rescue. Tamarind paste (see p.247) and pomegranate molasses are wonderful ways of delivering the sweet/sour balance.

Sweet flavours play a vital role in many kitchens, particularly South-East Asian. You will find that they highlight the savoury flavours. Try adding palm sugar, jaggery, honey or maple syrup.

Beans, chickpeas and lentils are fantastically good for you because they are packed with fibre and very low in fat, but they taste terribly worthy and dull until you throw some fat into the mix. This might be healthy fat such as cold-pressed rapeseed oil or extra-virgin olive oil, or it could be butter, pork or duck fat. The fact is – you won't eat much of the fat because the pulses are so filling, and quite honestly it's got to taste good otherwise what's the point?

STORING COOKED PULSES

People are often put off cooking legumes from scratch because of the time involved. However, preparing pulses in larger quantities can save you both time and money. It's just a question of getting into a regular pattern. Soaking is hardly a stressful business: it's not like you need to watch your beans as they swell. The simmering pot doesn't need much attention either, it can bubble away while you cook Sunday lunch, read the newspapers or watch a film.

If you prepare a potful of pulses, you have the basis for numerous meals for the week. It needn't seem repetitive, I promise. Taking chickpeas as an example, you could have hummus (see p.30) for sandwiches, Moroccan chickpeas and meatballs (see p.208) one day and Punjabi chickpea curry (see p.187) later in the week. Borlotti beans could turn up in a soup, a lunch box salad, a Tex-Mex chilli, and then reinvent themselves as a creamy mash. Cooked pulses are so versatile that having a supply of them in the fridge can mean an easy supper on the table in minutes.

In the fridge Simply cooked pulses will keep in their cooking liquid (which is a wonderful stock too) in a covered container for 5–6 days. Let them cool thoroughly before popping them in the fridge. Ladle out your beans and/or liquid as required.

Beans that have been cooked with onions, meats, stocks, bones or fats are best used within 3 days.

In the freezer Freezing legumes has been a revelation to me. It makes sense to freeze a few when you cook up a large pot. It's up to you whether you freeze them in or out of their cooking liquid, both methods work.

Usually I just freeze them in their cooking liquid in medium-sized bags that will be ideal to whip out for a side dish, a jar of hummus or a fabulous purée.

I've also had good results from draining the beans, laying them out on a tray, covering and then freezing them. The frozen beans can be transferred to resealable plastic bags so you can help yourself to as many as you want.

PERFECT PARTNERS

With the exception of soya beans, most pulses don't contain all the essential amino acids that provide us with the 'complete protein' we need to survive. However, the missing amino acids can be found in many grains, seeds and nuts. Combining legumes and grains is vital for vegans and vegetarians who are looking for non-animal sources of protein, and it's also important for anyone trying to lose weight, reduce cholesterol or eat a higher-fibre diet.

It seems incredible that the ancient vegetarian cultures of the world can have understood the miraculous effect of combining pulse and grain – and yet the classic combination of dal and rice or bread has sustained the vast Indian Hindu population for millennia. Similar pairings can be found all over the world: Mexican beans and tortilla, Caribbean rice and peas, Middle Eastern lentils and rice, even hummus – the combination of chickpeas and tahini in which the tahini's sesame seeds provide the missing amino acid. Baked beans on toast are the most regularly consumed example of a pulse and grain pairing in Britain.

You don't have to eat your legumes and 'partners' at the same meal – on the same day is fine – but the combinations of texture and flavour are great anyway.

Many of the recipes in the book quite naturally combine pulses with a complementary source of protein, but the following – by no means an exhaustive list – may help when planning salads and side dishes, so that you really get the most out of your legumes.

Bread

Most of us consume a large proportion of our cereals as bread, made from finely ground grains, commonly wheat. I do love a bit of white bread, such as baguette, ciabatta and a good old English bloomer. These breads are delicious alongside a soup and toast up beautifully for crostini – and, for me, pitta just has to be white. However, wholegrain breads contain so many more nutrients, not to mention the fibre. So by all means vary the bread that you eat, but as a general rule try to choose wholemeal loaves or flatbreads, or the traditional sourdoughs that often contain spelt and rye.

Rice

White rice, particularly **basmati**, is fabulous in fluffy pilafs and alongside many a vegetable curry, but when it comes to most salads and side dishes, the chewier texture and nuttier taste of a wholegrain **brown rice** is often preferable. There's obviously the nutritional upside too, with all the bran and germ intact.

Brown rice and, my absolute favourite, **red Camargue rice** are easy to find nowadays. Both take about 35–45 minutes to cook and lack white rice's irritating propensity for clogging and sticking.

Wild rice is a *very* distant relation of Asian rice; it is a wild grass that grows around the edges of lakes and rivers. Most of today's wild rice comes from around the Great Lakes of North America, and it is cultivated commercially in Minnesota. With its almost smoky depth of flavour and a really good chewy texture, I love to add wild rice to pulses. One problem I often encounter with vegetarian food is a lack of something to chew on and wild rice provides the answer. But do cook the grains until they begin to burst, which will take about 45 minutes, otherwise it's like having a pile of pine needles on your plate.

Whole grains, groats and berries

The whole grains of **wheat, barley** and **spelt** (farro), often known as groats or berries, can scream of those rather worthy salads that look like something ready for the guinea pig cage. However, when combined in a perfect balance of pulse, vegetable, dressing or sauce with plenty of aromatic flavour, they are truly delicious. You'll find these whole grains in health food shops, ethnic stores and, increasingly, in supermarkets.

It's a good idea to soak these whole grains for a few hours, or overnight along with your beans; this will not only speed up the cooking time but will make them easier to digest too. Cook them as you would your beans: put them in a pan with plenty of water or broth, bring to a boil and simmer until tender (you may need to top up the water as they tend to drink it up). This may take anything from 45 minutes to 2 hours.

Pearled grains

Pearl barley and **pearled spelt** are having a bit of a renaissance at the moment and quite rightly so. They have a wonderful nutty texture and flavour and are quicker to cook than the whole grains: simmer for between 20 and 40 minutes. The only downside is that the 'pearling' process removes the germ and bran, so you lose nutrients and fibre from the grain. However, if you're combining the grains with pulses packed with fibre and loads of fresh vegetables, you've got little to worry about.

Cracked or rolled grains

These are super-convenient since, as well as being smaller than the whole grains, they have often been parboiled or steam-treated so that cooking times are minimal. These are the ones to go for when you're throwing together a quick supper with a can of drained beans, a few veg and herbs. I love to use **bulgur wheat** and **couscous** as salad ingredients and accompaniments to moist, stewy meat or vegetable dishes.

Cracked wheat, or bulgur wheat, is highly nutritious since it includes much of the original bran and the germ of the grain. Bulgur is best known in tabbouleh, the Turkish fresh herb salad, and will usually need only about 10 minutes soaking in boiling water or on a low simmer. Cracked wheat has not been parboiled and will take longer to cook.

Traditional couscous takes hours to prepare and cook, but the commercial couscous we can buy today is often quite simply a matter of adding boiling water or stock. Barley couscous has an extra dimension of flavour and lots of fibre, while the **giant Palestinian wholegrain couscous** can add amazing texture as well as nutritional value.

Millet

We in the West tend to think of millet as little more than birdseed, but it's one of the world's most ancient cereal crops. It has been a staple in central India for thousands of years, although wheat, which is seen as a more versatile ingredient, has recently been taking its place. Millet is gluten-free, leading to the characteristic flat roti breads of India. In America and Europe, with rising levels of gluten intolerance, it's those gluten-free credentials that are drawing more attention to millet.

Try dry-roasting it in a pan and then adding just under twice its volume of water or stock. Cover and simmer for about 15 minutes, then switch off and leave the lid on for 5 more minutes. Fluff up with a fork and use in place of couscous.

Quinoa

Not a cereal but the seed of a plant closely related to spinach. Quinoa is the Spanish spelling of an ancient Inca crop with the name *kinwa* (and that's how it's pronounced too). Quinoa is often hailed as one of the world's 'superfoods' as, unusually among plant foods, it provides a complete protein. And, while I don't get too caught up in calculating my daily intake of vitamins and nutrients, it is wonderful to eat something that tastes great and is really good for you too.

Quinoa is fabulous in salads, and can basically be substituted in most recipes for couscous or bulgur wheat with obviously different, but delicious results. It is incredibly easy to cook: boil in water, stock or fruit juice for 15 minutes until each seed plumps up to reveal its own little halo.

Nuts and seeds

There are many other ingredients that can supplement your pulses, ensuring that vegetarians and vegans have a good protein intake. The following nuts and seeds are particularly valuable: **sesame seeds, sunflower seeds, pumpkin seeds, Brazil nuts, cashews, pine nuts and pistachios.**

Oats

While they might make a wonderful nutritional partnership with pulses, I just can't imagine a stodgier combination! However, you don't need to consume your perfect partners at the same meal in order to obtain your complete protein. So eat a good bowl of porridge in the morning, or snack on oatcakes before your lentil soup, and you'll have a seriously high fibre intake as well as that necessary protein.

SPROUTING

Until recently, the only sprouted bean you were likely to find outside specialist health food shops was the bean sprout (a sprouted mung bean) in your Chinese stir-fry. The myriad of other fabulous sprouts such as peas, chickpeas, lentils and peanuts were considered the domain of the earthy folk.

I have to admit, a few years ago I'd have been as likely to take up macramé as sprout my own legumes. But why not? As children we all witnessed the wonders of nature with a tray of cress on the school window sill. Sprouting is like an instant vegetable patch. It's so easy, cheap and ridiculously exciting, not just for toddlers but for frustrated would-be gardeners with no land to nurture or no time to dig. All you need is a large jar. You don't need to clutter your kitchen with trays of stagnating, damp cotton wool or to invest in a smart, tiered sprouter (although I do have one, and find it great when I'm after a bumper crop).

There's nothing new about sprouting: the Chinese have been doing it for thousands of years. Sprouting beans, nuts and seeds were grown aboard Captain Cook's ship to help ward off the scurvy that took so many sailors' lives in the eighteenth century. And in the First World War, sprouts were fed to British forces on the front line when fresh fruit and veg were unobtainable.

Today many nutritionists believe that consuming raw, living food leads to better digestion, higher energy levels and even rejuvenation (oh, yes please). Once sprouted, a seed has far higher levels of vitamins, proteins and minerals than in its dormant state. So those little sprouts that look and taste so good have entered the realms of the 'superfood'.

Sprouts of all kinds are magic sprinkled on top of almost any salad, adding amazing texture and flavour. In fact, they are one of the few salad ingredients that my six-year-old daughter actually seems to relish. Try adding a handful into a sandwich or a stir-fry too.

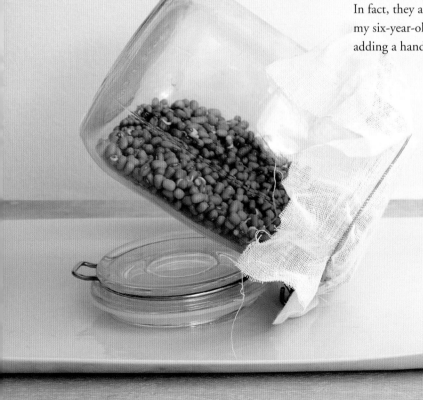

How to sprout

The simplest way to sprout is in a glass jar; I use a Kilner jar, which come in various sizes. Soak your pulses, nuts or seeds in the jar, in plenty of cool water, for a few hours. This is when the seed comes back to life.

The sprouts need to breathe, so secure a piece of muslin with an elastic band over the end of the jar. (I've read that some people use micromesh tights, but that really doesn't appeal to me.)

Carefully tip the water out through the muslin and allow the pulses to spread out along the length of the jar.

Leave the jar at an angle to continue draining onto a tray (this is where the lid of a Kilner jar forms a perfect stand). Place the jar somewhere at room temperature, out of direct sunlight.

Now all you need to do, leaving the muslin in place, is fill the jar with cool water, give it a swirl and drain your beans at 12-hourly intervals until they have sprouted.

Once the sprout is as long as the seed, it's time to tuck in, but you can leave it to grow longer if you prefer. Sprouting times will vary according to the age of your seeds and your room temperature, but you have a rough guide on p.22.

Storing

Give the sprouts a good final rinse and then let them drain. They need to be quite dry if you are storing them for more than a day in the fridge, so use a salad spinner or drain them on kitchen paper.

Most sprouts will keep in the fridge for at least a couple of weeks in a sealed container or resealable plastic bag. Sprouted chickpeas and peas, however, lose their fabulous crisp texture and are better eaten within a couple of days.

Avoiding hiccups

The joy of sprouting is that it's very straightforward and you're not going to wake up to discover that an army of slugs has devastated your crop. However, there are a few things to keep in mind:

- Sprouts need to be well rinsed, drained and able to breathe, otherwise mould may develop.
- Wash the jar or sprouter thoroughly between crops. It's a good idea to sterilize it from time to time.
- Don't overpack the jar: the seeds should lie in a layer no more than two deep.
- Get your pulses from a reputable source (I always use organic for sprouting), and don't even think of using garden seeds, which might have been treated with chemicals.

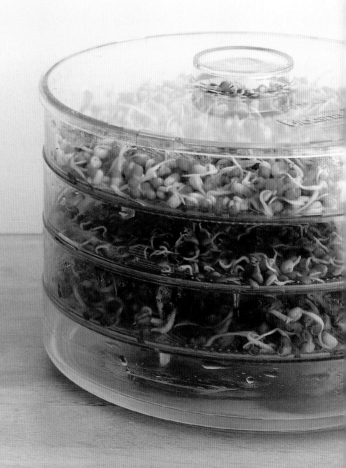

What to sprout

A pulse, just like a nut, is a dormant seed. It does seem bizarre to think of all those bags of dried beans, chickpeas and lentils in the supermarkets as bags of seeds just waiting to burst into life, but that's exactly what they are. Given moisture, air and the right temperature, they will miraculously sprout and grow.

Many health food shops and online suppliers can sell you seeds that are perfect for sprouting, although when it comes to mainstream lentils and chickpeas, I just use what I have. Ignore all the New World beans (including butter beans, kidney beans, haricots, flageolets, borlotti, cannellini, pinto beans – see pp.261–265), which have potentially serious allergy/toxicity/digestibility issues.

The following is a list, by no means comprehensive, of legumes that are ideal to sprout. Once addicted, I'm sure you'll be sprouting everything from radish seeds and brassicas to almonds and mustard. There are so many options, but they're not pulses, so I'll stop here.

Bean	Soaking time	Sprouting time	Characteristics
Alfalfa	4 hours	3–4 days	Yes, it is a legume! The superfood hero, bursting with vitamins and minerals.
Adzuki beans	8–12 hours	3–4 days	Gorgeous bright colour, sweet nutty flavour.
Moth beans	8–12 hours	12–24 hours	Super quick, very tasty; the beginners' sprout.
Mung beans	8–12 hours	3–4 days	The ubiquitous bean sprout, but so much more exciting when eaten as a very fresh, immature sprout.
Chickpeas	12–14 hours	2–3 days	Great in salads, or use the sprouts for a different take on hummus and felafel.
Lentils	8–12 hours	1–2 days	Perhaps my favourite of the lot. The lentils must be intact (not split such as red lentils). Smaller lentils seem to be quicker off the mark. All varieties add a nutty, earthy flavour to salads, snacks and sandwiches and could be thrown into a stir-fry.
Peas	12–14 hours	2–3 days	Sweet like baby peas straight from the pod, children love them. I prefer green peas; yellow ones have a stronger flavour, and of course split peas won't work at all.
Peanuts	12–14 hours	2–4 days	Peanuts are botanically legumes and not nuts. Sprouts are best eaten when the peanut has just started to germinate, with a large bulge rather than an actual sprout at its tip (when they can taste bitter).

USING THE RECIPES

Wherever possible, I've given a choice between using home-cooked and canned pulses. I recognize the need for dishes that you can fling together in a few minutes after work and the fact that boiling up an entire pot of beans just doesn't make sense if you're cooking for one. However, where dishes absolutely rely on the pulses absorbing stocks or flavours, I have only suggested using dried.

Note: When using canned pulses, be sure to drain and rinse them thoroughly.

I would love to think that this book will convince you that cooking your own pulses from scratch is worthwhile. Dried legumes are an absolute bargain and if you cook up a large pot, you can keep them in the fridge or freezer (see p.17) and dip into them during the week for many quick-fix meals.

If you're not an experienced bean cook, you may want to consult the soaking and cooking sections (see p.14–17) before starting the recipe. Very soon, you will know exactly how to soak, cook, flavour and store each type of legume. It's very straightforward.

I've divided the recipes into sections, in the order that we tend to eat things, to help you when looking for ideas. However, there are no rules here: many of the sides will happily play starring roles, salads can become light lunches and hearty soups a main course. Many vegetarian recipes include simple suggestions to transform them into carnivorous delights, so that mixed-diet households don't have to cook two meals.

Within each section, the recipes are grouped into chickpea, lentil, pea and bean recipes. Chickpeas are cosy couples, two to a pod, and their recipes tend to suit chickpeas and nothing else. Lentils, like little lovebirds, come in pairs too and, while recipes can often be interchanged between lentil types, they are usually not suitable for other legumes. Lastly come the peas and beans, packed like happy families in their pods. Many of the beans in these recipes can be interchanged, even if the bean police (and they are out there) get a bit upset about it. The Check Your Pulse section (see pp.252–265) will help you select suitable contenders.

There are a few cooking techniques that I use repeatedly, such as poaching eggs and roasting peppers, which you'll find in the Basics section (see pp.248–251). I've also included some sauces, salsas and seasonings that you'll find useful time and time again.

Most recipes will feed four people. However, some are just too time-consuming, or too fiddly, to bother making such small quantities and I will have given instructions for making a larger amount. Pulse dishes freeze very well and any leftovers can be stored successfully.

Above all, this is meant to be a springboard into the pulsating world of legumes. So get your finger on the pulse and start spilling the beans to all your friends – and I'll promise not to mention any other legumey clichés for the rest of the book.

NIBBLES, DIPS AND PURÉES

Fresh, steamed or roasted, peas and beans are truly moreish and a healthy alternative to crisps. Pulses make incredibly versatile purées too, ideal for canapés, dips, sandwiches, dolloped onto salads for light lunches and even highly nutritious baby food. Paired with interesting bread, your purée can be transformed into an elegant bite-sized croûte or a substantial supper bruschetta.

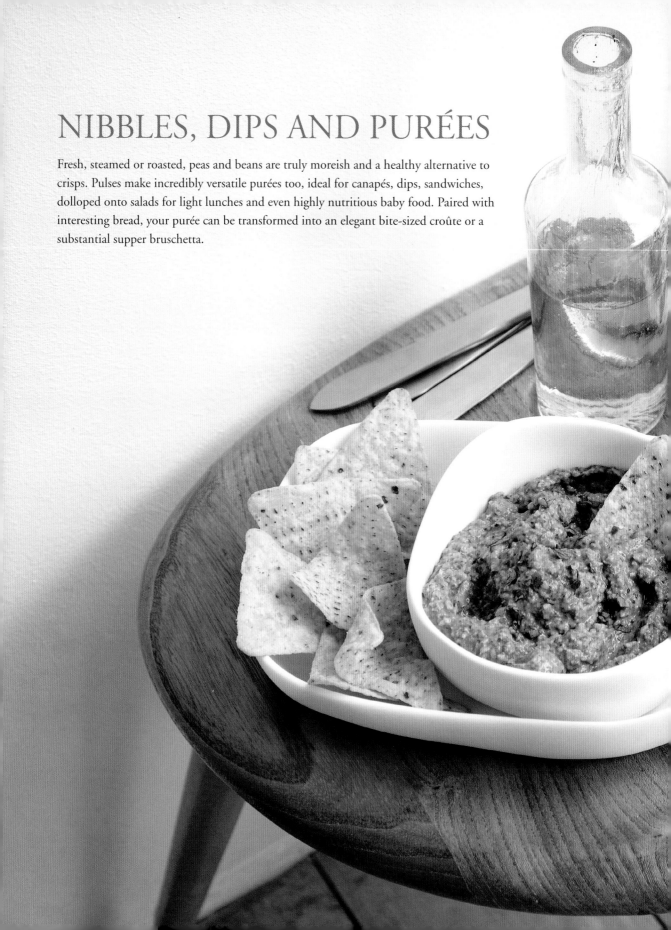

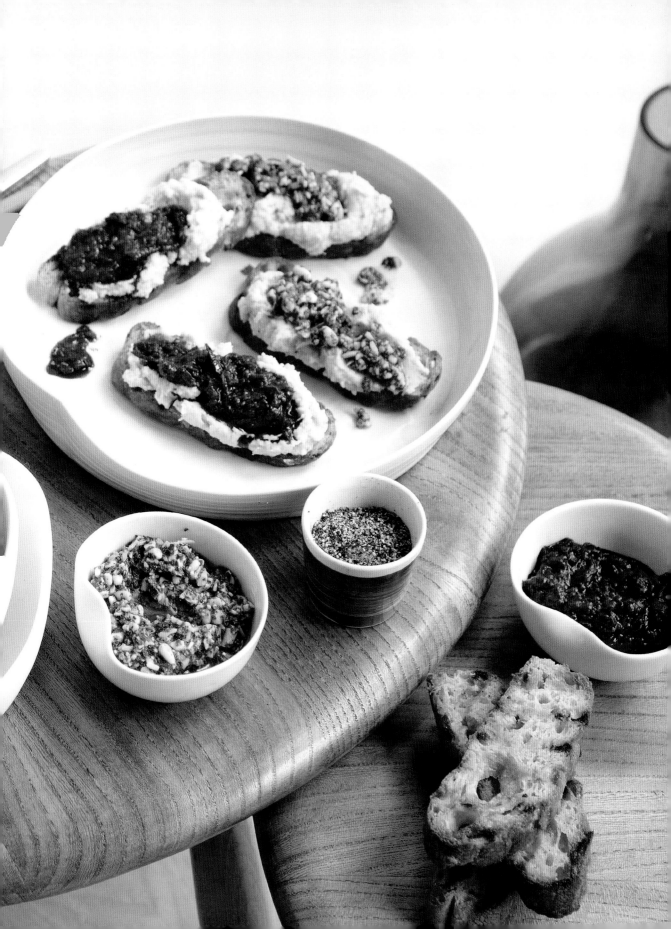

Japanese edamame: the glamorous, got-to-have-it bean of the day. The route to a size-zero figure (Victoria Beckham apparently lives on them), the first thing you make a grab for on the Yo! Sushi conveyor belt, the sell-out lunchtime supermarket snack teamed up with crunchy sea salt. It's madness, but I have to admit I'm addicted.

Edamame are a strain of fresh green soya beans and are usually popped straight from pod to mouth. If you can't find them fresh, then many Asian supermarkets stock frozen ones.

STEAMED EDAMAME

Serves 4

200 g/7 oz edamame beans (in their pods),
    frozen will do but fresh are best
1 tsp Maldon or other flaked sea salt

Place the beans in a steamer over a pan of boiling water and steam for 2 minutes.

Sprinkle with salt and serve, with an extra bowl to collect the discarded pods.

HOW ABOUT?

... kick-starting your beans. Try frying a diced red chilli in a spoonful of sesame oil and then stir-frying the beans in the oil for a few seconds before serving.

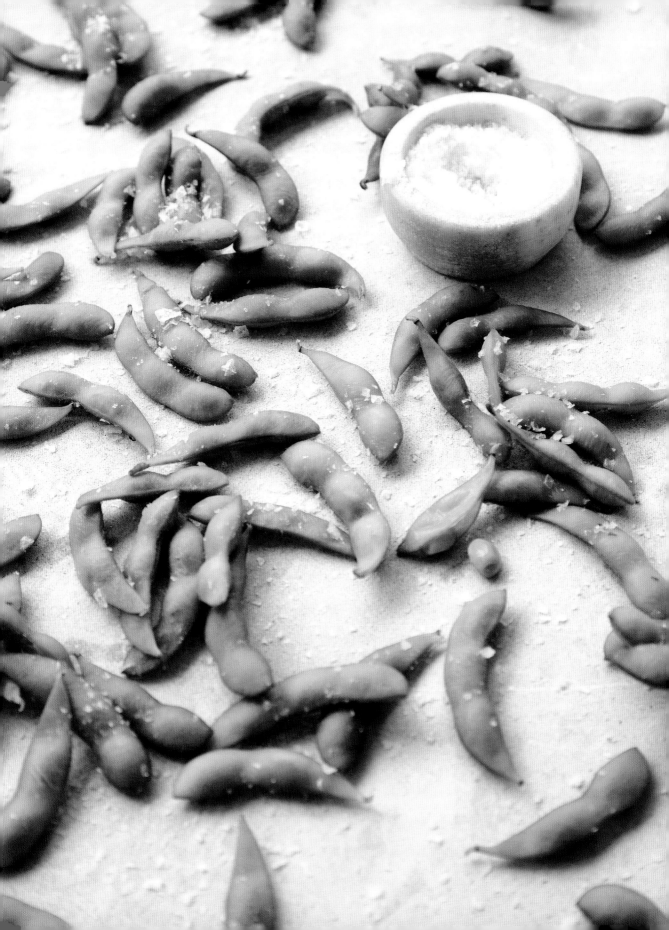

There are so many amazing Indian snacks made with pulses, but it was the pure simplicity of this recipe that caught my eye. It is traditionally served outside the temples of southern India during the Hindu festival of Navratri. Once eaten never forgotten, these chickpeas make a great little nibble to serve before a curry. The dark brown desi chickpea would be most traditional, but more readily available white (Kabuli) chickpeas are just fine.

It can be tricky tracking down whole coconuts, and you can use desiccated coconut, but if you do find a fresh one in an ethnic store, it is so much tastier.

SOUTHERN INDIAN CHICKPEAS AND COCONUT
SUNDAL ACCRA

Serves 4

1 tbsp vegetable oil, such as rapeseed, sunflower, groundnut (peanut)
   or coconut oil
1 tsp black mustard seeds
1 green chilli, very finely diced
1 tsp very finely chopped fresh ginger
5 curry leaves (optional)
½ tsp salt
1 tbsp urad dal, or – very unorthodox – red lentils (optional)
250 g/9 oz home-cooked chickpeas (garbanzo beans)
   or 1 x 400g/14 oz can of chickpeas
4 tbsp freshly grated coconut or 2 tbsp unsweetened desiccated coconut
handful of fresh coriander (cilantro), finely chopped

Heat the oil in a large frying pan over a medium heat, add the mustard seeds and wait until they begin to splutter.

Throw in the chilli, ginger, curry leaves, salt and raw dal or lentils, if using. When the aromas burst out of the pan and the lentils begin to crisp up, then stir in the chickpeas. Remove from the heat and stir well. Add the coconut and coriander and dive in – scrumptious warm or cold.

Crisp, roasted chickpeas, or *leblebi,* are a popular snack in Turkey. They also turn up in all sorts of Indian *chivda*, or what we often call Bombay mix. An incredibly healthy and delicious alternative to peanuts or crisps, they are an absolute bargain too, especially if you have cooked a large batch of chickpeas yourself. *Leblebi* are great to nibble at alongside a drink or could be sprinkled over a salad to give a bit of crunch. These will keep happily in an airtight container for a few days.

ROASTED CHICKPEAS

Serves 8–10

2 x 400 g/14 oz cans of chickpeas (garbanzo beans)
    or 500 g/1 lb 2 oz home-cooked chickpeas
2 tbsp extra-virgin olive oil or vegetable oil, plus 1 tsp to coat
1 tsp salt
2 tsp of your chosen spice mix (see below)

Preheat the oven to 200°C/400°F/Gas mark 6.

Drain the chickpeas and pat them dry with kitchen paper. Now toss them into a bowl with the oil: I would use olive oil if my spicing had a Mediterranean character and a vegetable oil such as sunflower or rapeseed for Asian flavours, but it's not crucial.

Place the chickpeas on a baking sheet and roast for about 30–40 minutes, giving them a little shake every 10 minutes or so to roll them over. Roast until crunchy; test a couple. I like them to be totally crisp, but you may prefer a little give, which will save on the dentist's bill.

Add 1 teaspoon of oil to give the salt and spices something to cling to and then toss with the salt and your chosen flavouring. Return to the oven for a couple of minutes and then leave to cool.

HOW ABOUT?

... using a ready-blended spice mixture, such as Moroccan *ras al hanout*, Indian *garam masala* or Ethiopian *berbere.*

... adding a handful of roasted nuts such as pistachios, peanuts, hazelnuts or almonds to the chickpeas along with the spices.

Try any of the following combinations:
• 1 tsp hot smoked paprika and ½ tsp dried thyme
• ½ tsp ground coriander, 1½ tsp ground cumin, pinch of cayenne pepper
• za'atar (see p.246), made with 1 tbsp toasted sesame seeds, 1 tsp dried thyme, 1 tsp sumac and a pinch of salt

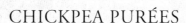

CHICKPEA PURÉES

Hummus is the Arabic word for chickpeas and has, in its various spellings, come to mean the purée. Over the last few decades, hummus has taken us by storm. Nowadays you are just as likely to find hummus as ham in any school lunch box. Fabulous as a dip with crudités or pitta, as an accompaniment to felafel or as a sandwich filling with roast vegetables, it is truly versatile.

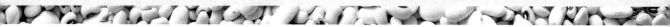

Most of the hummus sold commercially is *houmous bi tahini*, the rich, smooth variety made with tahini (sesame seed paste). It is quite a challenge to create the creamy texture of this Middle Eastern purée with home-cooked chickpeas. I would definitely add a teaspoon of bicarbonate of soda to the soaking water, cook until really soft, and ensure I removed as many skins as possible after cooking them. I have found that canned chickpeas give a silkier result; and for the very best texture of all, the jars of Spanish chickpeas are fabulous.

The richness of the tahini takes the place of olive oil in traditional recipes and a drizzle of extra-virgin olive oil is reserved for the customary garnish.

HUMMUS WITH TAHINI
HOUMOUS BI TAHINI

Serves 4 as a starter, 8 as a dip

300 g/10½ oz home-cooked chickpeas (garbanzo beans)
    or 1 x 400 g/14 oz can of chickpeas
juice of 2 lemons
2 garlic cloves, crushed
4–6 tbsp tahini
salt and black pepper or cayenne pepper
2 tbsp extra-virgin olive oil
1 tsp paprika
1 tbsp freshly chopped parsley

Place most of the chickpeas (keeping a few aside for the traditional garnish) in a food processor with the lemon juice and garlic. Give the tahini a good stir and then add 4 tbsp to the food processor, along with 2 tbsp water (preferably the cooking water if the chickpeas are home cooked).

Blend until the mixture is really smooth and then add more water to thin it down if necessary. Taste and adjust the seasoning: you will need some salt; you can zip the dish up with cayenne or just use black pepper; to enrich the purée, add more tahini; or lift the purée with more lemon juice.

Serve in a wide bowl. Stir the oil and paprika together and then swirl over the surface of the hummus. Sprinkle over the parsley and the reserved chickpeas.

HOW ABOUT?

… replacing the tahini with peanut butter, an unlikely but delicious trick.

For an additional garnish, try:
- za'atar (see p.246)
- pomegranate seeds and fresh coriander (cilantro)
- toasted pine nuts and slow-cooked caramelized onions

This makes a welcome change from the more familiar *houmous bi tahini*. The slightly rougher texture of home-cooked chickpeas is preferable in this recipe.

HUMMUS

Serves 4 as a starter, 8 as a dip

300 g/10½ oz home-cooked chickpeas (garbanzo beans)
    or 1 x 400 g/14 oz can of chickpeas
2 garlic cloves, crushed
juice of 1 lemon
250 ml/9 fl oz extra-virgin olive oil
salt and pepper

Place the chickpeas in a food processor with the garlic and lemon juice. Blend for a moment or two before adding most of the olive oil. Pulse the mixture, adding more oil as needed, until you have a nicely textured, rather than smooth, paste. Season to taste.

Try adding:
2 tsp freshly roasted and ground cumin seeds
1 hot chilli pepper, finely diced
handful of chopped fresh parsley
    or coriander (cilantro)

Supermarkets offer a wealth of hummus variations these days, and while I prefer the unadulterated version, roast vegetable combinations can be a very useful way of extending or tarting up yesterday's leftover hummus. *Illustrated on pp.32–33.*

ROAST VEGETABLE HUMMUS

Serves 6 as a starter, 10 as a dip

For each of the 3 variations below, you will need to start with the hummus recipe given on the left. Whizz the roasted vegetables in a food processor until fairly smooth. Add the hummus and whizz to combine. Taste and adjust the seasoning.

RED PEPPER HUMMUS
2 roasted red peppers (see p.249), peeled and deseeded, and 1 tsp smoked hot Spanish paprika, or cheat with some Spanish piquillo peppers from a jar.

ROAST PUMPKIN OR CARROT HUMMUS
Preheat the oven to 200°C/400°F/Gas mark 6. In a roasting pan, toss 600 g/1 lb 5 oz peeled and roughly chopped pumpkin or carrot with 2 tbsp olive oil and 1 tsp cumin seeds. Roast for about 40 minutes, until the vegetables are very tender.

ROASTED GARLIC
5 peeled garlic cloves could be added to the roasting pan with the peppers or pumpkin/carrots; remove once golden but not burned.

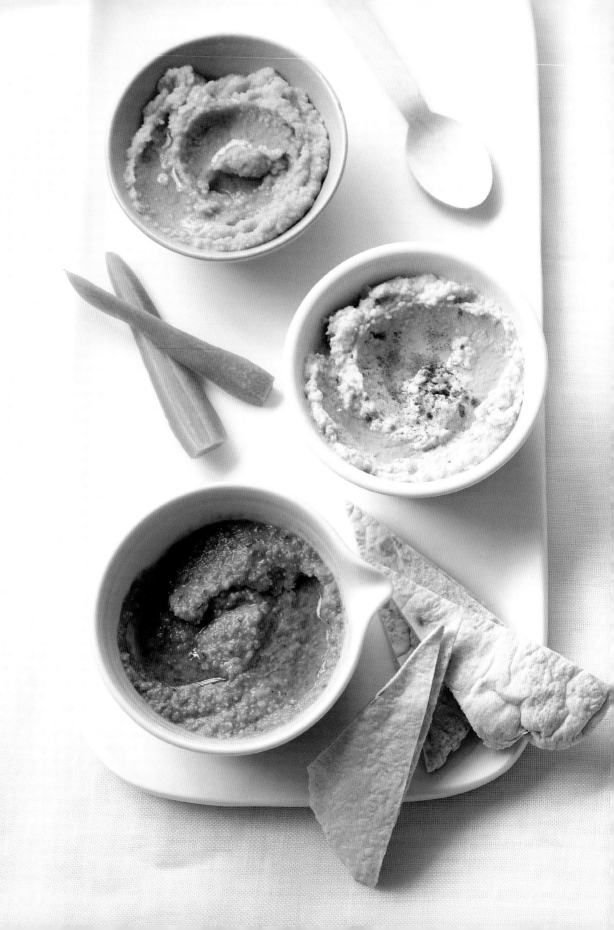

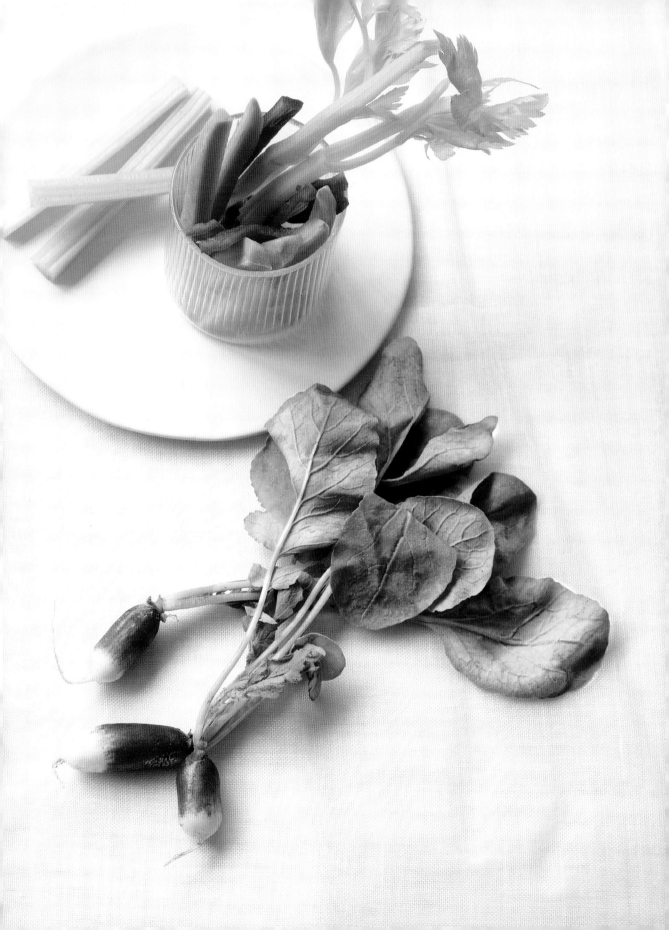

A fabulous blend of earthy lentils with smoky roast aubergine. The slippery texture that I often associate with the classic aubergine dish *baba ghanoush* is replaced with a more substantial creamy purée.

Charring the skin of the aubergine is crucial, otherwise you will lose out on the smoky flavour that absolutely makes the dish. No gas hob? Where's your inner Boy Scout? Open fire, wood burner, barbecue, grill, ridged griddle; you'll find a way.

PUY LENTIL AND SMOKED AUBERGINE PURÉE

Serves 4 as a starter, 8 as a dip

1 aubergine (eggplant)

5 garlic cloves, skin on

150 g/5½ oz/¾ cup Puy lentils, rinsed

4 tbsp extra-virgin olive oil

juice of ½–1 lemon

6 sun-dried tomatoes, finely chopped

salt and pepper

2 tbsp finely chopped parsley

Preheat the oven to 200°C/400°F/Gas mark 6.

Pierce the aubergine in a couple of places to prevent minor explosions and place directly over a gas flame to blacken the skin. After a couple of minutes, turn the aubergine over, using tongs. Most of the skin should be charred and crispy by the time you have finished.

Put the charred aubergine on a small baking sheet along with the garlic and roast in the oven for about 20 minutes or until the flesh has become soft and completely collapsed. You may need to whip the garlic out after about 15 minutes – the cloves should feel squashy and creamy when you squeeze them, but take care not to burn them or they will taste terribly bitter.

Meanwhile, put the lentils in a saucepan and cover by about 5 cm/2 in of cold water. Bring to the boil and then simmer for about 20–30 minutes until really tender; this not a moment for the *al dente* touch. Drain the lentils and add the olive oil.

Put the lentils and half the lemon juice in a food processor. Now remove the skin from the aubergine, squeeze the creamy paste from the garlic cloves and add to the lentils. Whizz to form a rough paste.

Add the tomatoes, some salt and pepper and the parsley. Pulse the mixture very briefly, as it's good to keep a little of the texture of the tomato. Taste and adjust the seasoning, adding salt, pepper, more lemon juice or an extra dash of olive oil. Just don't eat it all in the process.

HOW ABOUT?

... replacing the parsley with mint or coriander.

... using fresh garlic instead of roasted, probably just 3 cloves unless you need to keep the vampires at bay.

... throwing in a few toasted cumin seeds and a dash of pomegranate molasses.

Try this on crostini topped with:

• chopped hard-boiled egg, sea salt, fresh parsley and a dash of extra-virgin olive oil.

• slices of tiny plum tomato, some rocket and extra-virgin olive oil.

A great combination that I stumbled upon in my kitchen one day – only to discover later that *elaiosalata* is a regular on the Greek *meze* table. Whereas the Greeks use their distinctive oregano, I prefer to add plenty of rosemary. Delicious served on crostini with roasted red peppers, mixed with some tinned tuna and spread on a sandwich, or as a stuffing for Spanish piquillo peppers.

GREEN LENTIL TAPENADE

Serves 4 as a starter, 8 as a dip

150 g/5½ oz/¾ cup green lentils, rinsed

2 garlic cloves, crushed

1 large sprig of rosemary, stem removed and leaves finely chopped

3 tbsp capers, rinsed and drained

100 g/3½ oz pitted Kalamata olives

4 anchovy fillets in oil, drained

4 tbsp extra-virgin olive oil

juice of ½–1 lemon

salt and pepper

Put the lentils in a saucepan and cover with a good 10 cm/4 in of cold water. Bring to the boil and then simmer until tender; this may take anything from 20 to 45 minutes, depending on the lentils.

Drain and immediately, while the lentils are still warm, pulse together everything except the lemon juice and seasoning. I prefer to use a hand-held blender in the saucepan, keeping washing up to a minimum, but you could put everything into the food processor or blender. Taste and add salt, pepper and lemon juice as required.

HOW ABOUT?

… using fresh basil or dried oregano instead of the rosemary.

… omitting the anchovies, halving the olives and throwing in a good handful of sun-dried tomatoes.

… a speedy shortcut – use ready-cooked lentils and a few spoonfuls of shop-bought tapenade.

Not strictly speaking a dip or purée, more of a mush really, but this humble dish is truly moreish and always seems more than the sum of its parts. It makes a great addition to any *meze* selection and is wonderful scooped up with flatbread for a light lunch. You could make a meal of these lentils by serving them with rice, in which case you are getting close to the traditional Middle Eastern dish of *mjaddarah*.

SYRIAN-STYLE LENTILS

Serves 4 as a starter
4 tbsp olive oil
2 brown onions, sliced finely
6 garlic cloves, finely chopped
1 tsp cumin seeds, toasted and then ground
pinch of chilli flakes, or better still 2 tsp sweet Aleppo chilli flakes
200 g/7 oz/1 cup brown or green lentils, rinsed
salt and pepper
juice of ½–1 lemon
small bunch of coriander (cilantro), roughly chopped

Heat the oil in a large saucepan and add the onions. Keep the temperature fairly low and allow the onions to soften, sweeten and turn golden; this may take about 20 minutes. Be patient.

Take out half of the onions from the pan and set aside. Turn up the heat and throw in the garlic, cumin and chilli. Stir and, as soon as you can really smell the garlic, add the lentils and enough water to cover them by about 5 cm/2 in.

Bring to the boil and then turn down to a simmer. Cover the pan and cook until the lentils soften and begin to break down. You may have to add a little extra water from time to time if they are getting dry but go carefully, remember that you don't want to drain away any delicious juices later. Once the lentils are really soft, and this can take over an hour, taste and adjust the seasoning with salt, pepper and enough lemon juice to freshen the dish up. Stir in the coriander leaves and garnish with the remaining fried onions.

Serve with flatbread and perhaps a dollop of creamy Greek yogurt if you are feeling indulgent.

HOW ABOUT?

... stirring in some finely sliced Swiss chard leaves a few minutes before the end of the cooking time.
... adding a dash of pomegranate molasses along with the lemon juice.
... serving with tzatziki (see p.246).

This white bean purée would work well with other creamy beans such as haricots or flageolets too. The Italian flavours drew me to the cannellini bean. I love to serve this piled onto bruschetta with ripe cherry tomatoes and a few salad leaves for a simple lunch dish. You could also serve it as canapés on tiny croûtes (see p.44).

CANNELLINI, BACON AND SAGE PURÉE

Serves 4

2 tbsp olive oil

1 onion, finely diced

2 rashers of smoked bacon, finely chopped

3 garlic cloves, crushed

6 sage leaves, finely chopped

250 g/9 oz home-cooked cannellini beans
    or 1 x 400 g/14 oz can of cannellini beans

2 tbsp bean cooking water, water or stock

2–3 tbsp extra-virgin olive oil

juice of ½–1 lemon

salt and pepper

Heat the oil in a large saucepan and cook the onion until soft. Throw in the bacon and cook until it begins to turn brown and crisp at the edges. Add the garlic and sage, stirring until the garlic begins to turn golden but not burn.

Tip in the beans and a couple of tablespoons of stock or water. Stir and mash the mixture with the back of a wooden spoon. I like to leave this purée quite rough, but you could whizz it in the food processor or use a hand-held blender.

Add enough extra-virgin oil to give a rich and creamy consistency along with lots of lemon juice to add some fresh zip. Season well with salt and pepper.

HOW ABOUT?

... trying this purée with **rosemary, chilli and lemon zest**. Leave out the bacon and add 1 tsp finely chopped rosemary and a good pinch of chilli flakes along with the garlic. Zest your lemon before squeezing and add the zest a pinch at a time as you season the beans.

... **serving as a dip:** you will need to add a little extra liquid, ideally some of the bean cooking liquid or just stock or water.

Unless you harvest your own or have a great local greengrocer, frozen broad beans are often the best option. Fabulously fresh, or quickly frozen, baby beans taste sweet and almost creamy, unlike those mealy, bitter brutes that plagued my childhood. The natural sugars in broad beans are rapidly converted to starch; most of those on sale are at least a couple of days old and tend to be on the large side. Should you be so lucky as to have some fresh broad beans growing, for heaven's sake pick 'em young.

I always keep a bag of frozen baby broad beans in my freezer specifically for this recipe. I am happy to leave the skins on them here, as I enjoy the added texture. If using more mature beans, you will need to pop them out of their leathery skins after blanching.

BROAD BEAN AND MINT PURÉE

Serves 4

400 g/14 oz fresh or frozen baby broad
    beans (fava beans)
2 tbsp olive oil
1 onion, finely diced
3 garlic cloves, crushed

1 sprig of mint
juice of ½–1 lemon
3–4 tbsp extra-virgin olive oil
salt and pepper

If using frozen beans, make sure that they are fully thawed. If using fresh, blanch them in boiling water for a couple of minutes until just tender.

Heat the oil in a large frying pan and cook the onion until soft and golden. Add the garlic and stir until its unmistakable aroma really hits you. Throw in the beans and stir over a medium heat for a couple of minutes; they require very little cooking but need to absorb the wonderful garlicky oil.

Now begin to blend the mixture in a food processor or using a hand-held blender. Add a few mint leaves, some lemon juice, extra-virgin olive oil, salt and plenty of freshly ground black pepper. Whizz, taste, and then carefully balance the flavour if necessary with more mint, lemon, oil, salt or pepper. Keep in mind that if it's too minty and smooth, you will end up with something reminiscent of toothpaste.

HOW ABOUT?

... substituting the mint with basil or dill.

Try this on crostini topped with:

• a thin slither of salami, chorizo or cured ham or, for a bit more panache, shards of crisp *jamón serrano* (see p.250)
• shavings of pecorino cheese
• a dollop of fresh ricotta cheese

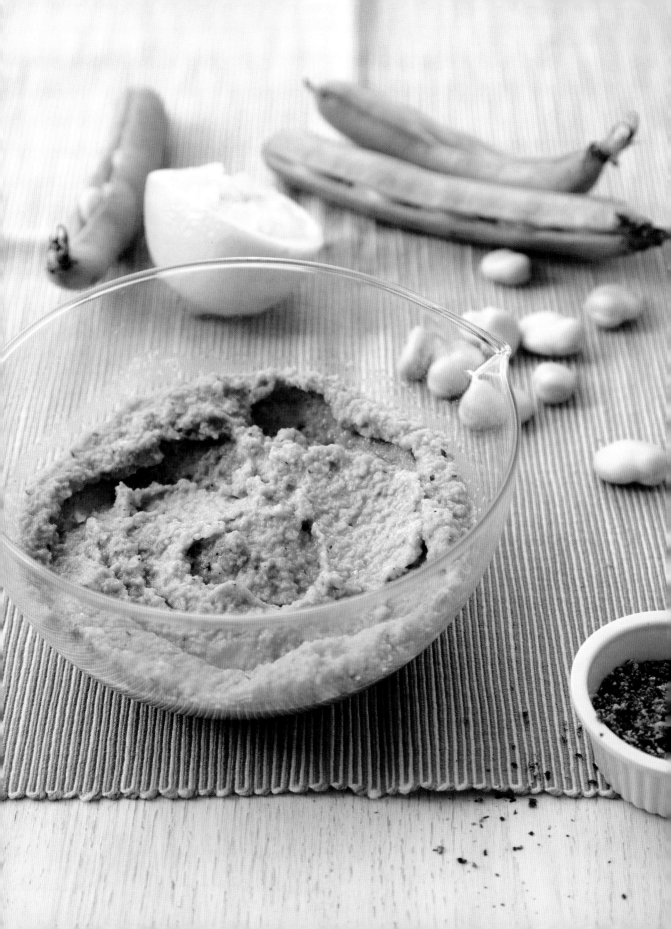

For those in a hurry or with absolutely no inclination to cook. *Illustrated right.*

CHEAT'S CREAMY BEAN CROSTINI

Serves 4 as a starter, or 20 as crostini

1 x 400 g/14 oz can of cannellini, haricot (navy) or flageolet beans
2 garlic cloves, roughly chopped
4 tbsp olive oil
juice of ½ lemon
salt and pepper
a few leaves of parsley, basil or marjoram (optional)

Whizz the beans, garlic, oil, lemon juice, salt and pepper in a food processor or with a hand-held blender. Taste the purée and adjust the seasoning. The creamed beans will be subtle but need to be balanced.

Put a tablespoon of purée on each crostini, pop on a leaf or two of your chosen herb and then top with a teaspoon of any of the following, straight from the jar or home-made:

• tapenade (leave out the lentils from the recipe on p.35)

• harissa (see p.245)

• pesto (see p.244)

• salsa verde (see p.242)

• romesco (see p.243)

When working on boats, a lot of time is spent in boatyards, and I spent several months based in Lavagna on the stunning Ligurian coast of Italy. Lunch was a ritual – and not a sandwich box in sight. We often piled into a tiny, dimly lit dockside restaurant with the workers from the yard, where everything (except pasta) was eaten directly from the waxed brown paper 'tablecloths'. Some days we started with *bianchetti* (tiny whitebait), other days it was *farinata* (a chickpea flatbread), but the most memorable of all were the few days of the early broad bean season. The boss simply threw down a pile of raw broad bean pods and a few shavings of pecorino and everyone dived in.

If you grow your own beans and can pick them when they're tiny, then you are in for one of the most exquisite antipasti imaginable.

RAW BROAD BEANS AND PECORINO

Per person

large handful of immature broad beans (fava beans) in pods
about 50 g/1½ oz pecorino cheese

Pile the beans into a large bowl, have another on hand for the discarded pods, and serve with a hunk of cheese alongside for everyone to help themselves.

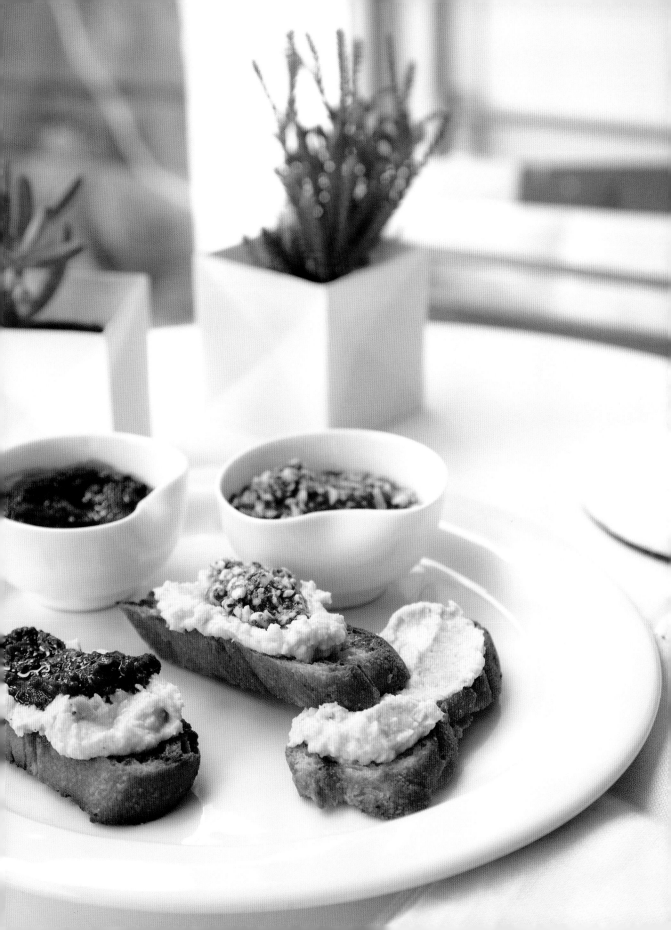

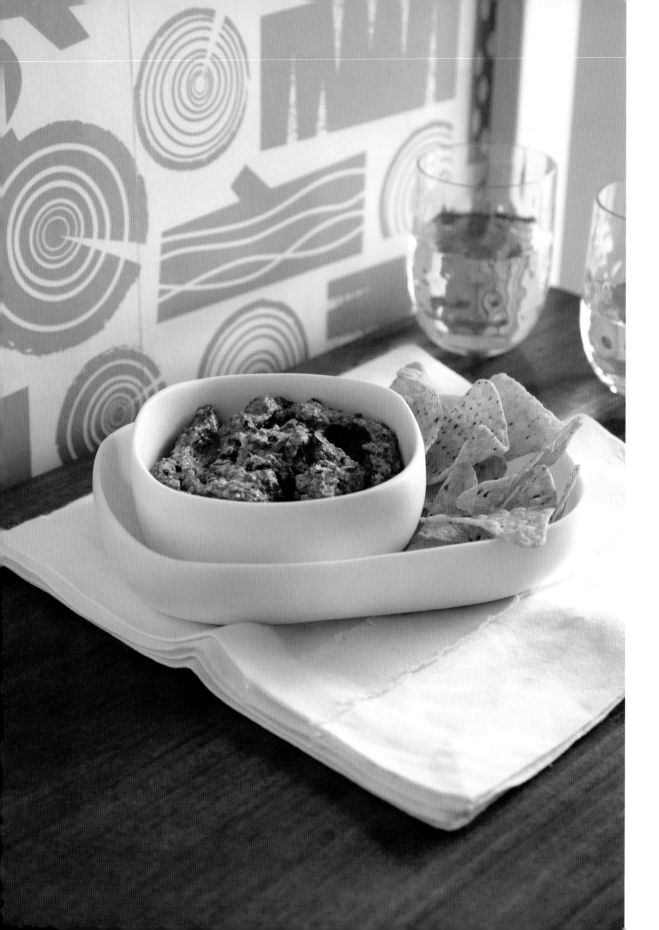

Chipotles are smoked jalapeño peppers, traditionally sold dried or in adobo, a spicy sauce made up predominantly of tomato and onion. You could use the chipotle paste or ketchup that is increasingly available in supermarkets. No chipotles at all? A spoonful of smoked Spanish paprika and a few hot chillies will taste great too.

Here's a Tex-Mex winner to serve alongside guacamole, tomato salsa and a few corn chips. Crack open an ice-cold bottle of beer, slide in the wedge of lime and let the fiesta begin.

BLACK BEAN AND CHIPOTLE DIP

Serves 4 as a starter, 8 as a dip

2 tbsp olive oil

1 onion, finely diced

3 garlic cloves, finely diced

1 tsp ground cumin

1 x 400 g/14 oz can of black beans or 250 g/9 oz home-cooked beans

2 chipotle chillies in adobo sauce, stalks removed

2 tbsp sour cream

juice of 1–2 limes

salt

1 tbsp chopped fresh coriander (cilantro)

Tabasco sauce (optional)

Heat the oil in a pan and cook the onion until soft and golden. Add the garlic and cumin and continue to cook until it smells wonderful.

Put the onion mixture into a food processor with the beans and half of your chipotles (it's always wise to tread carefully with any chilli). Whizz to a purée and then add the remaining chillies, sour cream, lime juice and salt by degrees until the dip is balanced.

Stir in most of the coriander, check the seasoning again, and add a dash of Tabasco if you're feeling fiery. Serve with a swirl of sour cream and a sprinkling of coriander.

HOW ABOUT?

... spreading over a wrap or tortilla with all, or any of the following: grated cheese, chopped tomatoes, green salad, guacamole, cooked chicken. Roll up tightly and slice for a snack or pop the whole thing in your lunch box.

... eating any leftovers with a baked potato and grated cheese.

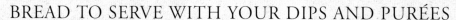

BREAD TO SERVE WITH YOUR DIPS AND PURÉES

You could of course opt for crisp sticks of raw vegetables, leaves of Gem lettuce, corn chips or potato crisps, but I usually serve my creamy pulse purées with bread. The right bready accompaniment can transform a simple hummus into an elegant canapé, stylish antipasti or a light lunch.

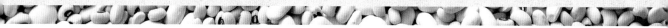

CROSTINI

Toast slices of ciabatta bread, 1–2 cm/about ½ in thick, under the grill. While the bread is still warm, rub it with a cut garlic clove, sprinkle with a pinch of salt and a drop of extra virgin olive oil.

VERY QUICK CROSTINI FOR THE MASSES

Cut the ciabatta loaf in half lengthwise (as if you were making one huge panini).

Toast the two halves, rub with garlic, sprinkle with oil and salt, and pile on your topping.

Now cut the ciabatta into individual servings and garnish.

BRUSCHETTA

A more substantial crostini, best made with a sourdough or good rustic bread. Toast the slices on a ridged griddle pan or on the barbecue. Rub with a cut garlic clove and sprinkle with salt and extra-virgin olive oil. Now pile on a hummus or purée and top with goodies such as cured meats, salsa or grilled vegetables.

Serve with a salad and you have a perfect starter or simple supper dish.

CROÛTES

Little French crispy toasts. Here's the moment to use up yesterday's leftover baguette or to purchase a slim *ficelle* loaf if you want more diminutive canapés.

Preheat the oven to 180°C/350°F/Gas mark 4. Slice the bread into very thin rounds, place on a baking sheet and drizzle with a tiny amount of extra-virgin olive oil. Place in the oven for about 10–15 minutes (depending on thickness) until dry and brittle. Cool on a wire rack and keep in an airtight container for up to 4 days.

Once topped with your chosen purée, these will stay crisp for a couple of hours.

HOW ABOUT?

... making two or three different purées and serving on crostini garnished with tiny tomatoes, boiled quails' eggs, olives or fresh herbs. Display them artistically on a large slate (provide plates, as they tend to collapse) and serve with drinks.

TARTINES

The French answer to bruschetta; bistros make all sorts of wonderful combinations that often end up being flashed under the grill.

Toast your bread (ideally something with a bit of substance such as a sourdough). Top with your purée and then perhaps some grated cheese, grilled vegetables or even a canned sardine. Place under the grill to melt or caramelize the topping and serve warm.

PITTA

Pitta makes an ideal packaging for any creamy dip or purée, along with plenty of fresh salady accompaniments. Just open up the pitta like a pocket, stuff everything inside, and you have the perfect candidate for the lunch box or picnic.

Pitta bread, be it white or wholemeal, is a really useful standby to keep in the freezer. You can toast it from frozen and in a matter of moments you have an ideal accompaniment.

PITTA CRISPS

A healthy alternative to potato crisps or corn chips for dipping.

Preheat the oven to 160°C/325°F/Gas mark 3.

Cut the pittas into 2.5-cm/1-in ribbons using a pair of scissors. Open the 'loops' of bread to give you thin fingers. Place these on baking sheets. There always seems to be a thinner and thicker side to the bread, so I use one baking sheet for the thinner, quicker-cooking, crisps and another for the thicker pieces.

Drizzle over a few drops of extra-virgin olive oil and season with a little salt. You can add dried herbs or spices at this point too. Toss the bread around to coat in the seasoning and arrange in a single layer. Bake in the oven for about 10–20 minutes, until dried out and crisp.

Cool on a wire rack and keep in an airtight container for up to 4 days.

WRAPS

Wheat tortillas or flatbreads wrapped around a soft juicy filling of puréed pulses along with a few scraps from yesterday's roast can make a great lunchtime alternative to the sandwich. Place your filling in the lower two-thirds of your bread, tuck in the sides and roll up.

I love to use *lavash* (a Middle Eastern flatbread) if I can get hold of it; it's a bit thinner than most tortillas. Just make sure that you are generous with the filling, otherwise the wrap can be a rather stodgy, bready affair.

HOW ABOUT?

... stiffer pulse mixtures will allow you to cut the rolled-up wrap into slices on the diagonal, turn on their side and serve as finger food, or part of a children's party spread.

BABY FOOD

Pulses provide valuable protein, iron, zinc and many other nutrients in a baby's diet, as well as giving a fantastic creamy texture to purées. It's a great idea to cook a batch of lentils or beans and freeze them in ice cube trays, or tiny pots. Each cube or pot can be thawed individually and combined with a vegetable purée, where the vitamin C will enable the body to absorb the iron effectively. Coupled with grains, pulses will provide all the essential amino acids so vital to a child's early development.

For the first couple of months of weaning, commonly from about 6 to 8 months, your baby will still be consuming large amounts of breast milk or formula and just beginning to sample simple fruit and vegetable purées. Mixing these with easily digestible baby rice can help the transition to solid food.

At about 8–10 months, as the baby's digestive system develops, you can begin introducing some pulses. The split, skin-free, faster-cooking lentils and beans are the ones to go for initially. Try:

- yellow split peas
- red lentils
- moong dal (skinned and split mung beans)

At this stage, you don't want to introduce the thicker-skinned beans and peas as they have high levels of fibre and are more tricky to digest, which could lead to discomfort and wind.

Smooth purées

Before you cook them, check pulses for the odd bit of gravel or stone. Tip the pulses on to a tray and give them a good look over. Rinse and drain.

Cover the pulses with about double their volume of water and boil for anything between 20 and 40 minutes, until they have totally collapsed to a creamy purée. Add more water if they seem dry and give them a stir from time to time so that they do not stick or burn on the bottom of the pan.

A pinch of ground ginger, turmeric or cumin, added as you begin cooking, will aid the digestion too while introducing new flavours.

In the early weaning stages, you may have to purée the pulses further to get a totally smooth result, but very soon the natural creamy texture is just perfect added to any vegetable purée. Try with an equal quantity of cooked and puréed carrot, pumpkin, parsnip or sweet potato (root vegetables are naturally sweet and go down well). You can freeze both cooked pulses and vegetable purées in ice cube trays or small pots, so that you can thaw any number of different combinations when you're too busy to cook from scratch.

Later on, your purée base can be mixed with a bit of leftover chicken or meat from the Sunday roast, fish, any root or green vegetables, and many of the other dishes the rest of the family are eating. The key is not to add any salted or sugary food.

Textured food

By about 10–12 months, the natural texture of soft, collapsed pulses is a great way to move forward from the silky-smooth purées of the first stage. You can begin to incorporate some of the thinner-skinned, more easily digestible whole beans. Try:

- mung beans
- adzuki beans

You can include more interesting flavours now too. I find it astounding that parents often give their babies tasteless food that they wouldn't dream of eating themselves.

Here is a very basic legume casserole that can be constantly reinvented to keep little ones interested (and you'll probably end up eating half of it yourself).

BASIC LEGUME CASSEROLE

knob of butter
100 g/3½ oz diced onion, shallot or leek
50 g/1¾ oz diced celery and/or red pepper
200 g/7 oz carrot, parsnip or sweet potato, diced
100 g/3½ oz red lentils, yellow split peas, moong dal,
    mung beans or adzuki beans
1–2 tsp basil, thyme or parsley, finely chopped

Heat the butter in a heavy-bottomed saucepan and cook all the vegetables together until soft. Add the pulses and herbs. Cover with plenty of water and cook until soft. Initially you may purée this, but it's a great introduction to lumpier food.

Real food

At last your baby will reach the stage when he or she is eating slightly mashed-up versions of the family food. It's a great time to introduce plenty of different flavours. Your child will be able to enjoy any of the pulses by now, adding valuable fibre and providing slow-release energy in his or her diet.

So try out any of the dip recipes in this chapter; dal and rice (see p.154) and refried beans (see p.162) were also favourites in our house. Just remember to cut out the salt and any hot spices.

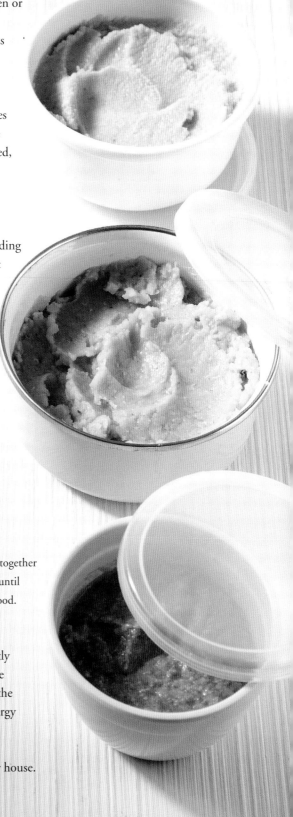

FRITTERS, PANCAKES AND PATTIES

Snacks, starters or the basis of a meal. Fried food is an undeniably delicious treat, but many of these little cakes and burgers can also be oven roasted.

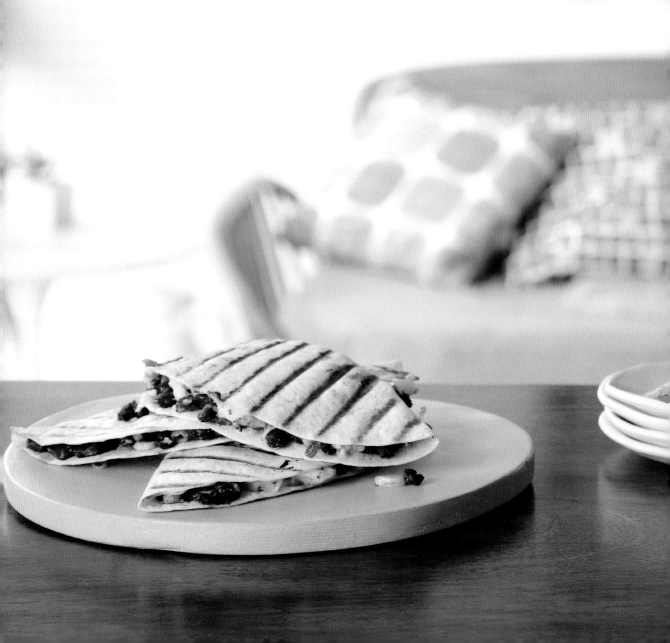

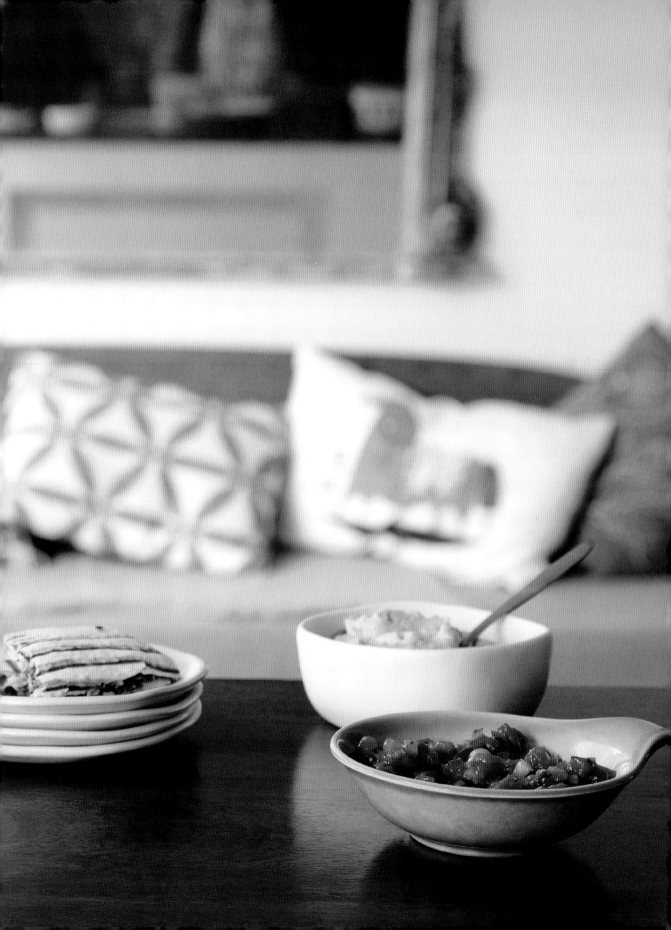

Felafel, the enduring stars of Mediterranean street food, are simple to make at home. These delicious little rissoles originated centuries ago in Egypt, where they are made with dried fava beans; elsewhere in the Middle East, chickpeas tend to be the main player. Do try tracking down some dry fava beans in Greek or Middle Eastern grocers. You could use some for the *ful medames* too (see p.181). I returned from my last trip to London's Edgware Road weighed down like a camel.

No time to soak? Skip to the next recipe, which breaks all the rules but is delicious nonetheless.

FELAFEL

Makes about 30

300 g/10½ oz/1½ cups chickpeas (garbanzo beans)
    or dried split, skinned fava beans or, better still, a 50/50 mixture,
    soaked in plenty of cold water for 24 hours
1 small fresh red chilli (see p.248), finely chopped,
    or a good pinch of cayenne pepper
½ red onion, finely diced
2 garlic cloves, crushed
2 tsp cumin seeds, roasted and ground
1 tsp coriander seeds, roasted and ground
large handful of parsley, chopped
large handful of fresh coriander (cilantro), chopped
½ tsp salt
½ tsp bicarbonate of soda (baking soda)
sunflower or olive oil for deep-frying

Drain the beans or chickpeas well and place them in a food processor with all the remaining ingredients (except the oil). Whizz to a green paste, stopping when you have a sticky but still slightly granular texture. (Pounding and mincing by hand is an option but you'd have to be very keen.) Taste and balance the seasoning and then leave the mixture to rest for about 30 minutes.

Now for the production line: scoop spoonfuls of the paste, roll it into walnut-sized balls, flatten them slightly and place on a tray. Continue until you have used all the mixture. Don't be tempted to upsize – the centre will never cook through.

In a large pan, heat the oil to 180°C/350°F, or until a cube of bread sizzles and browns in 30 seconds. Deep-fry your felafel, a few at a time, for about 4–5 minutes, until deep gold. Drain on kitchen paper.

If deep-frying is not your thing, I have had reasonable success with shallow frying: you will have to turn the felafel and also extend the cooking time a little to ensure that the centre cooks through. Serve hot.

HOW ABOUT?

... serving with tzatziki (see p.246) or harissa (see p.245) to dip into.

... doing things traditionally. Open up a pitta bread and drop in the felafel with a salad of crisp lettuce, cucumber and tomato, some tarator sauce (see p.245) and a dash of chilli sauce.

... making a double quantity and freezing some of the mixture to shape at a later date. Shaped frozen felafel tend to break up in the pan but can be thawed, brushed with oil and baked in a hot oven (200°C/400°F/Gas mark 6) for 15–20 minutes.

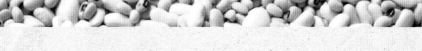

NEW-WAVE FELAFEL

The trend for roasted vegetable felafel has some traditional Middle Eastern cooks in a stew. Should these new kids on the block be termed felafel at all? Fritter, felafel, who cares? They taste divine, are quick to make and are virtuously baked rather than naughtily fried. These roasted vegetable and chickpea creations use cooked chickpeas rather than the traditional soaked raw pulses (see previous recipe), but unlike the homespun canned chickpea felafel, which becomes a pappy, crumbly mess, these are enhanced by the juicy vegetables. The mixture freezes brilliantly. You could even freeze trays of shaped felafel and place them in bags once frozen, ready to dip into on a busy night for a quick supper.

SHAPING YOUR NEW-WAVE FELAFEL

The best way, assuming that you don't own a Middle Eastern felafel scoop, is to make quenelles of the mixture using 2 dessertspoons. Take a small spoonful of felafel and pass it from spoon to spoon until you end up with a three-sided rugby ball shape (see picture on p.53). It's worth perfecting this technique for all sorts of purées, creams and even ice cream, when you feel like adding that extra bit of panache.

SWEET POTATO AND CORIANDER FELAFEL

Makes about 16

2 sweet potatoes, about 500 g/1 lb 2 oz
250 g/9 oz home-cooked chickpeas (garbanzo beans)
    or 400 g/14 oz canned chickpeas
2 garlic cloves, crushed
1 tsp cumin seeds, roasted and ground
1 tsp coriander seeds, roasted and ground
large pinch of cayenne pepper

½ tsp salt
2 tbsp roughly chopped fresh coriander (cilantro)
2 tbsp roughly chopped parsley
juice of ½–1 lemon
4 spring onions (scallions), finely sliced
2 tbsp olive oil

Preheat the oven to 200°C/400°F/Gas mark 6. Roast the sweet potatoes for about 45 minutes, or until they are soft. Cool a little before scooping out the flesh.

Blitz two-thirds of the chickpeas in a food processor with the garlic, spices, salt and herbs. Add the potato and pulse until fairly smooth. Taste and balance with lemon juice and more cayenne and salt if necessary.

Tip the mixture into a bowl and stir in the spring onions and the remaining chickpeas. This could all be blitzed together too, but I like a bit of extra texture.

Chill the mixture for an hour if you can (I've managed straight away but it is a bit of a sticky job) before shaping into small quenelles (see picture on p.53).

Place the felafel on a baking sheet lined with baking parchment, drizzle with a little oil and bake for about 15 minutes.

HOW ABOUT?

... adding a dash of extra-virgin olive oil to the mixture and serving as a vegetable purée alongside a roast.

BUTTERNUT SQUASH AND MINT FELAFEL

Makes about 16

450 g/1 lb butternut squash, peeled and cubed

3 tbsp olive oil

250 g/9 oz home-cooked chickpeas (garbanzo beans)
    or 400 g/14 oz canned chickpeas

2 garlic cloves, crushed

1 fresh red chilli (see p.248), finely chopped

1 tsp cumin seeds, roasted and ground

½ tsp ground cinnamon

½ tsp salt

10 mint leaves, ripped into small pieces

juice of ½–1 lemon

4 spring onions (scallions), finely sliced

Preheat the oven to 200°C/400°F/Gas mark 6.

Place the butternut squash in a roasting pan and toss with 1 tablespoon of the oil. Roast for about 30 minutes until tender and just starting to caramelize.

Blitz two-thirds of the chickpeas in a food processor with the garlic, chilli, spices, salt and about 5 mint leaves. Add the squash and pulse until the mixture begins to come together. Taste and balance with lemon juice, more salt and a touch more chilli if necessary.

Tip the mixture into a bowl and stir in the spring onions, and the remaining mint and whole chickpeas. This could all be blitzed together too, but I like a bit of extra texture.

Chill the mixture for an hour if you can (I've managed straight away but it is a bit of a sticky job) before shaping into small quenelles.

Place the felafel on a baking sheet lined with baking parchment, drizzle with the remaining oil and bake for about 15 minutes.

HOW ABOUT?

... roasting a whole butternut squash and using any leftovers in a salad, soup or mashed up with a few cannellini beans, garlic and olive oil on toast.

BEETROOT AND FETA FELAFEL

Makes about 16

450 g/1 lb beetroot (beets), washed and leaves trimmed

3 tbsp olive oil

250 g/9 oz home-cooked chickpeas (garbanzo beans)
    or 400 g/14 oz canned chickpeas

100 g/3½ oz feta cheese

2 garlic cloves, crushed

1 tsp cumin seeds, roasted and ground

large pinch of cayenne pepper

½ tsp salt

2 tbsp roughly chopped parsley

juice of ½–1 lemon

4 spring onions (scallions), finely sliced

Preheat the oven to 200°C/400°F/Gas mark 6.

Leave the beetroot whole, drizzle with 1 tablespoon of the olive oil and wrap in a foil parcel. Roast until a knife glides into the flesh easily: this could take anything between 30 minutes and 1 hour, depending on the size and freshness of the beetroot. Leave to cool and then peel; the skin should just slip off.

Blitz the beetroot in a food processor with two-thirds of the chickpeas, the feta, garlic, spices, salt and parsley.

Scrape the mixture into a bowl and stir in the spring onions and the remaining chickpeas.

Chill the mixture for an hour if you can (it makes it easier to handle), before shaping into small quenelles.

Place the felafel on a baking sheet lined with baking parchment, drizzle with the remaining olive oil and bake for about 15 minutes.

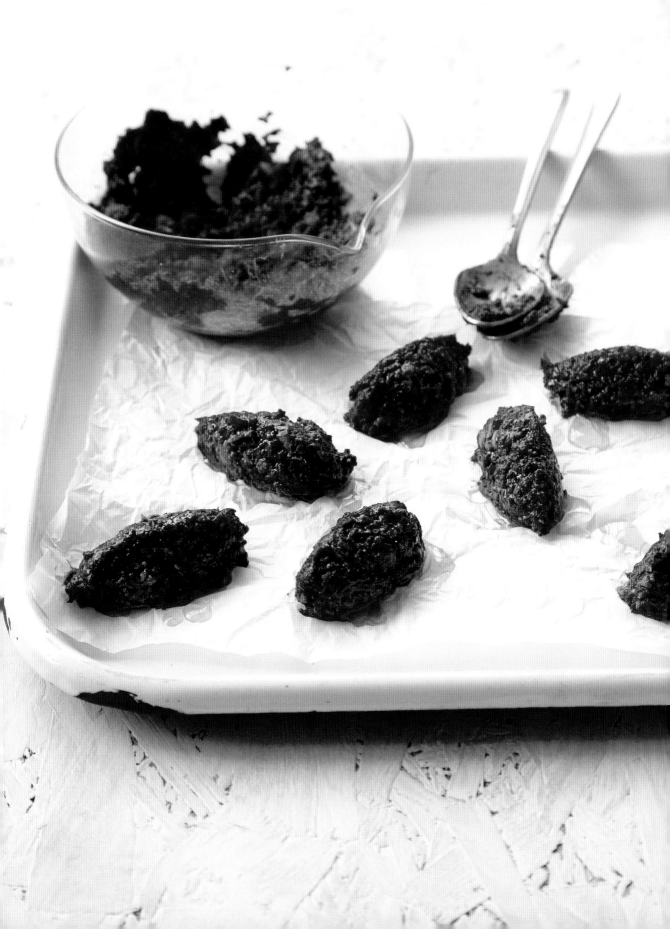

Italian *farinata*, *cecina*, *torta de ceci* (depending on where you're from), or *socca* from just over the French border in Nice, is a flatbread made from chickpea flour. Trattorias and bakeries the length of the Riviera draw regular lunchtime queues, and back in my Italian yachting days I became a fan too.

The bakery in Chiavari had a sign scrawled up in the window announcing the time the hot *farinata* was on sale, straight from the wood-fired oven. I remember zipping back to the boatyard on my moped with a meticulously tied greaseproof parcel of steaming *farinata* for the crew.

A wood-fired oven is obviously not on the cards for most of us, but you can create something approximating *farinata* in a very hot domestic oven. It's usually served simply with plenty of black pepper but I love to pile some slices of cheese or cured meat on the top.

CHICKPEA FLATBREAD
FARINATA

Serves 4
200 g/7 oz/2 cups chickpea flour (gram flour, besan)
½ tbsp finely chopped rosemary (optional)
salt and pepper
400 ml/14 fl oz water
3 tbsp extra-virgin olive oil

Tip the chickpea flour, rosemary and 1 teaspoon salt into a large bowl and gradually whisk in the water until you have a loose, lump-free batter. Rest the batter for at least 1 hour and up to 12 (strict timing instructions vary from town to town, although I've noticed little difference in the results).

Preheat the oven to 220°C/425°F/Gas mark 7.

Take a large flat tin or ovenproof frying pan (the professionals have a huge round pan specifically for the purpose) and heat it up in the oven or over a medium-high heat.

Skim off any froth from the top of the batter and then stir in most of the olive oil.

Add the remaining oil to the hot pan, swirling it to create a non-stick surface, just as you would for a pancake. Now tip in the batter to a depth of about 1 cm/½ in and place in the oven. Bake for 15–20 minutes or until the surface is crisp and bubbling. I also give it a quick blast under the grill for some extra colour.

Give it a few turns of the pepper mill, slice up with a pizza cutter and serve right away.

HOW ABOUT?

... serving with:
fried onions and Gorgonzola cheese,
or mozzarella, tomatoes and basil,
or Taleggio cheese and prosciutto.

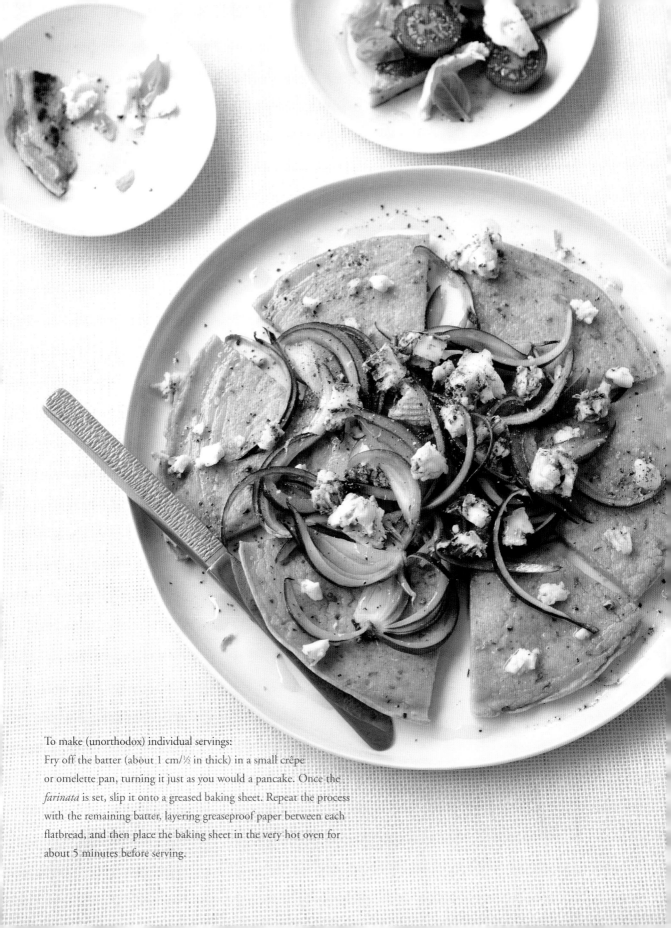

To make (unorthodox) individual servings:
Fry off the batter (about 1 cm/½ in thick) in a small crêpe
or omelette pan, turning it just as you would a pancake. Once the
farinata is set, slip it onto a greased baking sheet. Repeat the process
with the remaining batter, layering greaseproof paper between each
flatbread, and then place the baking sheet in the very hot oven for
about 5 minutes before serving.

Indian pakora, delicious deep-fried titbits in a light crisp batter, are similar
to Japanese tempura. But whereas tempura batter is made with wheat flour,
the Indian version uses chickpea flour, or besan. The batter can be lightly spiced
too. These are traditionally made in a karahi (or kadhai), a deep, wok-shaped
cooking pan.

A plate of mixed pakora with some zingy fresh mango pickle (see p.246) and
raita (see p.246) is an absolute treat.

SPICED VEGETABLE FRITTERS
PAKORA

Serves 4 as a pre-dinner nibble or starter

FOR THE BATTER

150 g/5½ oz/scant 1½ cups chickpea flour
   (gram flour, besan)

½–1 tsp salt

½ tsp ground turmeric

1 tsp ground coriander

1 tsp garam masala, shop-bought or home blend (see p.247)

½ tsp chilli powder or cayenne pepper

about 150 ml/5 fl oz/⅔ cup water

¼ tsp bicarbonate of soda (baking soda)

2 tbsp poppy seeds or 1 tsp nigella seeds (optional)

vegetable oil for deep-frying

1 lemon or lime cut into wedges, to serve

About 500 g/1 lb 2 oz prepared vegetables, such as:
   onion rings
   cauliflower or broccoli florets
   potato skins
   aubergine (eggplant), sliced and cut into crescents
   sweet potato or pumpkin, cut into thin chips
   mushrooms

Put the chickpea flour, ½ teaspoon salt and the spices into a large bowl and
gradually whisk in the water until you have a thick, smooth batter. Leave to
stand for about 10 minutes.

Just before using the batter, stir in the bicarbonate of soda and the poppy or
nigella seeds, if you are using them.

Pour the vegetable oil, to a depth of about 20 cm/8 in, into a large pan, deep-fat
fryer or heavy-bottomed wok. Heat the oil to 180°C/350°F. Test with a piece of
vegetable dipped in the batter: it should sizzle and rise to the surface. Cook for
about 8 minutes, then drain on kitchen paper, leave to cool slightly so you don't
burn your mouth, and taste; you may want to add extra salt or spices to the batter.

Dip 3 or 4 pieces of vegetable into the batter and then drop them carefully into
the hot oil; carry on dipping and adding until the surface of the oil is full but not
crowded. Cook for about 8 minutes, carefully stirring now and then, until the
vegetables are crisp and golden. Using a slotted spoon, lift them out of the oil and
drain on kitchen paper. Repeat until all the pakora are cooked. Serve hot, with
lemon or lime wedges.

HOW ABOUT?

… dipping a few shelled, raw prawns
in the batter.

… adding a teaspoon of cumin seeds
to the batter.

… giving the batter extra zing with a
little grated fresh ginger, a handful of
coriander leaves and a couple of green
chillies – all chopped extremely finely.

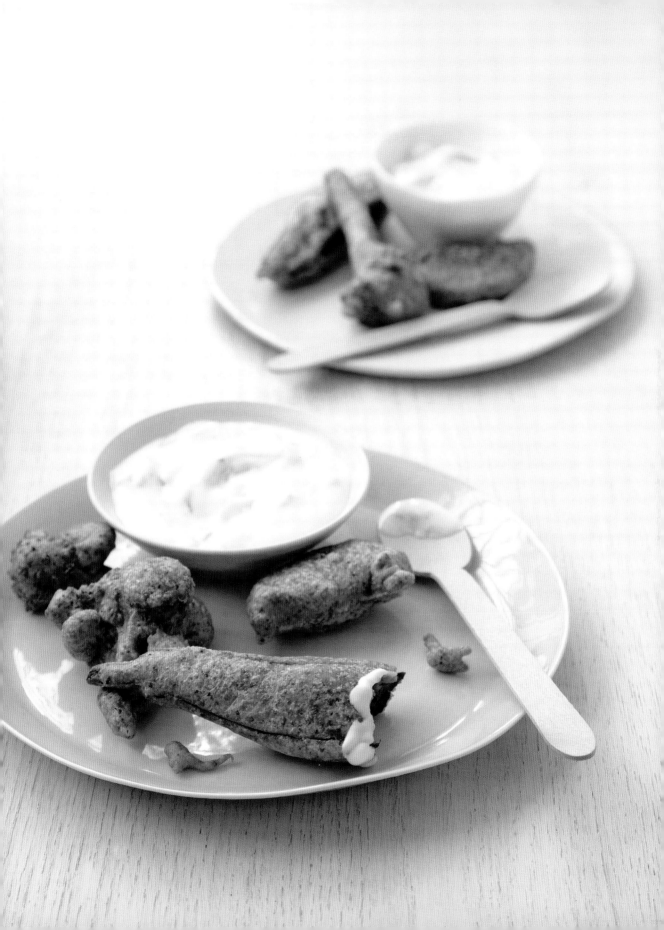

Balls, rissoles, burgers, cutlets; none of these culinary names exactly sing, especially when paired with the rather unglamorous lentil. Somehow '*albóndigas*', with all their tasty tapas connections, promise so much more. *Albóndigas* are usually meatballs, but the name derives from the Arabic word for hazelnut, so I have no qualms about using it here.

My great friend Mercé, who has a cookery school in the mountains to the north of Barcelona, once threw these together for our supper as we chatted over a glass of wine. The nuts are key to the wonderful texture. Once you have the basic formula for these *albóndigas*, you can switch the flavours to suit your mood or the contents of your fridge. Any leftovers will be ideal for your lunch box.

LENTIL AND HAZELNUT ALBÓNDIGAS

Makes 20

200 g/7 oz/1 cup brown lentils, rinsed

1 tbsp vegetable bouillon powder, ½ a vegetable stock cube or a bouquet garni

olive oil for frying

1 onion, very finely diced or grated

2 garlic cloves, crushed

2 carrots, very finely diced or grated

1 tsp ground, roasted cumin seeds

1 tsp paprika

handful of flat-leaf parsley, finely chopped

handful of hazelnuts, roughly chopped

salt and pepper

juice of ½–1 lemon

1 egg, lightly beaten

3–4 tbsp chickpea flour, rice flour (or plain/all-purpose flour at a pinch)

tzatziki (see p.246), to serve

Put the lentils in a pan and cover by about 5 cm/2 in of cold water. Add a little flavouring: bouillon powder, vegetable stock or a bundle of herbs. Bring the water to a simmer and cook until the lentils are really tender but not collapsed. Keep an eye on them, as you may need to top up with a little boiling water.

Meanwhile, heat 1 tablespoon olive oil in a small pan and cook the onion until soft. Add the garlic, carrots, cumin and paprika and stir for a minute or two until you're engulfed in fabulous smells. Tip the mixture into a large bowl.

Drain the lentils well, otherwise you will have a very sloppy mixture. Use a potato masher or a hand-held blender to mash about a third of the lentils so that the mixture will hold together, then add all the lentils to the vegetable mixture. Stir in the parsley and nuts and season well with salt, pepper and lemon juice. Cool.

Stir in the egg and just enough flour to bind the mixture. Roll the mixture into large walnut-sized balls (it helps to have damp hands as you do this) and lay them out on a tray. The balls will feel quite soft, but don't worry, they will hold together well.

Heat a little olive oil in a frying pan and shallow-fry the *albóndigas* until golden all over. Serve hot, with tzatziki.

HOW ABOUT?

... Moroccan style: adding chopped fresh coriander (cilantro) and cayenne pepper, replacing the hazelnuts with pine nuts, and serving with spiced tomato and chickpea sauce (see p.208).

... Indian style: throwing in grated fresh ginger, finely diced fresh chilli and 1 tsp curry powder, and making the cashew your chosen nut. Serve with raita and pickles.

This unorthodox approach to a southern Indian classic was inspired by a Jamie Oliver recipe. Traditional dosa batter is made with urad dal and rice, and, as Jamie points out, requires a couple of days to ferment; his version using chickpea flour is more accessible. Chickpea pancakes, or *chilla besan*, are traditional too, but are rarely stuffed as they are thicker (more American pancake than thin, lacy crêpe).

Dosa are often served for breakfast in their homeland but I'd happily eat this as a starter or light lunch. *Illustrated on pp.60–61.*

INDIAN STUFFED PANCAKES
DOSA

Makes 8

FOR THE FILLING
3–4 large potatoes, peeled and quartered
salt
2 tbsp vegetable oil
1 tsp mustard seeds
10 curry leaves
3–4 green chillies (see p.248), finely diced
2.5-cm/1-in piece of fresh ginger, finely chopped
2 tbsp cashew nuts, roughly chopped
1 tbsp split urad dal (optional)
3 red onions, sliced
1 tsp ground turmeric
juice of 1 lime or lemon

FOR THE BATTER
150 g/5½ oz/scant 1½ cups chickpea flour
    (gram flour, besan)
50 g/1¾ oz/7 tbsp plain (all-purpose) flour
large pinch of bicarbonate of soda (baking soda)
½ tsp salt
1 tsp mustard seeds
300 ml/10 fl oz/1½ cups water

TO SERVE
raita (see p.246)
mango chutney or mango pickle (see p.246)

First make the filling. Boil the potatoes in salted water until tender, drain, mash and set aside. Heat the vegetable oil in a frying pan and add the mustard seeds. As soon as they begin to pop, add the curry leaves, chillies, ginger, cashew nuts and urad dal. Cook until the room is filled with the magical smell of spices and the cashews are turning gold. Add the onions and turmeric and cook for a further 15 minutes, until the onions are soft and golden. Stir in the potatoes and season with lime juice. Taste and add salt and even a pinch of chilli powder if required.

Now make the batter. Put the chickpea flour, plain flour, bicarbonate of soda, salt and mustard seeds into a large bowl and gradually whisk in the water until you have a smooth batter.

Place a small pancake pan or non-stick frying pan over a medium heat and add a little vegetable oil. Swirl the oil around the pan and wipe away any excess with kitchen paper. Add a tablespoon of batter to the pan – these should be wafer thin – and spiral it quickly around, just as you would a crêpe. Once the surface begins to bubble and the bottom is crisp and golden, it's time to spoon some of the filling into the middle. Roll up and serve right away, with raita and chutney or pickle.

HOW ABOUT?

... mixing some cooked sweet potato, peas or pumpkin into the filling.
... no curry leaves? Add plenty of fresh coriander along with the lime juice.
... Shrove Tuesday with a difference: start with Indian pancakes and have the customary crêpes for pud.
... using the filling as a delicious side dish for spiced grilled chicken or fish.

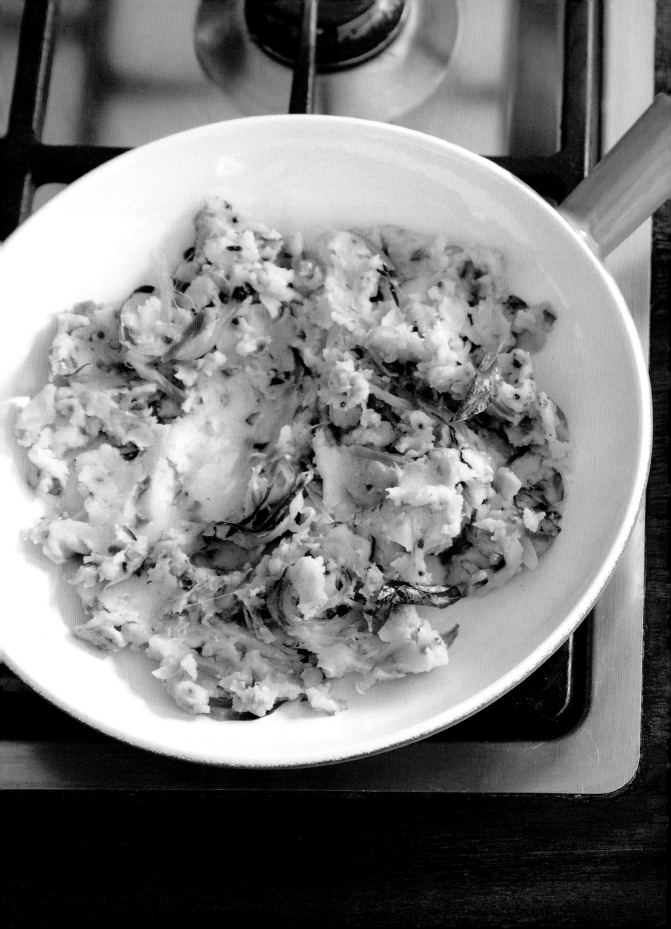

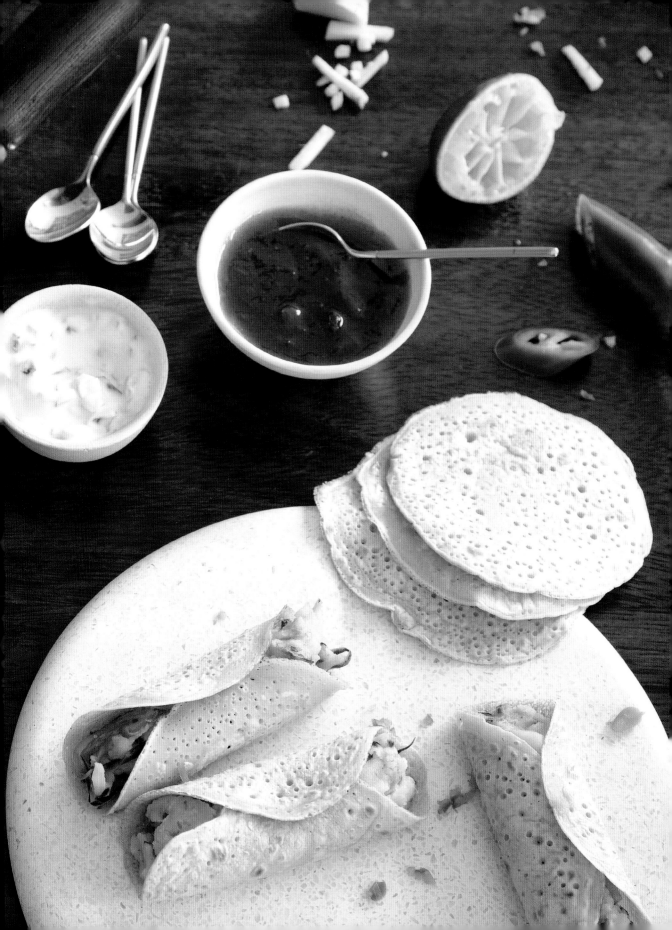

The Tex-Mex answer to a stuffed crêpe, this is a wheat-flour tortilla stuffed with cheese and whatever else comes to hand. American recipes call for Monterey Jack cheese, or sometimes Cheddar, but Wensleydale works wonderfully. The black beans make these quesadillas more substantial, great for a brunch with all the guacamole, salsa and sour cream trimmings.

BLACK BEAN QUESADILLAS

Serves 4 as a main, 8 as a starter or snack

150 g/5½ oz Wensleydale cheese, or Cheddar at a pinch, crumbled

6 spring onions (scallions), sliced

500 g/1 lb 2 oz home-cooked or 2 x 400 g/14 oz cans of black beans

4–5 pickled jalapeño peppers (from a jar), sliced (optional)

small handful of coriander (cilantro) leaves, finely chopped

salt and pepper

8 soft tortillas

olive oil

TO SERVE

tomato salsa (see p.244)

guacamole (see p.243)

150 ml/5 fl oz/⅔ cup sour cream

Mix together the cheese, spring onions, beans, jalapeños and coriander leaves. Season to taste with salt and pepper.

Divide the mixture among the tortillas and fold them over to form a half moon shape. You can do this ahead of time.

Heat a ridged griddle or heavy-bottomed frying pan, no oil required, and then cook the quesadillas two at a time.

Serve immediately or keep warm in the oven while you finish cooking the remaining quesadillas.

HOW ABOUT?

... replacing the black beans with refried beans (see p.162).

... adding some chopped *chipotles en adobo* (see p.248) or chipotle relish.

... using corn tortillas, as they do in Mexico where the quesadilla originated. Try tracking down some fabulous fresh ones.

... throwing in some cooked chicken, beef or ham.

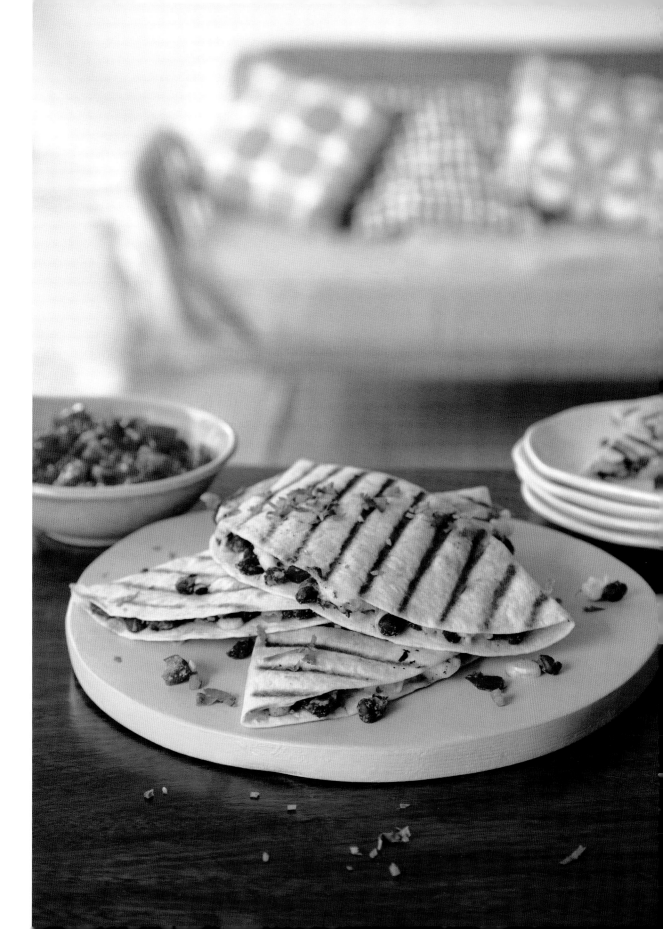

Creamy white beans with plenty of cheese, seasoning and herbs make fabulous little fritters that virtually melt in your mouth. The mozzarella helps to hold the fritters together. I wouldn't dream of using the blocks of solid mozzarella in a salad, but the texture works well here (the remainder can be used for pizza or frozen until you make more fritters).

Bite-size *frittelle* topped with a spoonful of piquant salsa verde are heaven for pre-dinner nibbles. Larger fritters can be served with a zippy salsa, crisp green salad and some crusty bread as a summery lunch.

CANNELLINI, PARMESAN AND BASIL FRITTELLE

Makes 8 large or 16–20 canapé size

olive oil for frying

1 onion, diced

2 garlic cloves, crushed

500 g/1 lb 2 oz home-cooked cannellini beans
    or 2 x 400 g/14 oz cans of cannellini beans

75 g/2¾ oz Parmesan cheese, grated

100 g/3½ oz mozzarella, very finely chopped

zest of ½ lemon

juice of ½ lemon

2 tbsp fresh breadcrumbs

1 egg, lightly beaten

large handful of basil leaves, ripped

salt and pepper

3–4 tbsp flour, for dusting

Heat 2 tablespoons of the olive oil in a large frying pan and cook the onion until soft and golden. Add the garlic and, as soon as you're engulfed in its wonderful smell, remove the pan from the heat and set aside.

Tip about two-thirds of the beans into a food processor, add the cooked onion and the garlic and all the remaining fritter ingredients. Pulse the mixture until it is fairly sticky but still has some texture. Remove the blade and stir in the whole beans. If mod cons aren't your thing, mash the beans with the back of a fork or a potato masher.

Now shape a small spoonful of the mixture into a small patty (it only need be the size of a large coin) and dust it with flour. Wipe the frying pan with a piece of kitchen paper and heat up a little oil. Cook the patty until deep gold, turning after a couple of minutes. Taste the cooked patty; you may need to balance the flavours of the bean mixture with more lemon, Parmesan, basil, salt or pepper.

Rest the mixture in the fridge for about 15 minutes to make it firmer and easier to handle.

Shape the mixture into equal-sized patties and shallow-fry a few at a time; keep them somewhere warm until you have cooked the lot. Serve at once, with salsa verde (see p.242) or Mediterranean tomato salsa (p.244).

HOW ABOUT?

... using pecorino in place of the Parmesan, finely chopped rosemary instead of the basil, and plenty of chopped fresh red chilli for a southern Italian version. Serve with a spoonful of Sicilian caponata (the sweet and sour Italian answer to ratatouille).

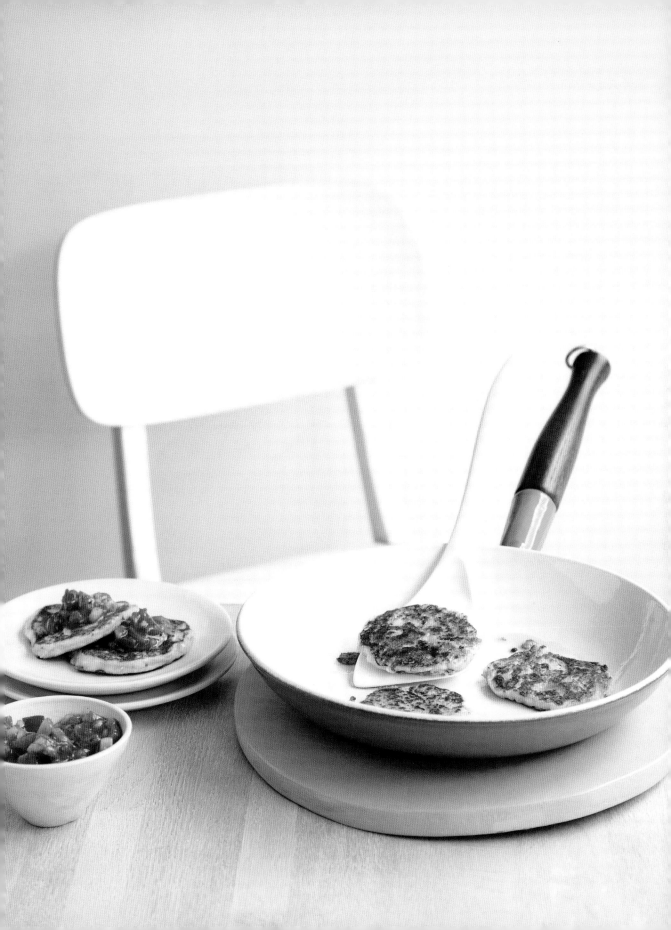

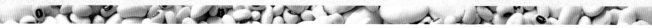

THE BEAN BURGER

These crispy-coated bean cakes can knock the socks off many a meaty burger. Serve them with dips, salsas or salads, but don't stuff them into burger buns, the result is just too starchy.

Once you have this basic mixture, you can play with any number of adventurous combinations. The formula works well with cannellinis, haricots, pintos, black beans, red kidneys, butter beans (all the New World beans in fact) and chickpeas too. Just remember to include a bit of texture with some whole beans, nuts or seeds, some zippy acidity such as lemon or vinegar and plenty of herbs or spicing.

MASTER RECIPE FOR BEAN BURGERS

Makes 6–8 burgers

2 tbsp olive oil

1 onion, roughly chopped

2 garlic cloves, crushed

2 x 400 g/14 oz cans of beans or 500 g/1 lb 2 oz
   home-cooked beans

2 eggs, beaten

5 tbsp dried breadcrumbs (see p.248)

salt and pepper

Heat the oil in a pan over a medium heat and cook the onion until just soft. Add the garlic (and any spices you are using) and cook until you're enveloped in wonderful smells. Set aside.

Purée three-quarters of the beans using a hand-held blender, whizz them in a food processor or just go wild with the potato masher. You want a slightly lumpy, creamy texture. Add the remaining whole beans and the onion and garlic mixture.

Stir in the eggs and breadcrumbs with whatever herbs, vegetables, nuts or seeds you are using. Season with salt and pepper to taste. Press the mixture into firm cakes. The size is up to you, but I usually make 6. A few hours' chilling in the fridge will firm up the burgers before cooking but is not absolutely necessary.

COOKING YOUR BURGERS

Pan-fry your burgers in olive oil over a medium heat. They will hold together fairly well but be gentle as you turn them over. About 5–6 minutes on each side will do the trick. You can keep them hot in the oven (160°C/325°F/Gas mark 3) for about 15 minutes; any longer and they dry out a little.

Alternatively, you can place the burgers on a greased baking sheet, drizzle with a little oil and bake in a hot oven (200°C/400°F/Gas mark 6) for about 20 minutes. I usually turn the burgers over to serve, as the underside crusts up nicely.

These take me back to my twenties, working as a cocktail waitress in San Francisco. There was a fabulous café down the road from our flat where I experienced my first really great vegetarian food. This flavour combination is well established in the Californian kitchen, with all its Mexican influences, and it's one I never tire of.

CALIFORNIAN BLACK BEAN BURGER

master burger recipe (opposite) made with black beans or a
    mixture of black and pinto
1–2 small fresh red chillies (see p.248), finely diced,
    or a large pinch of cayenne pepper
1 tsp ground cumin
zest of ½ lime
juice of 1 lime
1 tbsp chopped fresh coriander (cilantro)
2 tbsp sweetcorn kernels
3 tbsp roasted peanuts, roughly chopped (or sprouted
    peanuts, see p.265)

Add the chilli and cumin as you cook the garlic. Stir all the remaining ingredients into your bean mixture. Follow the cooking instructions opposite.

HOW ABOUT?

... serving with Mexican trimmings: salsa (see p.242), guacamole (see p.243) and perhaps a spoonful of rice with some *chipotle en adobo* stirred through (see p.43).

Crammed with fibre and vitamins, this really is a super-charged health hit. If you're trying to cut back on the calories, then you'd better skip the mustardy crème fraîche and make a fresh tomato salad instead, but do dress it with a mustardy vinaigrette (the mustard and tarragon combination is sublime). You can bake rather than fry the burgers too.

THE SUPER BURGER

master burger recipe (opposite) made with haricots (navy
    beans), cannellini, butter beans (large lima beans)
4 tbsp cooked quinoa (see p.19)
large handful of sprouting beans (see p.20)
1 tbsp balsamic vinegar
8 sun-dried tomatoes, very finely chopped
2 tbsp freshly chopped tarragon

TO SERVE
1–2 tbsp grainy French mustard
6 tbsp crème fraîche

Prepare the master recipe and stir in all the super burger ingredients. Season to taste. Follow the cooking instructions opposite.

Stir the mustard into the crème fraîche and serve with the burgers.

HOW ABOUT?

... serving with a mound of cooked spinach or a fresh tomato salad.
... replacing the sun-dried tomatoes with dried porcini mushrooms (soak and drain before chopping).

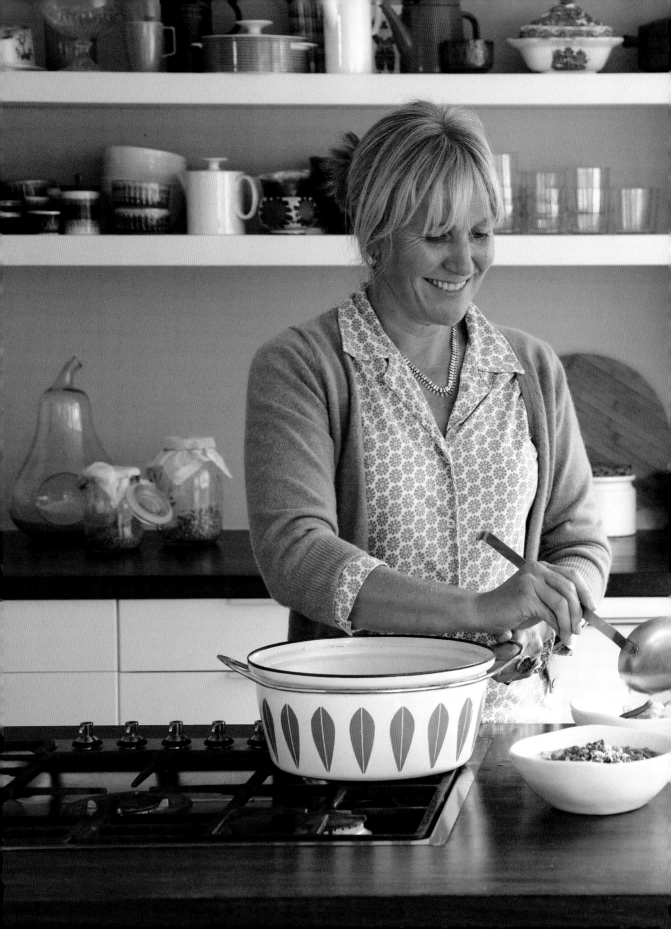

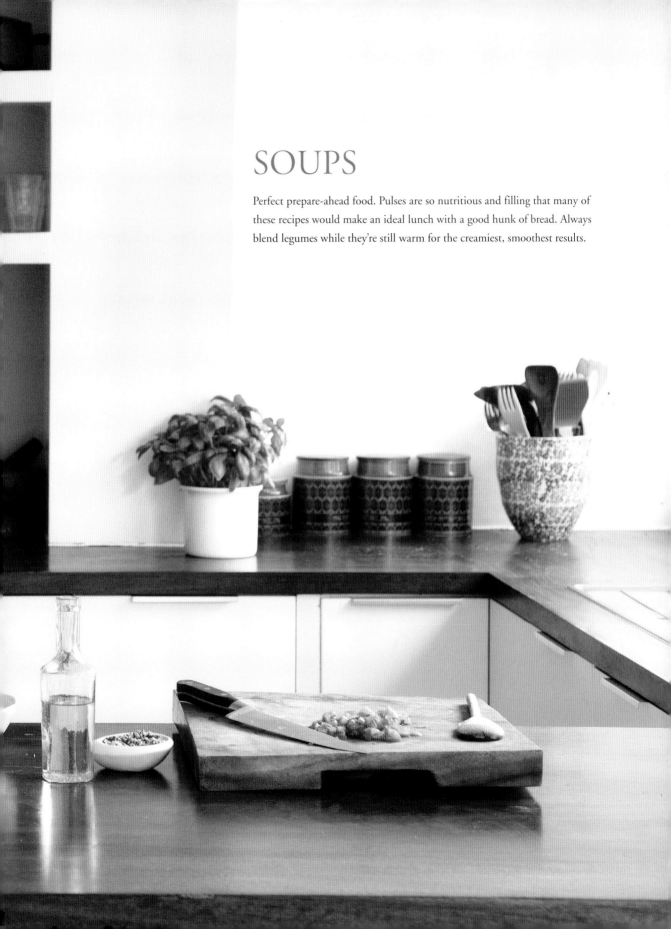

SOUPS

Perfect prepare-ahead food. Pulses are so nutritious and filling that many of these recipes would make an ideal lunch with a good hunk of bread. Always blend legumes while they're still warm for the creamiest, smoothest results.

Fast, easy, cheap and, above all, wonderfully, zippily delicious. This is a soup I always teach to teenagers on their student survival course. You can blitz it with a hand-held blender in the pan, so that's another plus – there's barely any washing up, but if you have the time, this becomes beautifully silky and creamy if well whizzed in a jug blender.

CHICKPEA, CHILLI AND MINT SOUP

Serves 4

3 tbsp olive oil

2 onions, diced

4 garlic cloves, finely chopped

2–3 red chillies (see p.248), finely chopped

2 x 400 g/14 oz cans of chickpeas (garbanzo beans)
   or 500 g/1 lb 2 oz home-cooked chickpeas

1 litre/1¾ pints/4 cups vegetable or chicken stock (a stock cube will do)

salt

juice of ½–1 lemon

about 12 fresh mint leaves, sliced

Heat the oil in a large saucepan and cook the onion until golden. Add the garlic and chillies and, as soon as you can really smell the sizzling garlic, add the chickpeas and the stock and simmer for about 10 minutes.

Blitz the soup, using a hand-held blender for convenience or a jug blender for a smoother result.

Taste. The soup will seem rather bland, but adding salt, plenty of lemon juice and the touch of mint will work wonders. Serve hot.

HOW ABOUT?

... serving with a dollop of Greek yogurt.

... adding lime juice and coriander instead of lemon juice and mint.

... frying up a few prawns or pieces of squid and popping them on the top.

A recipe from the unbeatably exuberant and passionate Italian food writer and teacher Ursula Ferrigno. I worked in a cookery school in Umbria with her many moons ago and will never forget opening the shutters at dawn to see her up a fig tree, harvesting breakfast for the students; she just never stops. Ursula's recipes are refreshingly simple and bursting with authentic Italian flavour.

A note on truffle oil. Many truffle oils are artificially flavoured, so do check the bottle before you buy.

CHESTNUT, CHICKPEA AND ROSEMARY MINESTRA WITH WHITE TRUFFLE OIL

Serves 4

4 tbsp olive oil

1 onion, finely chopped

1 carrot, finely diced

2 celery stalks, finely diced

4 garlic cloves, finely chopped

2 tsp rosemary, very finely chopped

850 ml/1½ pints/3½ cups vegetable or chicken stock

250 g/9 oz home-cooked chickpeas (garbanzo beans)
    or 1 x 400 g/14 oz can of chickpeas

200 g/7 oz cooked and peeled chestnuts – vacuum-packed are great

2 bay leaves

salt and pepper

white truffle oil, to drizzle

Heat the olive oil in a large saucepan and cook the onion, carrot, celery, garlic and rosemary very gently, stirring from time to time, until the vegetables are soft but not coloured. This will take about 15 minutes.

Add the stock, chickpeas, chestnuts and bay leaves and bring to the boil, then reduce the heat and simmer for about 20 minutes.

Season with salt and pepper to taste. Serve hot, drizzling with a little truffle oil at the table.

HOW ABOUT?

... not a fan of the pungent truffle aroma? Go for a good sprinkling of Parmesan instead.

A great comfort dish to have in your repertoire, as most of the ingredients are storecupboard staples.

If you can, seek out some pancetta rather than bacon, it really does make a difference. Traditionally, pancetta is not smoked but cured with salt and spices such as nutmeg, pepper and fennel and then aged for a few months. Don't trim off any fat: an Italian would be reduced to tears, as it's the best bit, adding fabulous flavour and fullness to your soup.

CHICKPEA, PANCETTA AND TOMATO SOUP

Serves 4

3 tbsp olive oil

100 g/3½ oz pancetta or unsmoked streaky bacon, finely chopped

2 onions, diced

about 5 sage leaves

3 garlic cloves, crushed

1 x 400 g/14 oz can of chopped tomatoes

1 x 400 g/14 oz can of chickpeas (garbanzo beans)
    or 250 g/9 oz home-cooked chickpeas

850 ml/1½ pints/3½ cups vegetable or chicken stock (a stock cube will do)

salt and pepper

200 g/7 oz cavolo nero, sliced really finely

extra-virgin olive oil and Parmesan cheese, to serve

Heat the olive oil in a large saucepan over a medium heat and cook the pancetta or bacon until the fat begins to render down.

Add the onions and cook until they are really soft and beginning to colour.

Stir in the sage and garlic and, once you are engulfed by their wonderful smell, it is time to tip in the tomatoes, chickpeas and stock. Season with a little salt and pepper to taste. Leave the soup to bubble away for about 10 minutes, then stir in the cavolo nero and cook for a couple of minutes.

Serve with a dash of extra-virgin olive oil and a sprinkling of grated Parmesan.

HOW ABOUT?

... throwing in a handful of tiny pasta shapes such as *stelle* or *ditalini* along with the chickpeas and making a meal of it.

... substituting the cavolo nero (Italian black cabbage, which is grown in the UK too) with some chopped spinach or baby spinach leaves.

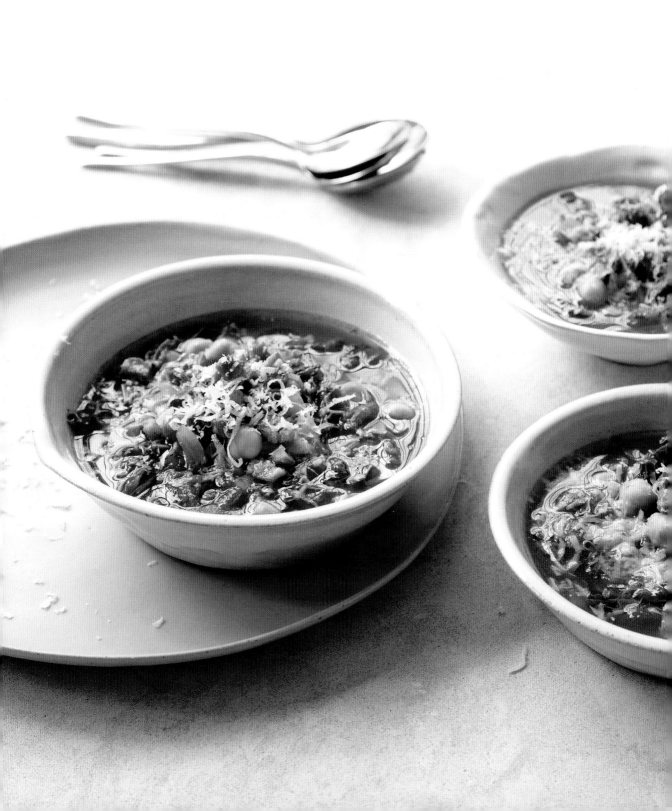

Lablabi is the traditional breakfast soup served up in virtually every Tunisian café. The magical combination of light, lemony broth with chickpeas, bread and poached egg will certainly set you up for the day.

This makes a perfect brunch dish. You could plate everything together as I've done or serve the basic soup and pass around small bowls with all the garnishes for your guests to add their own. Either way, it makes a fabulous, kaleidoscopic bowl of colour and flavour.

If you do get around to cooking your own chickpeas, their cooking water will really enhance the broth.

TUNISIAN CHICKPEA
AND LEMON BROTH
LABLABI

Serves 4

3 tbsp olive oil

1 large onion, diced

5 garlic cloves, crushed

700 g/1 lb 9 oz home-cooked chickpeas (garbanzo beans)
    or 3 x 400 g/14 oz cans of chickpeas

1 tsp ground cumin

1 tbsp harissa, bought or homemade (see p.245)

salt

850 ml/1½ pints/3½ cups vegetable stock
    or chickpea cooking water

juice of 1 lemon

2–4 slices of good, day-old rustic bread, ripped into
    large pieces

4 very fresh eggs, poached (see p.249)

1 tsp wine vinegar

TO GARNISH

4 tsp harissa

1 tbsp chopped fresh parsley

2 tbsp capers

12 black olives, chopped

2 roasted red peppers (see p.249), peeled, deseeded and
    cut into ribbons (optional)

dash of extra-virgin olive oil

1 lemon, quartered

Heat the olive oil in a large saucepan and cook the onion until soft and golden.

Add the garlic and, once your kitchen is filled with its fabulous smell, throw in the chickpeas, cumin, harissa, a pinch of salt and the stock. Simmer for 5 minutes.

Squeeze in the lemon juice and season with salt to taste.

Place the ripped bread in individual soup bowls, the wider the better. Ladle over the broth and some chickpeas and place a poached egg on top.

To garnish, I usually sit a small blob of harissa on top of the egg and serve some more at the table. Sprinkle all the other bits over the soup and serve with a wedge of lemon.

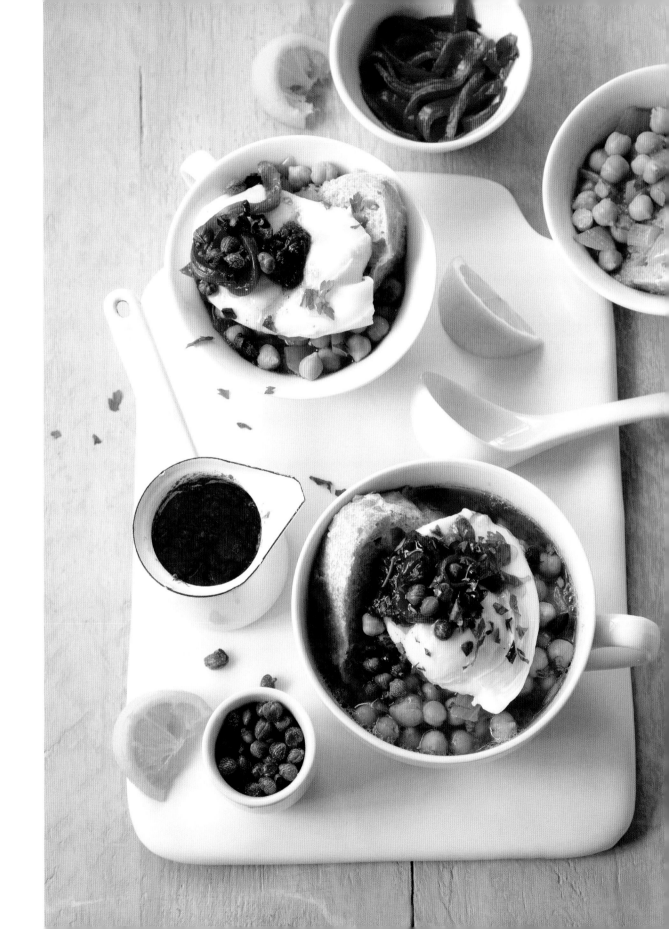

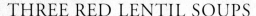

THREE RED LENTIL SOUPS

When it comes to soup, red lentils are supremely versatile. Their creamy texture and subtle taste provide a fabulous backdrop for a myriad of flavours, from the Mediterranean to the Bay of Bengal. Here are three recipes to get you started, but do alter and improvise according to what you have in your fridge, cupboard or, should you be so lucky, garden.

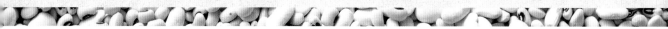

A favourite standby recipe, I can usually rustle this up without a trip to the shops. It came about in a boatyard in Provence, where I had to feed hungry deckhands a hearty lunch. Crisp blue winter sky and fresh baguette apart, it still tastes pretty wonderful.

TOMATO, ROSEMARY AND RED LENTIL SOUP

Serves 4

2 tbsp olive oil

1 onion, finely diced

2 garlic cloves, crushed

1 sprig of rosemary, leaves finely chopped

1–2 fresh chillies (see p.248), very finely chopped, or a good pinch of dried chilli flakes

225 g/8 oz/generous 1 cup red lentils, rinsed

1 x 400 g/14 oz can of chopped tomatoes

1.2 litres/2 pints/5 cups vegetable or chicken stock

salt

juice of 1–2 lemons

4 tbsp crème fraîche, sour cream or double (heavy) cream

Heat the oil in a large saucepan and cook the onions until soft and translucent. Add the garlic, rosemary and just enough chilli to give the soup a nice little kick. Once you can smell the garlic and rosemary, add the lentils, tomatoes and stock and simmer for about 30 minutes, or until the lentils are soft.

If you feel that the soup is too thick, add a little water or stock. Taste and balance with salt and enough lemon juice to lift the soup: it should be really fresh and zippy. Serve hot, topped with a spoonful of crème fraîche.

HOW ABOUT?

... adding some chopped cooked sausage to the soup just before serving – a traditional chipolata or a spicier Italian sausage.

... thyme, basil or parsley could be substituted for the rosemary.

A substantial soup inspired by the spicing of the traditional and much lighter broth, *rasam*, that's typically served as an aperitif in Chennai (Madras). Use a good curry powder or whip out your pestle and mortar and play around with the spices.

INDIAN SPICED LENTIL SOUP

Serves 4

2 tbsp vegetable oil

1 onion, finely diced

2 garlic cloves, crushed

5-cm/2-in piece of fresh ginger, chopped

1 tsp medium curry powder or your own Indian spice blend

225 g/8 oz/generous 1 cup red lentils, rinsed

1 x 400 g/14 oz can of chopped tomatoes

1.2 litres/2 pints/5 cups vegetable or chicken stock

1 tbsp tamarind paste (see p.247)

2 tbsp finely chopped fresh coriander (cilantro)

salt

juice of 1–2 limes

Tabasco or any hot chilli sauce

pinch of brown sugar or jaggery
    (a fudgy, unrefined palm or cane sugar from India)

4 tbsp plain yogurt

Heat the oil in a large saucepan and cook the onion until soft and translucent. Throw in the garlic, ginger and curry powder, stir for a minute or two and then add the lentils, tomatoes, stock and tamarind. Simmer the soup until the lentils are soft and beginning to collapse. Add more liquid if you would prefer a thinner soup.

Stir in the coriander, then taste and season with salt, lime juice and enough Tabasco/chilli to put a spring in your step. A good pinch of sugar or jaggery will do wonders for this soup. You want the perfect balance of sweet, sour, salty and spice. Serve hot, with a dollop of yogurt.

HOW ABOUT?

... halving the amount of stock in the recipe and serving this as a dal alongside rice or a curry.

... adding 2 parsnips, peeled and finely chopped, along with the lentils. The combination is sublime and the parsnips' natural sweetness will mean you need no sugar. You will need to add an extra cup or two of water to thin the soup.

Pumpkin gives this soup a wonderful velvety texture and when it comes to the flavour, the Thai balance of spicy, sweet, sour and salty is vital. The chilli provides the spicy heat, so just keep adding small amounts of fish sauce or soy, lime juice and sugar until you reach perfection.

PUMPKIN, COCONUT AND LENTIL SOUP

Serves 4

2 tbsp vegetable oil

small bunch of spring onions (scallions), finely sliced

2 garlic cloves, crushed

5-cm/2-in piece of fresh ginger, chopped

1–2 fiery chillies (see p.248), finely chopped

2 stalks of lemongrass, outer leaves removed and remainder finely sliced

225 g/8 oz/generous 1 cup red lentils, rinsed

500 g/1 lb 2 oz pumpkin or butternut squash, peeled, deseeded and
    cut into 2 cm/¾ inch dice

1.2 litres/2 pints/5 cups vegetable or chicken stock

400 g/14 oz can of coconut milk

1 tbsp tamarind paste (see p.247)

2 tbsp finely chopped fresh coriander (cilantro)

Thai fish sauce or tamari soy sauce

juice of 1–2 limes

pinch of brown sugar or palm sugar (optional)

Heat the oil in a large saucepan and add most of the spring onions (setting aside a tablespoon to garnish). Add the garlic, ginger, chilli and lemongrass and stir for a minute or two, until you are engulfed in fabulous smells. You will be wheezing if you have been generous with the chilli!

Add the lentils, pumpkin or squash and the stock, and simmer until the lentils are soft and the pumpkin flesh has collapsed.

Stir in the coconut milk, tamarind and most of the coriander. Now taste and balance the soup with fish sauce or soy sauce, lime juice and sugar.

Serve hot, sprinkled with the remaining spring onions and coriander.

HOW ABOUT?

... thinning the soup with a little extra stock or water and adding some sugarsnap peas for the last 2 minutes of cooking

... stir-frying some raw prawns with a little chilli and garlic and serving on top of the soup.

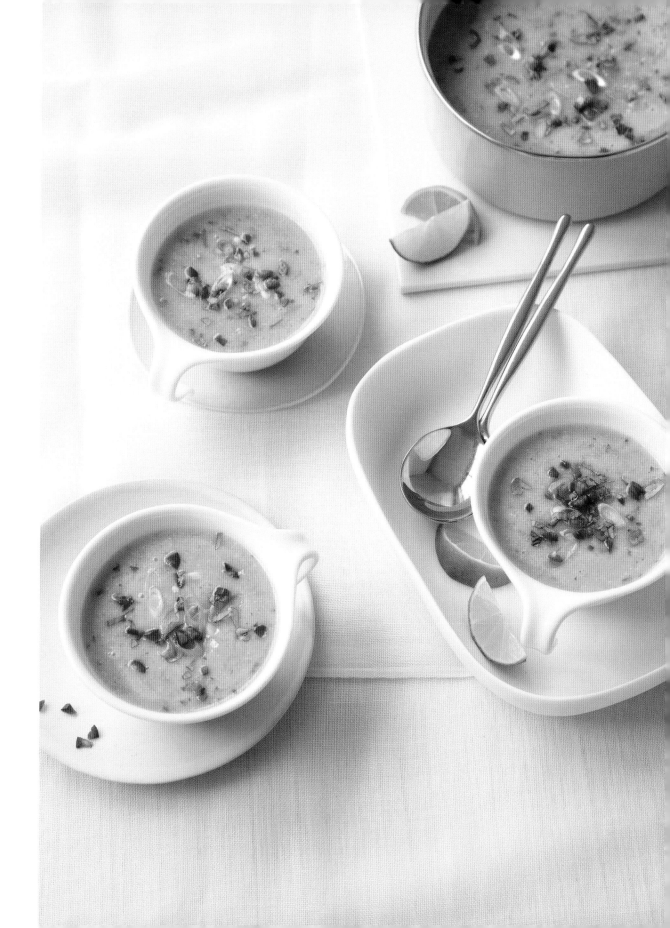

A combination to savour in the autumn. I've played around with some scribbled notes I made about a soup I ate in a woodsmoke-filled bistro, high in the French Pyrenees. The French are obsessive mushroom foragers, but you can use dried ceps (porcini) and whatever fresh mushrooms your greengrocer or supermarket offers.

Serving sautéed wild mushrooms on top of the soup elevates this from rustic kitchen pottage to something a little more elegant.

FRENCH WILD MUSHROOM AND LENTIL SOUP

Serves 4

15 g/½ oz dried porcini mushrooms

3 tbsp olive oil

1 onion, diced

1 carrot, diced

2 celery stalks, diced

2 garlic cloves, crushed

225 g/8 oz/generous 1 cup small green lentils such as Puy or Castelluccio, rinsed

1.5 litres/2¾ pints/6½ cups chicken or vegetable stock

1 bouquet garni

juice of ½ lemon

salt and pepper

FOR THE SAUTÉED WILD MUSHROOMS

300 g/10½ oz mixed wild mushrooms such as girolles, chanterelles, morels, horns of plenty, ceps

30 g/1 oz unsalted butter

2 shallots, finely diced

1 garlic clove, crushed

small handful of flat-leaf parsley, roughly chopped

Soak the dried mushrooms in enough hot water to just cover them and set them aside for 30 minutes. Once soft, squeeze out any excess water and chop them finely. Reserve the flavoured soaking liquid – it may need straining if it is gritty.

Heat the oil in a large saucepan over a low heat and cook the onion, carrot and celery until really soft but not coloured. Throw in the garlic and, as soon as you can smell it, add the chopped dried mushrooms and the lentils. Stir everything together and then add the stock, the mushroom liquid and the bouquet garni. Simmer for about 30 minutes until the lentils are really tender.

I like to purée a small quantity of the lentils with a hand-held blender to give a creamy base liquid. You may decide to skip this step, or alternatively purée the lot and make a smooth soup. Add a little water or stock if the soup seems very thick. Taste and adjust the seasoning with salt, lemon juice and plenty of black pepper.

Clean the wild mushrooms thoroughly with a brush or kitchen paper. If tricky to clean, you can rinse them briefly, but do not soak or they will become slimy.

Melt the butter in a large frying pan and cook the shallots over a low heat until translucent. Turn up the heat and toss in the mushrooms. After about 5 minutes, once the mushrooms have begun to caramelize and their liquid has evaporated, add the garlic and parsley and stir for a minute over the heat. Taste and season.

Serve the soup hot, with a mound of sautéed mushrooms in each bowl.

HOW ABOUT?

... stirring a few tablespoons of crème fraîche into the lentils for a richer result.

... economizing by using chestnut (cremini) mushrooms in place of the wild – but don't leave out the dried porcini mushrooms as they give depth of flavour.

... adding some chopped bacon along with the onion, carrot and celery.

The 'pea-souper' fogs that used to engulf England's capital gave this soup its other name, London Particular. It's fantastically hearty and comforting, just the thing for feeding a hungry crowd on a shoestring budget. This is cold-climate soup: the Scandinavians, Dutch, Germans, Poles, Canadians and North Americans all have their own variations.

Pea and ham soup is a great way to use up leftover ham on the bone or a good excuse to cook up a few ham hocks.

SPLIT PEA AND HAM SOUP

Serves 6

30 g/1 oz butter

1 onion, diced

1 carrot, finely diced

1 leek, washed, trimmed and finely chopped

1–2 cooked ham hocks and stock (see p.250) or a ham bone – you need about
   300 g/10½ oz ham scraps

300 g/10½ oz/1½ cups yellow split peas, rinsed

2 bay leaves

2–3 tbsp Worcestershire sauce (optional)

pepper

2–3 tbsp double (heavy) cream (optional)

Melt the butter in a large saucepan over a medium-low heat and cook the onion, carrot and leek until soft.

Meanwhile, remove the fat from the hocks and shred off most of the meat. Strain their cooking water to use too, but do give it a taste: it may be very salty and then you might decide to use half stock, half water.

Once the vegetables are soft, add the ham bones, split peas, bay leaves and about 2 litres/3½ pints of liquid: ham stock, water or combination of the two.

Simmer until the peas have softened and begun to collapse. Remove the bones and purée about a third of the soup. Use a blender or food processor and return to the pot or, better still, just plunge in a hand-held blender for a few seconds.

Top up with more water or ham stock if the soup is very thick, and then taste and season with Worcestershire sauce, if using, and pepper. You're unlikely to need more salt, especially if you add the Worcestershire sauce. Now you can choose whether to add the cream; rather unorthodox, but I love it. Heat through and add the shredded ham to the soup, leaving a little to sprinkle on the top.

HOW ABOUT?

... mixing plenty of finely chopped chives with some crème fraîche and stirring in at the table.

... going Dutch: add 3 handfuls of chopped celeriac with the vegetables, use green split peas and serve with slices of boiled *rookworst* (or another northern European smoked sausage), rye bread and mustard.

... going veggie: leave out the ham and Worcestershire sauce. Add 3 handfuls of chopped celeriac and some thyme along with the vegetables, use good vegetable stock and serve with a sprinkling of roast almonds and smoked paprika.

Here's a really quick soup that can be thrown together in minutes. I always keep a bag of peas in the freezer and most of the other ingredients will probably be lurking around your kitchen too.

It's a great idea to freeze leftover celery, ready diced, so that you always have some to hand. The trinity of onion, carrot and celery, known as a *mirepoix* in France or a *soffritto* in Italy, is the starting point for so many dishes.

GREEN PEA AND MINT SOUP

Serves 4

2 tbsp olive oil

2 onions, finely diced

2 carrots, finely diced

1–2 potatoes, peeled and diced

2 celery stalks, finely diced

1 garlic clove, crushed

500 g/1 lb 2 oz/3½ cups frozen peas

1 litre/1¾ pints/4 cups chicken or vegetable stock

salt and pepper

about 10 fresh mint leaves, chopped

juice of ½–1 lemon

4 tbsp crème fraîche

8 rashers of streaky bacon, fried or grilled and then diced (optional)

Heat the oil in a large saucepan and cook the onions gently until soft. Add the carrots, potatoes and celery, and cook for another 10 minutes, until the vegetables are soft but not browned.

Throw in the garlic, give it a stir, and then add most of the peas. Keep a couple of handfuls back to add to the soup later. Lots of recipes advise you to strain a pea soup after blending, but that increases the faff and the washing up. I prefer to toss a few whole peas in at the end, which somehow makes the slightly rough texture of the soup seem fine.

Add the stock, season with salt and pepper to taste, and bring to the boil for a minute or two. Now add half of your mint: mint and peas are a classic pairing, but too much mint can make the soup taste a bit toothpastey.

Blend the soup, ideally using a hand-held blender, but a regular blender or food processor are fine too. Add a little more stock or water if the soup seems too thick. Stir in the reserved whole peas. Taste and balance the flavours with salt, pepper, lemon juice and more mint if necessary.

Serve hot, in bowls, with a tablespoon of crème fraîche, and a sprinkling of crispy bacon.

HOW ABOUT?

... replacing the mint with a large bunch of watercress.

... using broad beans instead of peas. You will need to pop them out of their leathery skins but the soup will be a just reward.

... serving the soup cold, with yogurt instead of crème fraîche. In this case, I do think it is worth straining the soup for a lighter, more summery feel.

... garnishing with fresh pea shoots instead of bacon.

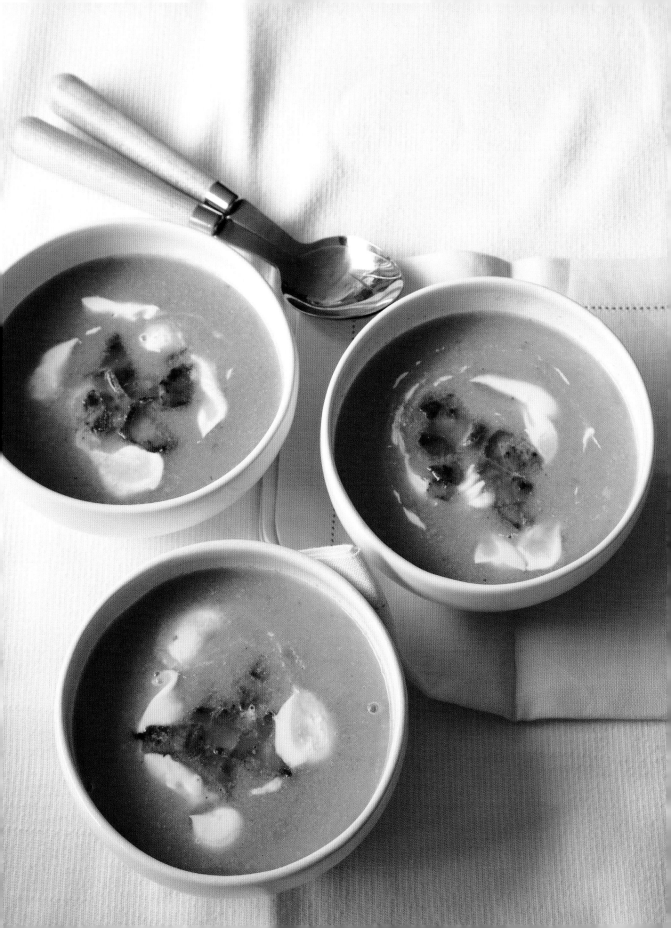

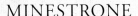

MINESTRONE

A classic from the Italian kitchen. Minestrone varies with the season, the region, the family recipe: wherever or whenever you go there will be a different variation. The key is creating a soup with the very best produce on offer, balancing light tender vegetables with more filling starchy ones for a substantial and incredibly healthy soup.

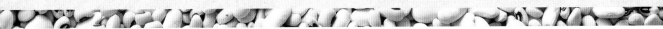

This is a legume showcase with borlotti, broad beans, green beans and peas. Do vary the vegetables – that's the idea. Finely sliced fennel or Swiss chard would be delicious instead of, or as well as, any of the other greens.

SUMMER MINESTRONE WITH PESTO

Serves 6–8

2 tbsp olive oil

1 onion, diced

2 carrots, diced

2 celery stalks, diced

handful of green beans, sliced into 2 cm/¾ inch pieces

handful of broad beans (fava beans), preferably skinned

handful of fresh or frozen peas

small bunch of asparagus, trimmed and sliced into
    2 cm/¾ inch pieces

1 courgette (zucchini), finely diced

salt and pepper

2 litres/3½ pints/2 quarts vegetable stock,
    or chicken stock for a richer result

250 g/9 oz home-cooked borlotti beans (cranberry beans)
    or 1 x 400 g/14 oz can of borlotti beans

2 potatoes, cut into 2 cm/¾ inch dice

100 g/3½ oz pasta, tiny shapes such as *ditalini* or *stelle*

2 tomatoes, peeled, deseeded and diced

pesto (see p.244)

Heat the oil in a large saucepan and cook the onion, carrots and celery for about 5 minutes, until soft. Now add about half of each of your green and broad beans, peas, asparagus and courgette, sprinkle with a little salt and stir around in the oil for a couple of minutes.

Add the stock and simmer for about 30 minutes. Don't worry about the texture of the vegetables, the idea is to flavour the soup.

Throw in the borlotti beans, potatoes and pasta, and simmer until the potato is beginning to soften.

Now add the remaining green vegetables and cook for about 5 minutes – you want these to remain fresh and *al dente*.

Taste and season with salt and pepper, then stir in the tomato. Serve the soup in bowls, with a large teaspoon of pesto in each.

HOW ABOUT?

... adding about 6 tablespoons of double cream to the soup just before serving.

... breaking up some fine spaghetti (wrap in a tea towel and snap away) instead of buying tiny pasta.

... leaving out the pasta and placing a piece of toasted, day-old country bread in the bottom of each bowl.

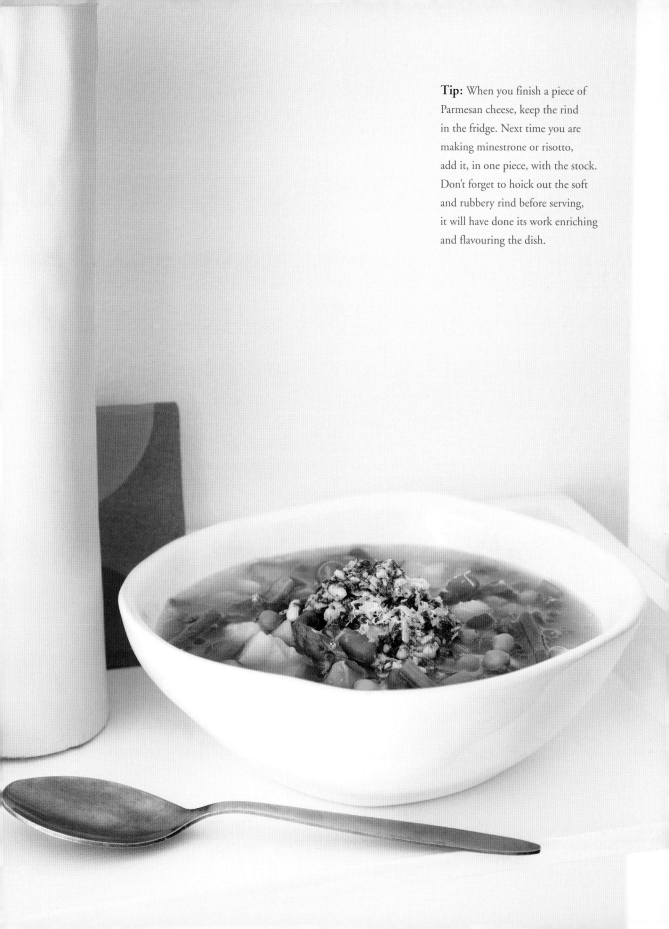

Tip: When you finish a piece of Parmesan cheese, keep the rind in the fridge. Next time you are making minestrone or risotto, add it, in one piece, with the stock. Don't forget to hoick out the soft and rubbery rind before serving, it will have done its work enriching and flavouring the dish.

Another version of the Italian 'big soup'. This is a fortifying comfort dish with a huge hit of vitamin C from the squash, cabbage and tinned tomatoes.

WINTER MINESTRONE

Serves 6–8

2 tbsp olive oil

1 onion, diced

2 carrots, diced

2 celery stalks, diced

250 g/9 oz pumpkin or squash, diced

about 6 leaves of cavolo nero or Savoy cabbage, sliced finely

salt and pepper

2 litres/3½ pints/2 quarts vegetable stock, or chicken stock for a richer result

400 g/14 oz can of chopped tomatoes

250 g/9 oz dried borlotti beans (cranberry beans)

   or 1 x 400 g/14 oz can of borlotti beans

2 potatoes, cut into 2 cm/¾ inch dice

100 g/3½ oz pasta, tiny shapes such as *ditalini* or *stelle*

3 tbsp chopped fresh parsley

3 tbsp freshly grated Parmesan cheese

extra-virgin olive oil

Heat the olive oil in a large saucepan and cook the onion, carrots and celery for about 5 minutes, until soft. Now add the pumpkin, the leaves and a pinch of salt and cook gently for about 5 minutes.

Add the stock and tomatoes and simmer for about 20 minutes. Add the beans, potatoes and pasta, and cook until the potato is tender and the pasta is *al dente*.

Season well with salt and freshly ground black pepper and serve with plenty of parsley, Parmesan and a swirl of extra-virgin olive oil.

HOW ABOUT?

... adding 100 g/3½ oz diced pancetta or bacon with the onions at the beginning, or shredding in some ham from a cooked hock (see p.250) at the end.

... using risotto rice instead of pasta for a Venetian version (it will take about 20 minutes to cook).

... throwing in some diced raw red peppers with the vegetables, or a hit of chilli (see p.248), and serving with grated pecorino as they do down south.

Years ago when I cooked on an Italian yacht, my guests always became delirious at the first sighting of fresh borlotti beans in their pink speckled pods and regularly asked for this soup. The idea of beans and pasta certainly seemed a hefty one, especially in a Sardinian heatwave. I soon learned the beauty of this soup is that you can leave the beans and pasta swimming in a light summer broth, while in winter you can blitz some of the beans to make a thick creamy base.

The soup is fabulous with fresh or dried beans. If using dried, remember to soak them for at least 4 hours, or overnight.

BORLOTTI AND PASTA SOUP
PASTA E FAGIOLI

Serves 4–6

4 tbsp olive oil	1 litre/1¾ pints/4 cups water or chicken stock
1 onion, finely diced	1 fresh red chilli (see p.248), chopped (optional)
1 carrot, finely diced	1 sprig of rosemary
1 celery stalk, finely diced	1 small sprig of basil
50 g/1¾ oz unsmoked pancetta, diced (optional)	1 tbsp tomato purée
4 garlic cloves, crushed	salt and pepper
250 g/9 oz dried borlotti beans (cranberry beans), soaked for at least 4 hours, or 1 kg/2¼ lb fresh pods to shell at home	150 g/5½ oz pasta, tiny shapes such as *tubetti* or *ditalini*
	extra-virgin olive oil

Heat the oil in a large saucepan and cook the onion, carrot, celery, pancetta (if using) and garlic until soft.

Drain and rinse the soaked dried beans, or shell the pods. Chuck the beans into the pan with the vegetables and stir to coat them in the oil. Add enough water or stock to cover the beans by about 5 cm/2 in and then add the chilli and herbs. It is an idea to put your rosemary in a muslin bag or Dick Whittington-style bundle so that the needles don't just fall into the soup. Bring the liquid to a boil and then simmer for anything between 30 and 90 minutes, depending on whether you are using fresh or dried beans. Add the tomato purée, salt and pepper once the beans begin to soften. Cook until really tender but still intact.

Now the choice is yours: for a lighter soup, leave all the beans whole or, for a thicker version, purée about half of the beans in their cooking liquid (I find it easiest to ladle out the beans that I want to keep whole and blitz the rest in the pot with a hand-held blender). You can make the soup in advance up to this stage.

When you're nearly ready to serve, bring the soup up to a simmer, add the pasta and bubble away until the pasta is cooked through. Stir from time to time as the beany liquid can catch and burn on the bottom of the pan.

Taste and adjust the seasoning and serve in bowls with a swirl of extra-virgin olive oil.

HOW ABOUT?

... some finely diced, peeled tomato and ripped basil to sprinkle over the summer version.

... sprinkling with some freshly grated Parmesan; acceptable in some circles but almost a keelhauling offence in my case. *'Non si fa'*, 'it's just not done', I was told.

Cannellini bean soup is a popular Tuscan dish, which becomes a delicacy in August when locals buy fresh beans in the markets. Thankfully the soup is great with dried beans too. This really is a time to cook your own rather than open a can; the beans need to soak up all the aromatics as they cook. It's worth cooking a double quantity (at least) at the same time and using the remaining beans for a salad or purée.

The pure simplicity of the soup means you really can savour the taste of the beans. It also makes a fabulously creamy base for dozens of variations.

CANNELLINI SOUP

Serves 4
2 tbsp olive oil
1 onion, finely diced
1 carrot, finely diced
1 celery stalk, finely diced
1 leek, finely diced
250 g/9 oz dried cannellini beans, soaked for at least 4 hours, or overnight
1.5 litres/2¾ pints/6½ cups chicken or vegetable stock
1 bay leaf
small bunch or muslin bag of sage, rosemary or thyme, or a mixture
salt and pepper
2 tbsp extra-virgin olive oil

Heat the oil in a really large saucepan and gently cook the onion, carrot, celery and leek until very soft but not coloured.

Drain the beans, add to the pan, and stir them around with the soft vegetables for a couple of minutes.

Add the stock, bay leaf and herbs and boil for 10 minutes, then reduce the heat and simmer for anything between 30 minutes and 1 hour, depending on the age of your beans. They need to be really tender and creamy.

Remove the bay leaf and herbs. While they are still warm, ladle the beans and some of the stock into a blender or food processor and purée until really smooth. It's sometimes good to keep a few whole beans for texture, so set a few aside if you like.

Return the soup to the pan and season well with salt and pepper. Serve in bowls with a swirl of extra-virgin olive oil and some warm ciabatta bread.

HOW ABOUT?

... blitzing in some roasted sweet potato, pumpkin or cauliflower when you purée the soup.
... leaving out the herbs and stirring a good dollop of fresh pesto into each bowl as you serve.
... adding some sautéed wild mushrooms (see p.80) to each bowl.
... frying a couple of crushed garlic cloves with some finely diced cherry tomatoes, a few semi-dried tomatoes (see p.249) and plenty of chopped parsley. Pile on top of the soup to serve.

Cannellini soup was given cult status by Gordon Ramsay with his white bean cappuccino, which has inspired many copycat recipes over the years. Here's another!

The butter and cream certainly up the calories here but, hey, we all need to throw caution to the wind once in a while. This is a great soup to serve from tiny cups at a drinks party. I collect espresso cups and a mixture of colours and styles looks really fun. *Illustrated on pp.90–91.*

CANNELLINI AND PORCINI CAPPUCCINO

Serves 6 as a starter, or makes about 24 espresso cups

cannellini soup (see opposite)

20 g/¾ oz dried porcini mushrooms

150 ml/5 fl oz/⅔ cup double (heavy) cream

30 g/1 oz unsalted butter

Soak the dried mushrooms in a few tablespoons of warm water while you begin to boil the beans for the soup. Once the mushrooms are soft, you can squeeze out any excess water and chop them finely. Add them to the bean pot along with their deeply flavoured soaking liquid, but take care – you may need to strain the liquid if it is gritty.

Purée the soup and then press it through a sieve, using a spatula or the back of a ladle to get a truly smooth result. Return the soup to the pan, bring up to a simmer and add the cream. Taste and adjust the seasoning. Chop the butter into three and whisk in a piece at a time. Now you can decide whether to serve this soup as it is or add a frothy cappuccino finish.

If you are going for the cappuccino look, then some rather patient whizzing with a hand-held blender for about 5 minutes, lifting up and down through the soup, will eventually get you there. I have a milk frother attached to my coffee machine, so I top off the aerated soup with a couple of spoonfuls of fluffy milk froth.

HOW ABOUT?

... toasting some really fine slices of ciabatta, cut on the diagonal, in the oven. Dot with truffle oil while still warm and serve alongside the soup.

... leaving out the porcini and adding a large handful of fresh tarragon leaves when you blitz the soup.

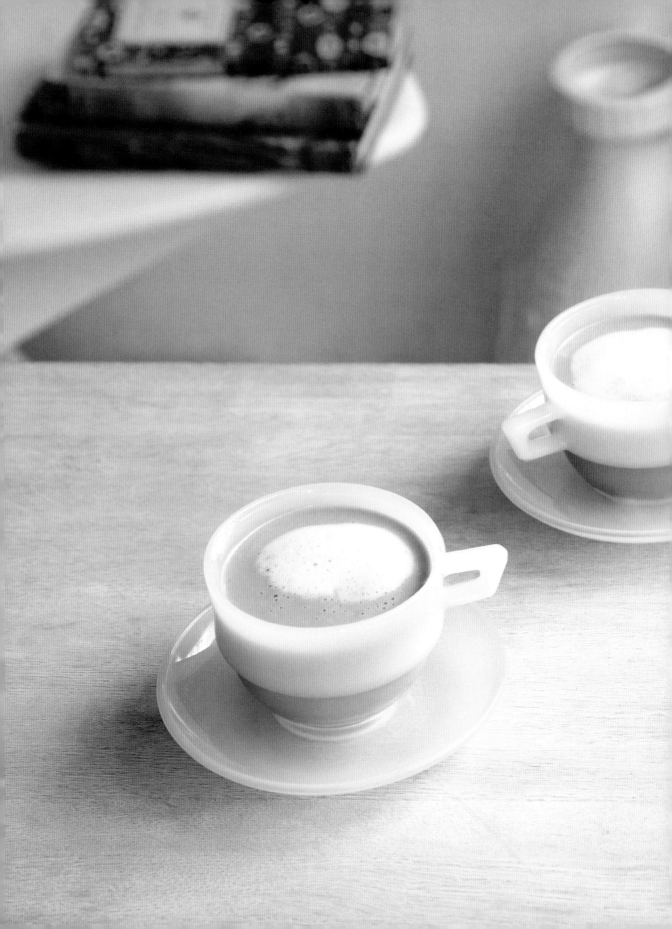

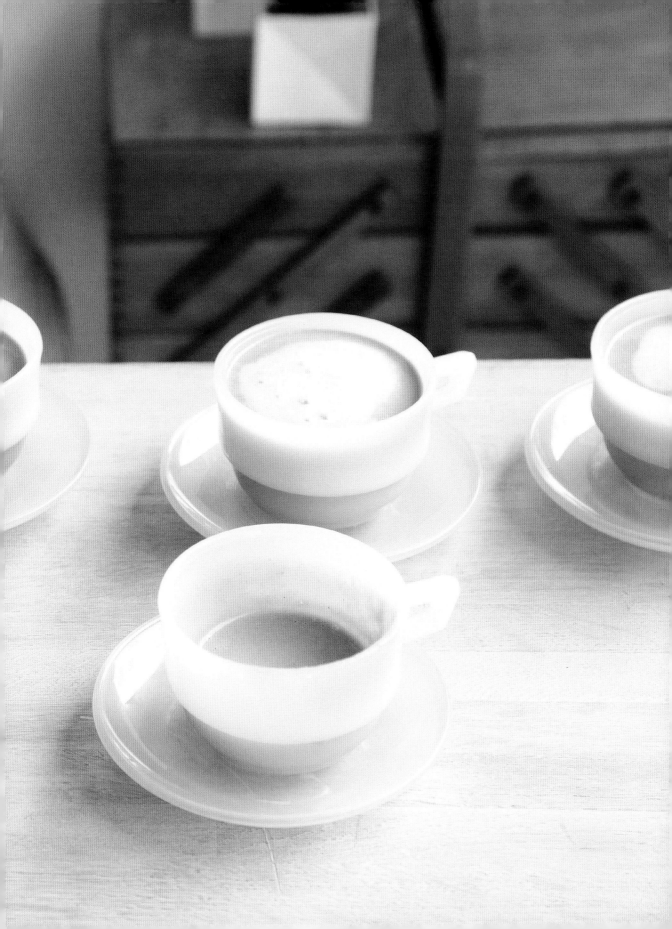

A hearty, satisfying soup with vibrant fresh flavours. Serve the soup with sour cream, guacamole, corn tacos or toasted tortillas and you have a meal in a bowl.

There's nothing new about this soup combination; variations exist throughout Latin America. Beans, corn and squash were the pillars of the ancient Central and South American diet. Just as beans and rice, or beans and bread, have been combined in other food cultures to provide precious protein, here it was beans and corn. The squash provided the essential vitamins and three humble crops became the mainstay of entire civilizations.

SQUASH, BLACK BEAN AND SWEETCORN SOUP

Serves 4

2 tbsp olive oil

1 onion, diced

450 g/1 lb butternut squash, peeled, deseeded and cut into 5 cm/2 inch chunks

2 garlic cloves, crushed

salt and pepper

1 tsp ground cumin

1 tsp sweet Spanish smoked paprika

½ tsp chilli flakes

400 g/14 oz can of chopped tomatoes

300 ml/10 fl oz/1¼ cups vegetable stock (a good cube or bouillon powder will do)

250 g/9 oz home-cooked black beans or 1 x 400 g/14 oz can of black beans

200 g/7 oz sweetcorn kernels

Tabasco sauce (optional)

juice of ½–1 lime, or 1 tbsp wine vinegar (optional)

handful of fresh coriander (cilantro), chopped

150 ml/5 fl oz/⅔ cup sour cream

Heat the oil in a large saucepan and cook the onion until soft and beginning to colour. Add the squash and stir around for a couple of minutes. Toss in the garlic, a pinch of salt and the spices, and stir for about a minute, then tip in the tomatoes and stock. Simmer for about 15 minutes or until the squash is just tender.

Scoop out about half of the squash with a little of the liquid, place in a deep container and purée with a hand-held blender. You could use a potato masher or blitz all the soup in the saucepan, but I like the contrast of the large intact chunks of squash with the velvety soup. Return the puréed squash to the soup. Add the beans and sweetcorn, and a little water if the soup is very thick, and simmer for 5 minutes.

Taste and balance the flavours with salt, pepper or Tabasco, lime juice or wine vinegar. Serve in bowls, with a scattering of coriander and a large spoonful of sour cream.

HOW ABOUT?

... making the soup in advance; the beans will soak up the flavours.

... crumbling some Wensleydale or Cheshire cheese into the soup instead of the sour cream.

... serving with guacamole (see p.243) and tortilla chips.

... creating a bit of table drama by grating over some dark chocolate as you serve.

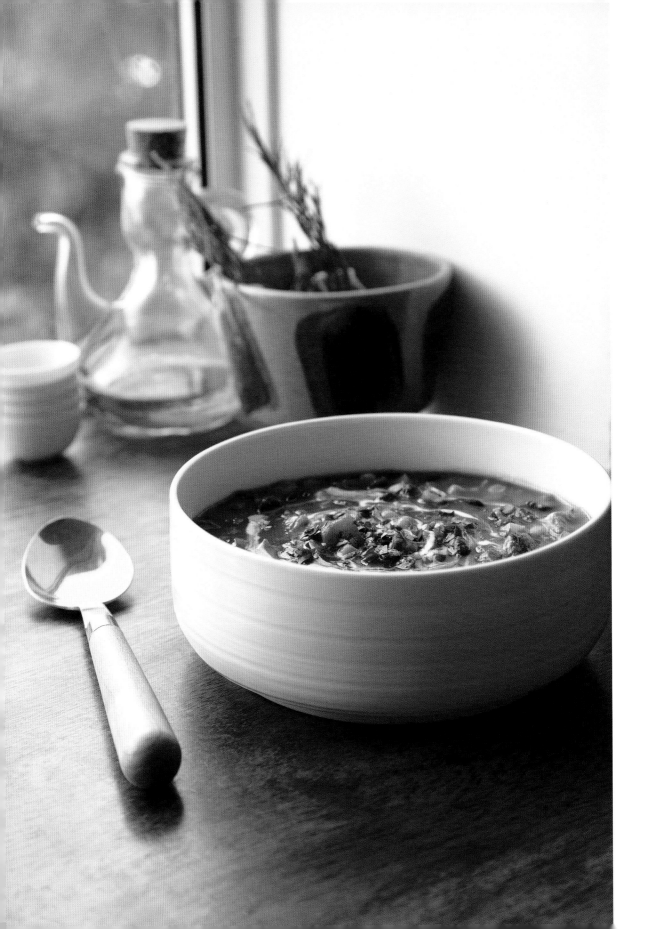

Peanuts, or groundnuts, are used liberally in the soups and stews of West Africa. There are recipes with smoked fish, chicken or beef, but this lightly spiced version with sweet potato is my favourite. It may not be totally authentic – I'm quite sure the locals aren't using peanut butter – but it certainly makes for a super-quick and scrumptious supper dish. Be sure to use unsweetened, organic peanut butter that has no additives, or alternatively grind your own roasted peanuts and add a good pinch of salt.

AFRICAN PEANUT SOUP

Serves 4

2 tbsp vegetable oil such as sunflower, groundnut or rapeseed

1 onion, roughly diced

2 garlic cloves, chopped

2.5-cm/1-inch piece of fresh ginger, finely diced

large pinch of chilli flakes or ¼ tsp cayenne pepper

1 tsp ground cumin

large pinch of ground cinnamon

2 orange-fleshed sweet potatoes, peeled and roughly chopped

400 g/14 oz can of chopped tomatoes

300 ml/10 fl oz/1¼ cups vegetable or chicken stock

3 tbsp organic smooth peanut butter

salt and pepper

juice of ½ lime

a few leaves of fresh coriander (cilantro), to garnish

Heat the oil in a large saucepan and fry the onion until soft. Add the garlic, ginger, chilli, cumin and cinnamon, and stir until you can smell the fabulous aromas.

Add the sweet potatoes and stir to coat in the spices, taking care not to let the garlic burn. Tip in the tomatoes and stock, and bubble away gently for about 10 minutes, until the sweet potato is soft.

Spoon the peanut butter into a small bowl, stir in enough of the soup broth to make a smooth cream and then add to the soup.

Using a hand-held blender or potato masher, purée some of the potato. I like to leave some lumps in the soup, but you may prefer to blitz the lot in a blender. Season with salt, black pepper and lime juice, sprinkle over some coriander and serve.

HOW ABOUT?

... adding a few red kidney beans and serving as a stew with rice.

... throwing in some chicken thighs along with the diced potato; they will flavour the soup beautifully. Once cooked, fish them out, remove the skin and bones and return the shredded chicken to the pot.

MISO SOUP

Quick, savoury, satisfying. Miso soup is the thing to reach for when the first signs of a cold set in; zipped up with plenty of ginger, it seems to fortify and restore. Throw in a few vegetables, noodles or tofu, and the miso soup becomes a light meal. You can buy sachets of instant miso soup, but it makes sense to have a jar of miso paste at the ready. As well as soup, you can use it in dressings, marinades and to add that umami depth of savoury flavour to many vegetarian dishes. The darker the paste, the more pronounced the flavour.

Traditional miso soup is based on dashi stock, made from kombu seaweed and dried bonito (a type of tuna) flakes. To make dashi stock, soak a 7.5-cm/3-inch piece of dried kombu in 1 litre/1¾ pints/4 cups cold water for 30 minutes. Bring to the boil, add a handful of bonito flakes and remove from the heat, leave to stand for 5 minutes, then strain. The simple soups below replace this with a vegetarian stock.

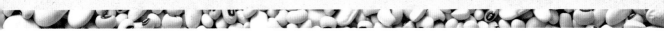

I adore this very simple vegetable stock base.

ALMOST INSTANT MISO SOUP

Serves 4
1-cm/½-inch piece of fresh ginger, cut into tiny matchsticks
1 shallot or ½ small onion, finely diced
½ carrot, finely diced
1 litre/1¾ pints/4 cups water
2–3 tbsp miso paste

Put the ginger, shallot and carrot in a saucepan with the water and bring to the boil for 3–4 minutes.

Ladle a few tablespoons of the stock into a small bowl (or a soup mug). Add the miso paste and stir to dissolve. Pour the miso back into the saucepan and warm through for a couple of minutes, but do not boil (or you will bump off all the friendly bacteria).

Pour into mugs or bowls. The vegetable bits will settle, but I can't resist spooning them out and eating them too.

Adding noodles turns this miso soup into a satisfying meal.

MISO WITH SOBA NOODLES

Serves 4
about 8-cm/3-inch pieces of dried kombu
1 litre/1¾ pints/4 cups water
4 dried shiitake mushrooms, covered in warm water and
    soaked for 15 minutes
1 carrot, sliced into matchsticks
150 g/5½ oz dried soba noodles
2–3 tbsp miso paste
300 g/10½ oz pak choy, sliced
4 spring onions (scallions), finely sliced
1 tbsp toasted sesame seeds

Bring the kombu and water to the boil in a large saucepan. Pick out the mushrooms from their soaking liquid. If the liquid is gritty, strain it, then add it to the saucepan. Remove the stalks and slice the mushrooms. Add the mushrooms and the carrot to the pan and simmer for about 10 minutes.

Cook the noodles in lightly salted boiling water until tender (4–5 minutes). Drain and rinse in cool water.

Discard the kombu from the stock pan. Put the miso paste in a small bowl, ladle over some hot stock and stir until the miso has dissolved. Add the pak choy to the stock pan and bring to the boil. As soon as the leaves have softened, turn down the heat and add the noodles and the miso.

Serve in bowls, topped with spring onions and sesame seeds.

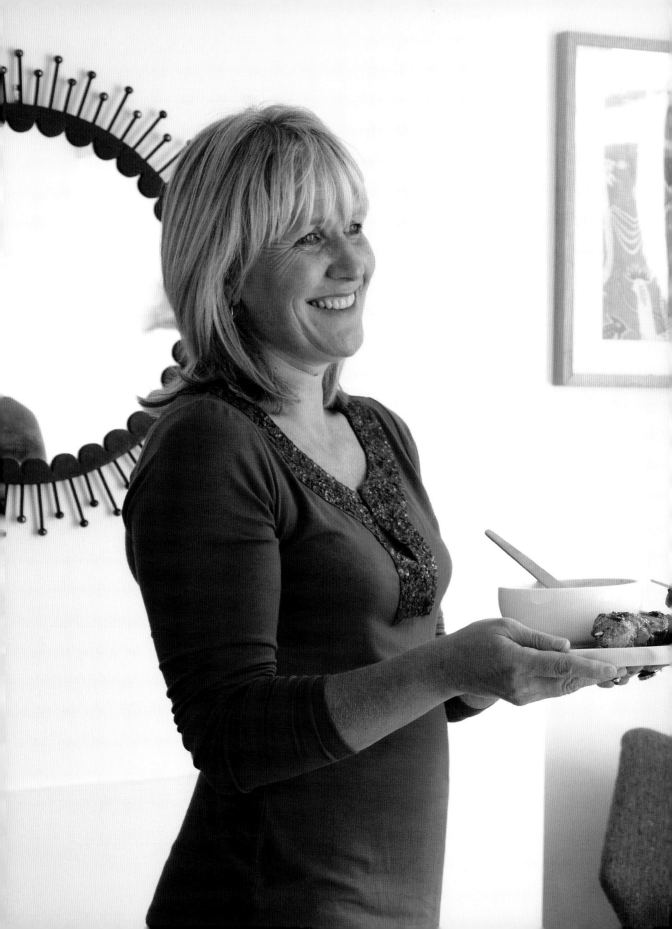

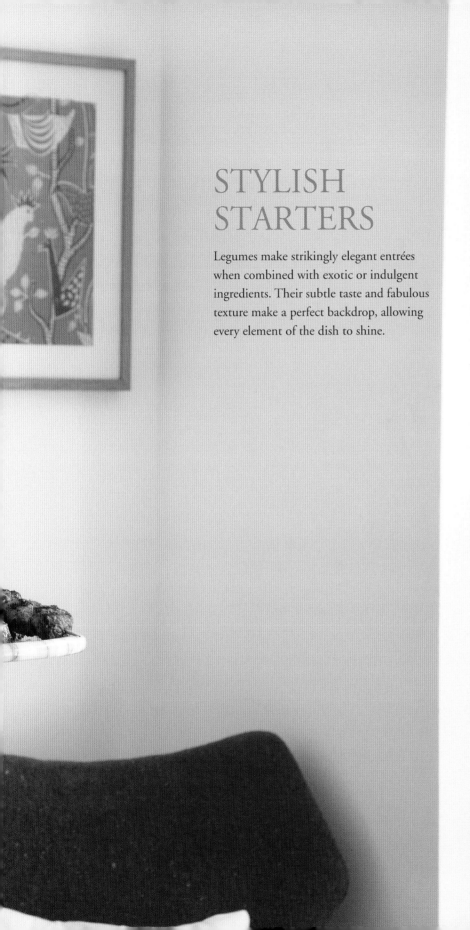

STYLISH STARTERS

Legumes make strikingly elegant entrées when combined with exotic or indulgent ingredients. Their subtle taste and fabulous texture make a perfect backdrop, allowing every element of the dish to shine.

The French answer to coleslaw, celeriac remoulade is a bistro classic. Here the lentils give extra texture and body, and, served with some good fresh bread, I'd be happy eating this for a light lunch.

CELERIAC AND PUY LENTIL REMOULADE

Serves 4

200 g/7 oz/1 cup Puy lentils, rinsed

1 bay leaf

1 celeriac, about 700 g/1 lb 9 oz, peeled and trimmed

juice of ½ lemon

salt and pepper

2 tbsp roughly chopped fresh parsley

2 tbsp capers, roughly chopped

FOR THE DRESSING

5 tbsp mayonnaise, bought or homemade (see p.242)

1–2 tbsp Dijon mustard

2 tbsp crème fraîche

Put the lentils in a saucepan with the bay leaf and add cold water to cover them by about 5 cm/2 in. Bring to the boil and then simmer for about 20 minutes, until tender but still intact. You may need to add a dash more water during this time, so do keep an eye on them.

Meanwhile, cut the celeriac into matchsticks, throw it into a bowl and toss it around in the lemon juice.

Drain the lentils if necessary (I sometimes find that I have miraculously added the perfect amount of water), remove the bay leaf and season with a little salt and pepper.

To make the dressing, mix together the mayonnaise, mustard, crème fraîche, salt and a good grind of black pepper. The dressing should be tart, creamy and thick enough to cling to the celeriac and lentils.

Stir the celeriac, lentils, parsley, capers and dressing together, taste and adjust the seasoning.

Serve within a few hours of making: the celeriac becomes soft and pappy after a while.

HOW ABOUT?

… stirring in some matchsticks of smoked ham.

… serving alongside smoked trout, salmon or mackerel.

… a lighter option. It's not a dieter's delight, it was never meant to be, but if calories are key, then replace the mayonnaise and crème fraîche with some extra-virgin olive oil and toss in a few toasted hazelnuts to keep things interesting.

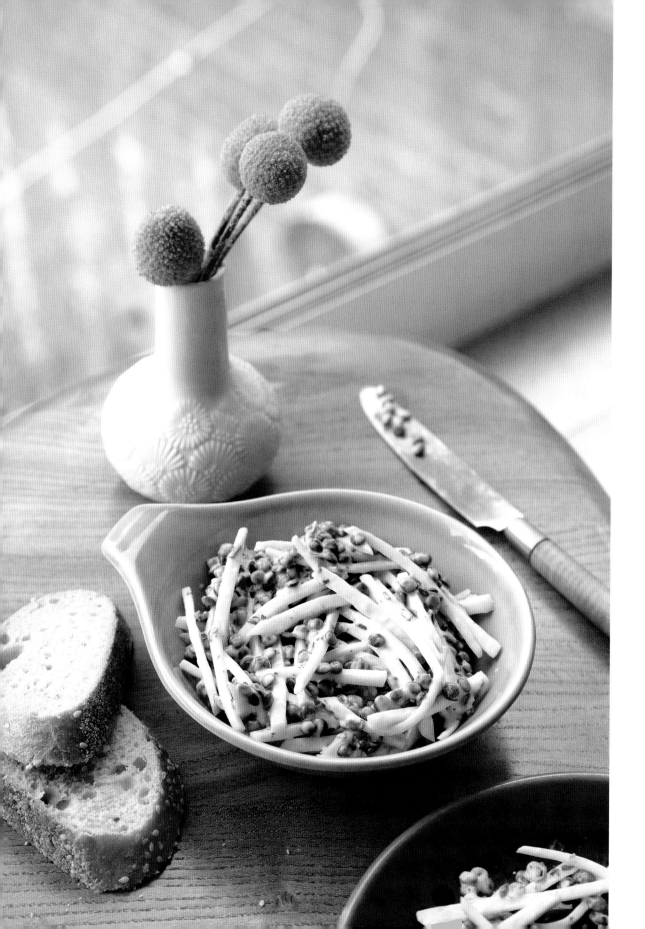

Wine may be Rioja's most famous export, but the region is also one of the biggest market gardens of Spain. Artichokes, asparagus, *pochas* (Spain's answer to the fresh borlotti) and Gem lettuces are all major crops but perhaps the most fêted vegetable of the lot is the piquillo pepper. The small, roasted, piquant peppers, sold in jars and cans, are the perfect size for stuffing and have a permanent place in my cupboard for last-minute entertaining. This dish can be prepared ahead and just heated through a few minutes before serving.

PIQUILLO PEPPERS WITH GREEN LENTIL TAPENADE AND GOAT'S CHEESE

Serves 4

225 g/8 oz jar of piquillo peppers – about 12–16 peppers

green lentil tapenade (see p.35) – purée half of the lentils and stir the whole lentils into the purée

3 tbsp olive oil

1 onion, finely diced

4 garlic cloves, crushed

2 sprigs of thyme, leaves removed

4 tbsp dry white wine

4 tbsp double (heavy) cream

salt and pepper

200 g/7 oz young creamy goat's cheese, such as the Welsh Pant-Ysgawn, cut into thin slices

2 tbsp extra-virgin olive oil

2 small crostini (see p.44) per person

Empty the peppers carefully onto a small tray and select a dozen (or just eight if they are large) of the peppers, checking that they are not ripped. Stuff the peppers carefully with the lentil tapenade. Set aside.

Heat the olive oil in a saucepan and cook the onion until soft. Add the garlic, half the thyme and the remaining peppers. Stir over a medium heat until you can smell the garlic and then pour in the wine. Let the wine come up to the boil and then add the cream. Remove from the heat and blend until smooth in a blender or food processor. Season with salt and pepper to taste, and set aside.

Preheat the oven to 190°C/375°F/Gas mark 5.

Divide the sauce among 4 individual oven-to-table dishes; the French white porcelain gratin dishes with ears are ideal or the tiny terracotta *cazuelas* from Spain. Divide the goat's cheese among the dishes and place the stuffed peppers on top, leaving a glimpse of the cheese. Sprinkle with the remaining thyme. When you are nearly ready to eat, place in the oven for about 10 minutes.

Serve right away, with a dash of extra-virgin olive oil to give the peppers a beautiful sheen, and with crisp crostini to dip into the melted cheese and peppery sauce.

HOW ABOUT?

... filling the peppers with hummus, creamy bean purée, lentil and aubergine purée or Syrian lentils (all these recipes are in the dips and purées chapter).

Use the tiniest broad beans you can find, literally the size of a fingernail. Any larger and you will need to remove the skins, although that's not such a hardship and it makes them look beautiful in any case. In Spain, you can buy jars of preserved '*habitas baby*' – at a price – but I'd rather use fresh or frozen. Once cut into, the quail's egg oozes its velvety yolk over the beans, providing a rich, ambrosial sauce.

BABY BROAD BEANS WITH JAMÓN AND QUAILS' EGGS
HABITAS CON JAMÓN

Serves 4

600 g/1 lb 5 oz podded broad beans (fava beans), skinned if large
    (frozen beans work well too)
2 tbsp olive oil
½ onion, diced
2 thick slices of *jamón serrano*, cut into small cubes, with the fat on
4 quails' eggs
2 garlic cloves, finely sliced
1–2 tsp sherry vinegar
pepper
about 6 fresh mint leaves, ripped up

Bring a large saucepan of water to the boil and have a bowl of iced water at the ready. Plunge the beans into the boiling water for a minute, drain and then tip them into the cold water. (If using frozen beans, you can skip this step as they were blanched before they were frozen.)

Heat the oil in a large frying pan over a low heat and cook the onion and the *jamón* gently until the onion softens and the ham fat begins to render down.

Now poach your eggs. The only tricky bit is breaking the rather stubborn shells: just saw through the shell very carefully with a serrated knife. Follow the poaching instructions on p.249 – quails' eggs will need only about 1 minute each. You can dunk them back into the hot water to ensure they're really hot just before serving.

Throw the garlic in with the onion and stir until it begins to turn golden and smells wonderful. Drain the beans and add to the pan, stirring to coat them in the oil. Sprinkle with the vinegar and taste: the ham will probably provide enough salt, but you may like to add a little freshly ground black pepper. Add the mint.

Serve warm with a poached egg on top and some rustic bread to soak up the juices.

HOW ABOUT?

... leaving out the *jamón* and egg; serve the beans with slithers of aged Manchego cheese instead, or on top of some ricotta or cream cheese on a crispy crostini.
... sprinkling some of the cooked ham and beans over a green salad.

Stunningly shiny, jet-black beluga lentils dull down and lose a bit of their sexy edge once cooked, so I suggest adding some squid or cuttlefish ink to the pot, which will inject the lentils with both dramatic colour and a little sea flavour. You could use any other tiny, firm lentil instead of beluga, as they will all turn black.

Squid is fantastically quick and simple to prepare, especially if you ask your fishmonger to clean it for you. Cut the tubes into large asymmetrical pieces rather than the customary rings (reminiscent of so many 'rubber band in batter' experiences) and take great care not to overcook.

The flavour combination was inspired by a wonderful *arros negre*, 'black rice', dish that I ate on the seafront in Sitges, just south of Barcelona.

BLACK LENTILS WITH CHARGRILLED SQUID AND AIOLI

Serves 4

150 g/5½ oz/¾ cup beluga lentils, rinsed

1 onion, halved

1 bay leaf

1 sprig of thyme

2 tbsp or 2–3 sachets of cuttlefish ink (available at
    most fishmongers)

salt and pepper

½ lemon

5 tbsp extra-virgin olive oil

450 g/1 lb cleaned squid, with tentacles

1 tbsp chopped fresh parsley

TO SERVE

1 lemon, cut into 4 wedges

aioli (see p.242) or 4 tbsp good-quality mayonnaise
    mixed with 1–2 crushed garlic cloves

Put the lentils in a saucepan with the onion, bay leaf and thyme. Cover with about 5 cm/2 in of cold water, bring to the boil and simmer for about 30 minutes, until tender. Keep an eye on them, topping up with a little more water if they begin to dry out, but you don't want to end up with a watery stock that you have to tip away. Once they are tender, remove the onion and herbs, strain off any excess liquid, stir in the cuttlefish ink and season well with salt, pepper, a squeeze of lemon and 2 tablespoons of the olive oil.

Open up the squid tubes by cutting down one side; lay them flat and score the inside without cutting right through the flesh. Score diagonally at 1-cm/½-in intervals and then across the other way to create a lattice pattern. This ensures that the squid cooks quickly and evenly without curling up. Cut the squid into a few large pieces. If the squid are large, you may want to cut the tentacles in half too, although I love the way they curl open like flowers when left whole.

Place the squid in a bowl with a little salt and pepper and 1 tablespoon of the oil. Massage it around so that the flesh is all lightly oiled. In another bowl, put the remaining 2 tablespoons of olive oil, the parsley and a squeeze of lemon.

HOW ABOUT?

… substituting cuttlefish for the squid. You'll certainly not need to buy an ink sachet if you prepare your own as they are bursting with the tar-black ink. Take care, removing the sac is a very satisfying but pretty messy business.

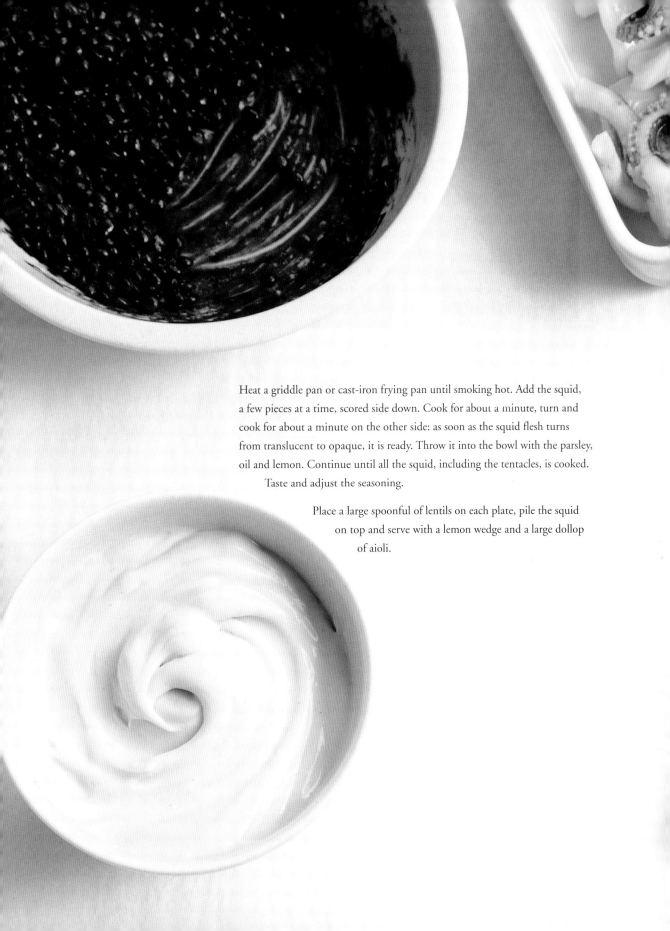

Heat a griddle pan or cast-iron frying pan until smoking hot. Add the squid, a few pieces at a time, scored side down. Cook for about a minute, turn and cook for about a minute on the other side: as soon as the squid flesh turns from translucent to opaque, it is ready. Throw it into the bowl with the parsley, oil and lemon. Continue until all the squid, including the tentacles, is cooked. Taste and adjust the seasoning.

Place a large spoonful of lentils on each plate, pile the squid on top and serve with a lemon wedge and a large dollop of aioli.

Scallops are, without a doubt, one of my desert island dishes. I'm so predictable, I just can't ignore them on a restaurant menu. The combination with pea purée is a classic and tastes even more wonderful with a bit of pork thrown in. Do try to find the soft cooking chorizo if you can, otherwise the result can be quite leathery (if you can only find the firmer, hard-cure chorizo, I would dice it finely before frying).

Seek out diver-caught scallops whenever possible: their harvesting is kinder to the seabed than those caught in drag nets. Fresh is best too, as many frozen scallops are plumped with huge amounts of water, which makes their texture pappy and the surface impossible to sear and caramelize.

PAN-SEARED SCALLOPS WITH CHORIZO AND PEA PURÉE

Serves 4

12 scallops – or 8 if they are particularly large

1 tbsp olive oil

salt and pepper

100 g/3½ oz mild, soft chorizo cut into 2-cm/¾-inch pieces

200 ml/7 fl oz/¾ cup chicken stock

250 g/9 oz/1¾ cups frozen peas, ideally petits pois

3 or 4 fresh mint leaves

1 tbsp extra-virgin olive oil

1 tbsp sherry vinegar

Remove and discard the white muscle and frill from around the outside of the scallops and cut off the crescent of orangey coral. Toss the scallops and coral in the olive oil and sprinkle with pepper. Set aside in the fridge.

Heat a large heavy-bottomed frying pan over a low heat and cook the chorizo gently for about 5 minutes. You won't need any oil if you go slow, as the fat in the sausage will render. Keep the chorizo warm in a low oven and leave the bright orange cooking oil in the pan.

Heat the chicken stock in a pan and throw in the peas with a good pinch of salt. Bring to the boil and then add the mint. Drain and then purée the peas in a food processor or using a hand-held blender, add the extra-virgin olive oil, taste and season.

Heat a griddle pan or a heavy-bottomed pan until smoking hot. Add the scallops and sear for about a minute on each side, resisting the temptation to poke and move them around. You may need to cook them in 2 batches (if too crowded they'll steam rather than fry). Sear the coral too.

Spoon some pea purée onto 4 warmed plates, top with the scallops, coral and the chorizo.

Add the sherry vinegar to the chorizo cooking oil along with a tablespoon of water, swirl over a high heat and then spoon over the scallops. Serve at once.

HOW ABOUT?

... using streaky bacon instead of the chorizo.

... adding some shards of crisped prosciutto (see p.250).

... serving the purée with grilled fish or lamb.

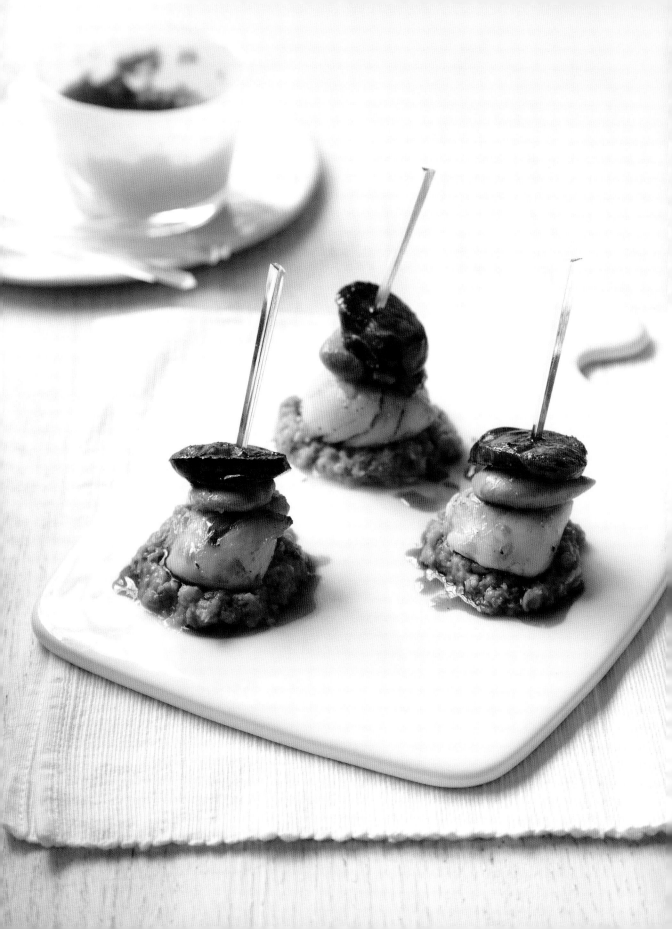

Pinchitos morunos, or Moorish kebabs, are often found in Spanish tapas bars. These little skewers of succulent, spiced lamb or pork are traditionally cooked over coals but a really hot ridged griddle pan works well too. Begin marinating the meat 12 hours in advance if possible.

The broad bean purée is fabulous with the lamb and elevates this delicious bar snack to elegant starter status. The purée can be prepared well in advance, leaving just a few minutes of searing to complete the dish.

SPICED LAMB PINCHITOS WITH BROAD BEAN AND ROAST GARLIC PURÉE

Serves 4

400 g/14 oz lean lamb leg meat, cut into 4 cm/1½ in cubes

FOR THE MARINADE

2 garlic cloves, crushed

3 tbsp olive oil

juice of ½ lemon

1 tsp ground coriander

1 tsp ground cumin

1 tsp paprika

½ tsp dried thyme

FOR THE BROAD BEAN PURÉE

1 small bulb of garlic, sliced in half equatorially

1 tbsp olive oil

200 g/7 oz/1¾ cups fresh or frozen baby broad (fava) beans

1 small sprig of rosemary, very finely chopped

2 tbsp extra-virgin olive oil

zest and juice of ½ lemon

salt and pepper

Mix the marinade ingredients together in a large bowl and add the meat. Cover and chill for up to 12 hours. Soak 12 wooden skewers in water for a few hours.

Preheat the oven to 180°C/350°F/Gas mark 4. Place the halved garlic bulb, cut side up, on a baking sheet and brush with the olive oil. Roast in the oven for about 20 minutes, until the cloves feel soft and squashy. Cool, then squeeze out the flesh.

Steam or boil the broad beans for about 3–5 minutes (just 1 minute will do for frozen beans), then dunk into cold water before popping each bean out of its pale green skin to reveal the fabulous bright green bean inside.

Blitz the beans in a blender or food processor with the garlic flesh, half the rosemary, the extra-virgin olive oil, most of the lemon juice and zest and a little salt and pepper. Taste and add more rosemary, lemon juice and zest, salt and pepper until the flavour is beautifully balanced. Just before serving, warm the purée through, either in a small pan with a splash of water added, or alternatively in the microwave.

Heat a griddle pan until smoking hot (you should have had the barbie going for a while if you've gone for that option). Thread the lamb onto the skewers, season with a little salt and char for a couple of minutes on each side. Serve the kebabs right away, with the warm broad bean and garlic purée.

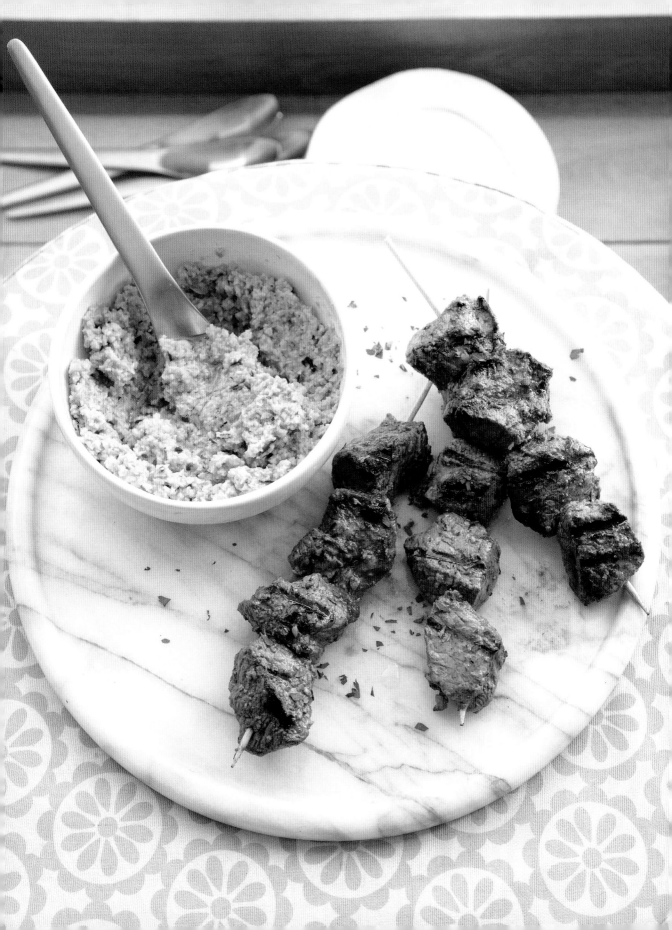

This recipe comes from Barney McGrath of Maitreya Social, a fabulous vegetarian restaurant on St Mark's Road in Bristol. The pistachios give this pâté its extravagant edge, pricey but delicious. Served with sweet and sour pickles, chutney and some tasty bread, it makes a great light lunch, you could even squeeze it into a sandwich box for an upmarket office snack.

SUN-DRIED TOMATO, BUTTERBEAN AND PISTACHIO PÂTÉ

Serves 6–8

250 g/9 oz/2 cups pistachios

2 tbsp olive oil

½ tsp sweet smoked paprika

salt and pepper

100 g/3½ oz sun-dried tomatoes

1 small red onion, diced

2 garlic cloves

1 large sprig of rosemary, leaves finely chopped

2 large sprigs of thyme, leaves finely chopped

1 tbsp balsamic vinegar

200 g/7 oz home-cooked butter beans (large lima beans) or 1 x 400 g/14 oz can of butter beans

small handful of fresh basil

50 g/1¾ oz/½ cup ground almonds

TO SERVE

sourdough toast

small jar of cornichons or gherkins

chutney or onion marmalade (see p.245)

Preheat the oven to 180°C/350°F/Gas mark 4. Tip the pistachios onto a baking sheet, toss them around in 1 tablespoon of the olive oil and the smoked paprika, and sprinkle with a pinch of salt. Roast for about 7 minutes (but check after 4 – this would be an expensive cremation calamity), until the nuts are lightly roasted.

Put the tomatoes in a small bowl, cover with boiling water and leave to soak.

Heat the remaining oil in a heavy-bottomed pan and cook the onion over a low heat until soft. Throw in the garlic and herbs and season. Once the onion is caramelized, add the balsamic vinegar and stir over the heat for a minute or two.

Drain the tomatoes and blitz in a food processor with the onion mixture, the butter beans and basil to make a rough purée. Remove and set aside.

Put about 50 g/1¾ oz of the pistachios in the processor and pulse quickly to chop them coarsely. Throw them in with the bean mixture and blitz the remaining pistachios as finely as possible.

Add the finely ground pistachios and the almonds to the bean purée and mix everything really thoroughly to combine. The pâté should seem really stiff. You can add a few more ground almonds if it seems too moist, keeping in mind that it will firm up a bit once chilled. Press the pâté into a terrine mould or loaf tin or simply roll it into a cylinder in some clingfilm. Chill for a couple of hours.

Serve with sourdough toast, cornichons and a good chutney or onion marmalade.

HOW ABOUT?

... experimenting with other nuts: cashews, whole almonds, peanuts or a combination of whatever you have in the cupboard.

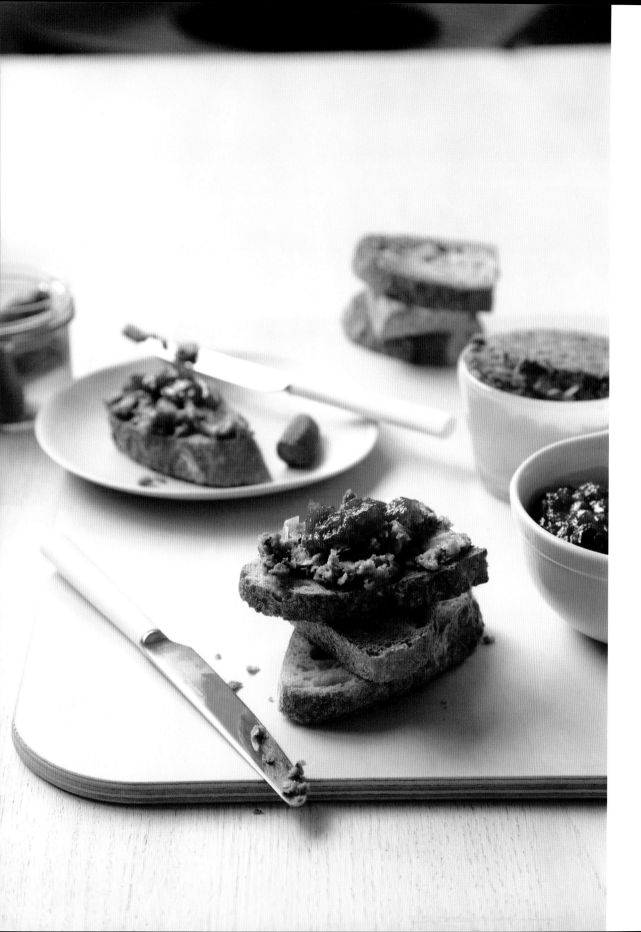

Up in the northern Spanish region of Asturias, they are truly passionate about their beans. There's the hefty pork-based *fabada* with chorizo, bacon, ham and black pudding that can really only be justified by a serious hike (and there's plenty of scope in the stunning Cantabrian mountains) and this much lighter, sublime seaside classic with clams.

Try to seek out the dried *alubias planchadas* if you can – Spanish specialists will stock these wonderfully buttery white beans – otherwise haricots will do very well. You can cook the beans hours in advance.

It's important to make sure that your clams are not at all gritty. Soak them for about 30 minutes in 2–3 changes of fresh water, swishing them around gently. Scrub them with a brush and discard any broken or open clams.

CLAMS WITH WHITE BEANS
FABES CON ALMEJAS

Serves 4–6

4 tbsp olive oil

2 onions, finely diced

1 carrot, finely diced

300 g/10½ oz/1½ cups dried *alubias planchadas* or haricot (navy) beans, soaked overnight

2 bay leaves

1 tsp salt

900 g/2 lb tiny clams such as carpet clams, well cleaned

150 ml/5 fl oz/⅔ cup dry white wine

3 tbsp extra-virgin olive oil

2 garlic cloves, finely chopped

1 tomato, peeled and diced

small bunch of parsley, roughly chopped

Heat the olive oil in a large saucepan and cook the onions and carrot until soft. Drain the beans and add them to the onions, along with the bay leaves and enough cold water to cover them by about 5 cm/2 in. Bring to the boil and skim off any scum, then turn down to a gentle simmer, cover and cook for about 1–1½ hours, until fabulously tender. Check the beans from time to time as the cooking times vary; add more water only if the beans are standing above the water. The liquid should have thickened but the beans should still be intact. Add the salt.

Once the beans are cooked, you can prepare the clams. Heat the wine in a large pan and tip in the clams, cover and steam for about 3 minutes, shaking the pan now and then, until the clams have opened.

Using a slotted spoon, lift out the clams and add them to the beans. Now check the wine and clam juices; if they are clear, then just slosh them in; if not, allow the grit to settle before carefully pouring three-quarters of the juices into the beans and discarding the rest.

Rinse the pan and then heat the extra-virgin olive oil with the garlic until the garlic just begins to colour. Throw in the tomato and most of the parsley. Stir and then tip over the beans. Serve at once, sprinkled with parsley, with some crusty bread.

HOW ABOUT?

... adding a good pinch of saffron to the beans about halfway through the cooking.

... cooking some prawns with the garlic and tomato and throwing these in too.

The combination of crab and ginger is spectacular and the glass noodles, sprouted mung beans, edamame and peanuts give this dish its pulsating credentials.

You could easily double the quantities and have this as a summer lunch. The noodles, beans and dressing can be put together a couple of hours in advance but leave the plating up until the last minute.

CRAB, EDAMAME AND NOODLE SALAD

Serves 4

100 g/3½ oz glass or cellophane noodles

large handful of cooked edamame beans (you can use the fresh podded, frozen cook-and-then-pod, or frozen slightly larger green soya beans)

250 g/9 oz mixed brown and white crabmeat – or just white if you prefer

small handful of home-sprouted mung beans (see p.20) or bean sprouts

2 tbsp roasted peanuts, roughly chopped

1 large sprig of coriander (cilantro), leaves removed

1 lime, quartered, to serve

FOR THE DRESSING

2 tbsp caster sugar

3–4 tbsp white wine vinegar

2 tbsp water

2 tbsp Thai fish sauce

2-cm/¾-inch piece of fresh ginger, very finely diced

1–2 bird's eye chillies, or other small hot chillies, very finely diced

5-cm/2-inch slice of cucumber, very finely diced

2 spring onions (scallions), very finely sliced

To make the dressing, heat the sugar with the vinegar and water until the sugar has completely dissolved. Leave to cool. Add the remaining dressing ingredients. Taste and balance the salt, sugar, heat and acidity. This is a classic Thai dipping sauce and it should really zing.

Put the noodles in a bowl. Blanch or steam the edamame, either way they'll only need a couple of minutes. Drain – and use the boiling water to pour over the noodles. Soak the noodles for 1 minute and then drain through a sieve and rinse them in cold water; you can throw in the edamame to keep them gloriously green too. Drain the noodles and beans and place them in a large bowl with the dressing.

Check the crabmeat over for any stray bits of shell. Divide the brown meat among 4 individual plates: it will sit under the noodles (if you stir this rich, creamy meat through the noodles they will lose their clean, fresh shine).

Toss half of the white crabmeat through the noodles along with the sprouted beans and divide among the plates. Sprinkle over the peanuts, coriander leaves, remaining crabmeat and any leftover dressing from the bowl. Serve with a slice of lime.

HOW ABOUT?

... making a veggie version with matchsticks of carrot and red pepper, mangetout and some marinated tofu (see p.199).

... replacing the crab with cooked tuna, salmon, rare steak or pink duck breast.

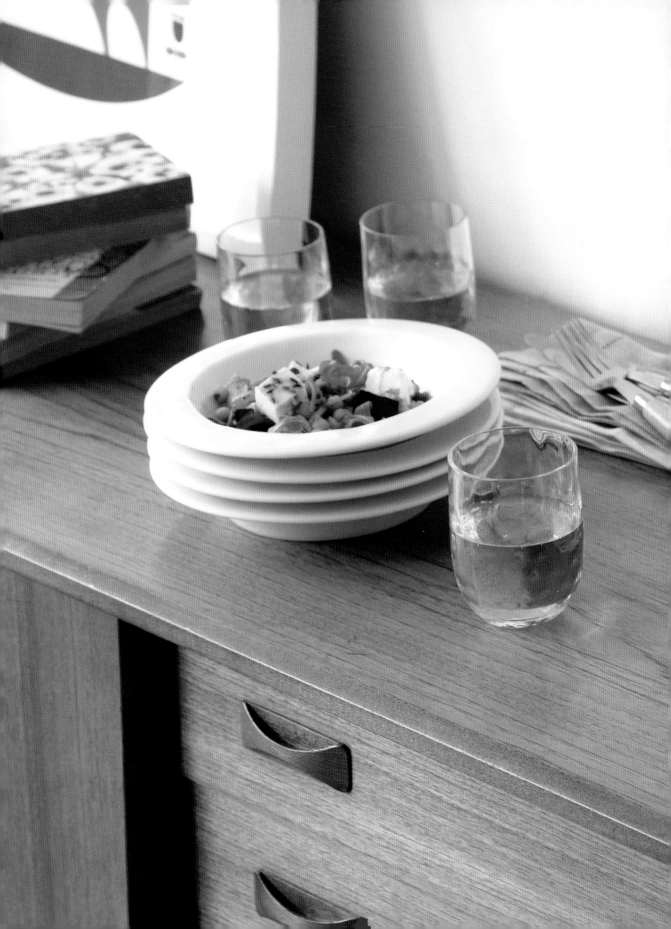

SALADS

A salad can be transformed from a side dish to a delicious main player with the addition of lentils, beans or chickpeas. Bean-based salads make brilliant packed lunches, filled with flavours that actually benefit from a few hours lurking in the lunch box and loaded with slow-release energy. Be sure to add plenty of oily, zippy dressing – the pulses will just drink it up.

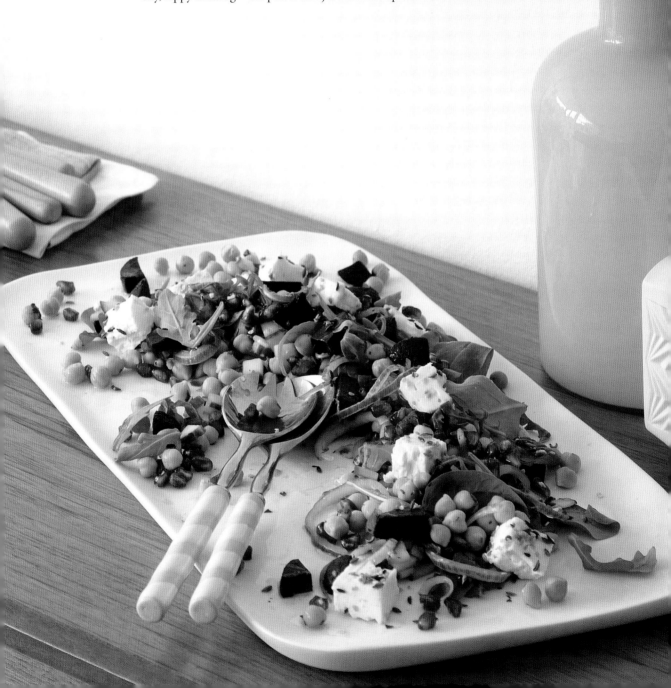

Chickpeas make this refreshing eastern Mediterranean salad substantial enough to eat as a main course along with toasted pitta.

Make sure that your cheese is authentic Greek brine-cured sheep's cheese (or less commonly a blend of sheep and goat's cheese) and not the similarly packaged, and desperately bland, cow's milk 'salad cheese', which lacks the characteristic tang and texture that you're after.

CHICKPEA, BEETROOT AND FETA SALAD

Serves 4

½ red onion, sliced

2 tbsp red wine vinegar

4 tbsp extra-virgin olive oil, plus extra to serve

3 garlic cloves, halved

500 g/1 lb 2 oz home-cooked chickpeas (garbanzo beans) or 2 x 400g/14 oz cans of chickpeas

salt and pepper

1 tbsp sesame seeds

1 tsp fennel seeds

200 g/7 oz feta cheese, cut into 2.5 cm/1 inch dice

100 g/3½ oz baby spinach or other salad leaves

½ cucumber, diced

large bunch of flat-leaf parsley, chopped

about 20 fresh mint leaves

2 small cooked beetroot, roughly diced

seeds from 1 pomegranate

Soak the sliced onion in the vinegar; it will turn a glorious fuchsia pink and become softer and more digestible.

Gently warm the olive oil and garlic in a saucepan for about 5 minutes. The idea is not to fry the garlic but to infuse the oil and soften the garlic's flavour. Remove the pan from the heat and take out the garlic, chop it finely and return it to the pan along with the chickpeas. Stir them around in the warm oil, season with a little salt and pepper, and then set aside to cool.

In a dry frying pan, toast the sesame and fennel seeds until the sesame seeds dance around and turn gold. Tip the seeds onto a plate and carefully toss the feta around to coat each dice in a speckled crust.

Put the onion with the vinegar, the chickpeas with their garlic oil, the salad leaves, cucumber, parsley and most of the mint in a serving bowl and mix carefully. Now add the feta and beetroot and toss carefully just a couple of times, otherwise the entire salad will turn a milky pink. Taste and adjust the seasoning if necessary.

Sprinkle with pomegranate seeds and a few mint leaves and serve with toasted pitta or sourdough bread and a dash of extra-virgin olive oil.

HOW ABOUT?

... adding a few pitted Kalamata olives.

... adding some roasted pistachios along with the pomegranate.

... adding grilled or chargrilled sliced aubergine.

... using fresh coriander instead of mint.

... serving this alongside grilled lamb cutlets, or lamb leg steaks. Marinate them in lemon juice, olive oil, oregano and grated onion for a few hours. Season with salt and pepper just before grilling.

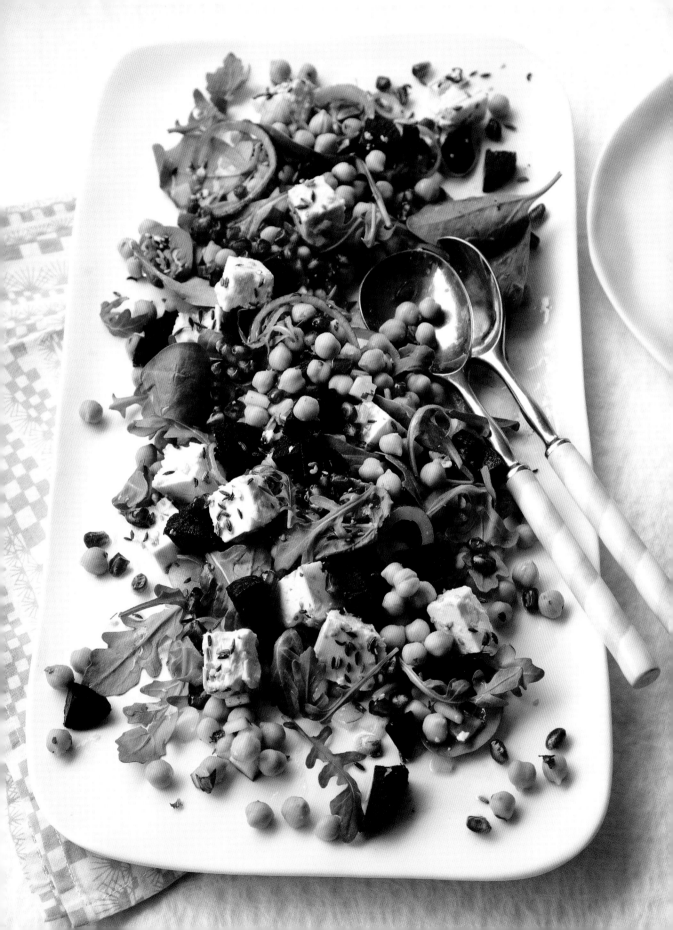

Fast food, the Indian way. All over India, small carts line the roadside selling delicious savoury snacks, or *chaat*, such as this hot and sour salad. The ingredients are usually mixed to order, keeping every customer happy. You can do the same at home, holding back on the chilli, lime juice and spices for the less adventurous.

Serve with yogurt and flatbread, ideally roti but toasted pitta will do fine.

ZIPPY INDIAN CHICKPEA AND POTATO SALAD
CHANA CHAAT

350 g/12 oz potatoes, cut into large pieces

250 g/9 oz home-cooked chickpeas (garbanzo beans)

    or 1 x 400 g/14 oz can of chickpeas

4 tomatoes, diced

10-cm/4-inch piece of cucumber, diced

2.5-cm/1-inch piece of fresh ginger, finely diced

½–1 red onion, finely diced

3–4 fresh green chillies (see p.248), finely diced

juice of 2 limes

1 tsp salt

1 tsp brown sugar or grated jaggery

1 tsp cumin seeds

1 tsp coriander seeds

1 tsp *amchur* (sour green mango powder), or perhaps a dash more lime juice

large handful of fresh coriander (cilantro), roughly chopped

OPTIONAL – ALL OR ANY OF THE FOLLOWING:

2 carrots, grated

1 small mango, diced (a 'raw' or unripe mango would be fabulous)

100 g/3½ oz raw beetroot, grated

Boil the potatoes in salted water until just tender and then dice roughly.

Meanwhile, rinse the chickpeas and place them in a large bowl with the tomatoes, cucumber, ginger and onion.

Traditionally this is a dish with a good kick, but taste the tip of one of the chillies and decide how much you want to add.

Stir in the lime juice, salt, sugar and spices. If you are using *chaat masala* (see right) instead of the spices, then go easy on the salt as the masala is salty too.

Stir in the potatoes, any fruit or vegetable options, and the coriander. Taste and adjust the seasoning: this should be mouth-puckeringly sour.

HOW ABOUT?

... seeking out some *chaat masala* (a sharp spice mix used to season savoury snacks) in an Indian grocer's. Substitute it for the cumin, coriander and *amchur*. *Chaat masala* would also be delicious sprinkled on the roasted chickpeas (see p.29).

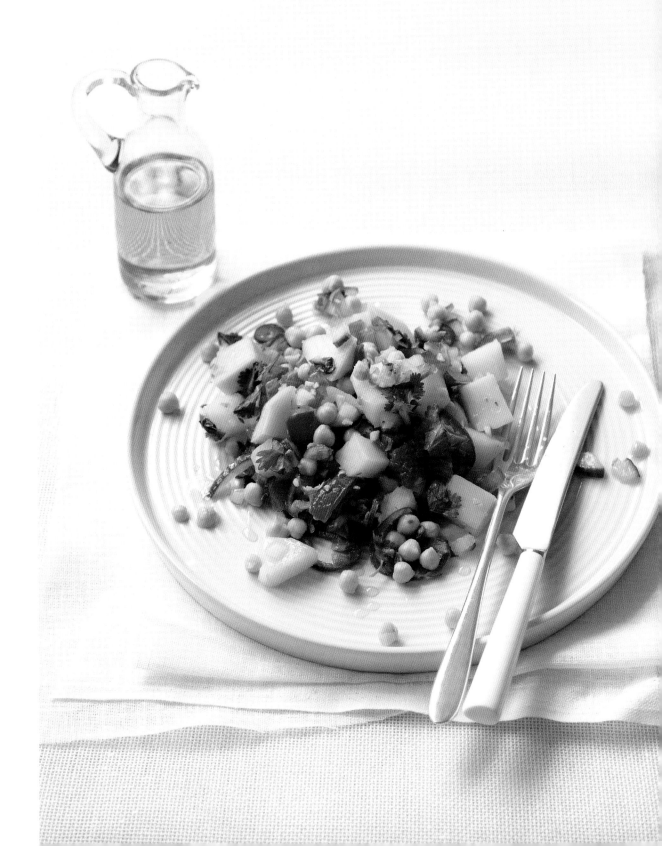

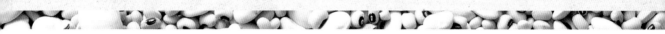

HERBY LENTIL SALAD WITH THREE VARIATIONS

Tiny marbled teal-grey Puy lentils, nut-brown Castelluccio or black beluga lentils are the best to choose for salads as they hold their shape beautifully. The idea is to cook until tender but still *al dente*; once overcooked, they turn into an unappetizing mush. It's always worth doubling the recipe and cooking up a decent-sized pot of these lentils even if you're not feeding a crowd; they will keep for a few days in the fridge and are incredibly versatile. Here are plenty of salad ideas, but you might like to stir them into a bowl of roasted vegetables, add them to a meat ragù, or even warm them with a little crème fraîche or tomato passata to serve as a side dish with grilled meat or fish.

This would be fabulous with a teaspoon of Dijon mustard stirred in and served alongside some cold ham or a good pork pie.

SIMPLE LENTIL SALAD

Serves 4

250 g/9 oz/1¼ cups Puy or Castelluccio lentils, rinsed

1 bay leaf

1 small red onion or 6 spring onions (scallions), finely sliced

2 tbsp red wine vinegar

1 garlic clove, crushed

4 tbsp extra-virgin olive oil

salt and pepper

4 tbsp chopped flat-leaf parsley

Put the lentils in a pan with the bay leaf and cover with about 5 cm/2 in of cold water. Bring to the boil and then simmer for about 20–30 minutes, until tender but still intact.

Meanwhile, if you are using red onion rather than spring onions, pour the vinegar over the onion and leave to soak. The onion will turn fuchsia pink and become softer in both texture and flavour.

Drain the lentils, reserving their cooking liquid, and while still warm, add the red onion or spring onions, vinegar, garlic and olive oil and season well with salt and pepper.

Leave to cool, then stir in the chopped parsley. If the salad seems dry, add a little of the lentil cooking liquid.

You'd be highly unlikely to find a lentil salad in Spain, in fact it's often impossible to find anything but the ubiquitous *ensalada mista* (that lettuce, tomato, tuna and egg medley that I happen to love). This combination of show-stopping Spanish ingredients is mine. It's a bit of an extravagance but fabulous for a treat. Montenebro, the smooth and tangy goat's cheese from the province of Avila, is my desert island cheese and the *jamón* gives some superb crisp texture.

IBERIAN LENTIL SALAD

Serves 4

150 g/5½ oz/1 cup baby broad beans (fava beans) – frozen are fine

1 tsp fresh thyme leaves

100 g/3½ oz piquillo peppers (from a jar or can), sliced

simple lentil salad (see opposite)

150 g/5½ oz Montenebro cheese or any really good creamy goat's cheese,
    diced or crumbled

100 g/3½ oz lamb's lettuce

2 tbsp extra-virgin olive oil

juice of ½ lemon

salt and pepper

50 g/1¾ oz *jamón serrano*, crisped (see p.250)

Blanch the broad beans for a couple of minutes in boiling water, refresh them under the cold tap and slip them out of their skins. If using frozen beans, you can just thaw them, give them a pinch and they will pop out of their skins.

Stir the thyme and most of the peppers into the lentil salad. then carefully mix in the cheese.

Toss the lamb's lettuce with the olive oil and lemon juice, then taste and season.

Place the leaves on 4 serving plates, pile some of the lentil salad on top, then garnish with the remaining peppers and the crispy *jamón*.

HOW ABOUT?

... tossing in some roasted almonds instead, or as well as, the *jamón*.
... using any leftover peppers for the stuffed piquillos (see p.100).

It's a good idea to cook a whole butternut squash and use the remainder in a soup or alongside your Sunday roast.

LENTIL, GOAT'S CHEESE, ROASTED SQUASH AND COURGETTE SALAD

Serves 4

2 tbsp olive oil

200 g/7 oz butternut squash, peeled and cut into large dice (prepared weight)

2 courgettes (zucchini), sliced into thick chunks

½ tsp dried chilli flakes

simple lentil salad (see p.118)

salt and pepper

extra-virgin olive oil

red wine vinegar

200 g/7 oz good, soft goat's cheese, roughly diced or crumbled

10–15 fresh mint leaves, ripped

Preheat the oven to 200°C/400°F/Gas mark 6.

Put the squash in a large roasting pan and roll it around in 1 tablespoon of the olive oil. Roast for about 20 minutes, or until beginning to brown and soften.

Now turn the squash dice over carefully, add the courgettes and sprinkle with the remaining olive oil and chilli flakes. Roast for a further 10 minutes.

Stir the vegetables into the lentil salad while they are still hot and taste the salad. It may need more salt, pepper, extra-virgin olive oil or vinegar.

Tumble the goat's cheese and mint through the salad and serve.

HOW ABOUT?

... putting the lentil and roast vegetable salad in an ovenproof dish and crumbling the goat's cheese over the top. Bake in a medium oven (180°C/350°F/Gas mark 4) for about 10 minutes, until the cheese melts and oozes through the lentils.

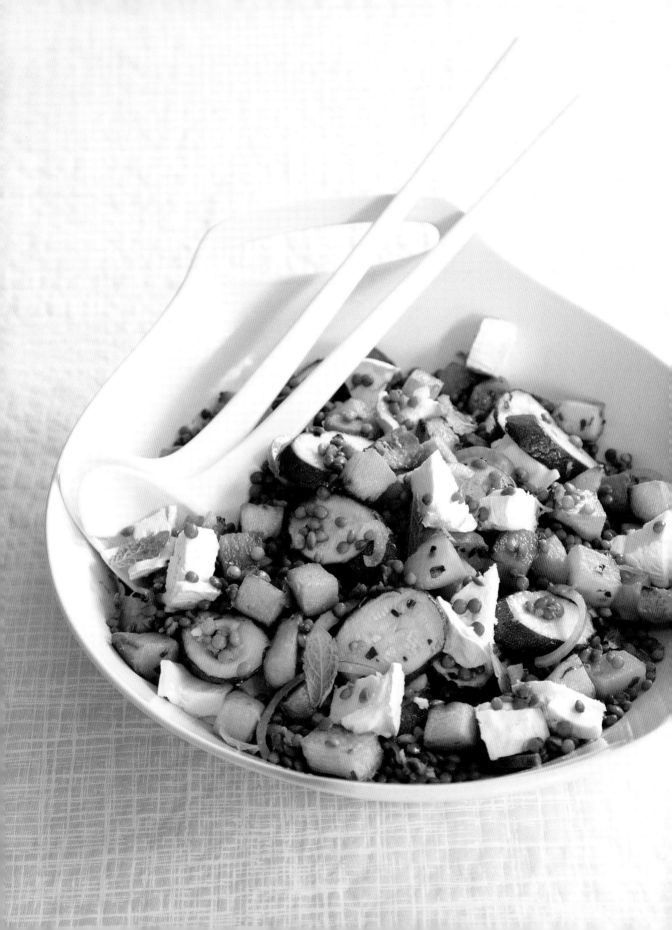

A wonderful light summer lunch. Everything can be prepared well ahead and then assembled just before serving.

Hot-smoked salmon has a great texture, more akin to poached salmon than smoked. Some adventurous cooks hot-smoke their own fish, but I'm keeping this quick and simple.

HOT-SMOKED SALMON, EGG AND LENTIL SALAD

Serves 4

200 g/7 oz fine green beans, topped but not tailed

4 cornichons or small gherkins, sliced

simple lentil salad (see p.118)

4 x 85 g/3 oz fillets of hot-smoked salmon, flaked into large pieces

3 eggs, boiled for 6 minutes (see p.249), shelled and quartered

FOR THE HERBY CRÈME FRAÎCHE

3 tbsp crème fraîche

1 tbsp finely chopped fresh dill

1 tbsp finely chopped fresh parsley

2 tsp grainy mustard

salt and pepper

Steam or boil the green beans until just tender and then refresh them under the cold tap to keep them crisp and bright. Drain well.

Stir the cornichons and green beans through the lentil salad, taste and check the seasoning.

Mix together the crème fraîche, herbs and mustard and season to taste. Crème fraîche is naturally slightly sour, but you might want to add a dash of vinegar or lemon juice.

Arrange the salmon and eggs on top of the lentils and serve with a spoonful of the crème fraîche.

HOW ABOUT?

... trying smoked trout or smoked mackerel instead of the salmon.

... using canned tuna instead of the salmon and adding some roasted red pepper (see p.249) – a salade Niçoise with a twist. Replace the creamy dressing with a good vinaigrette.

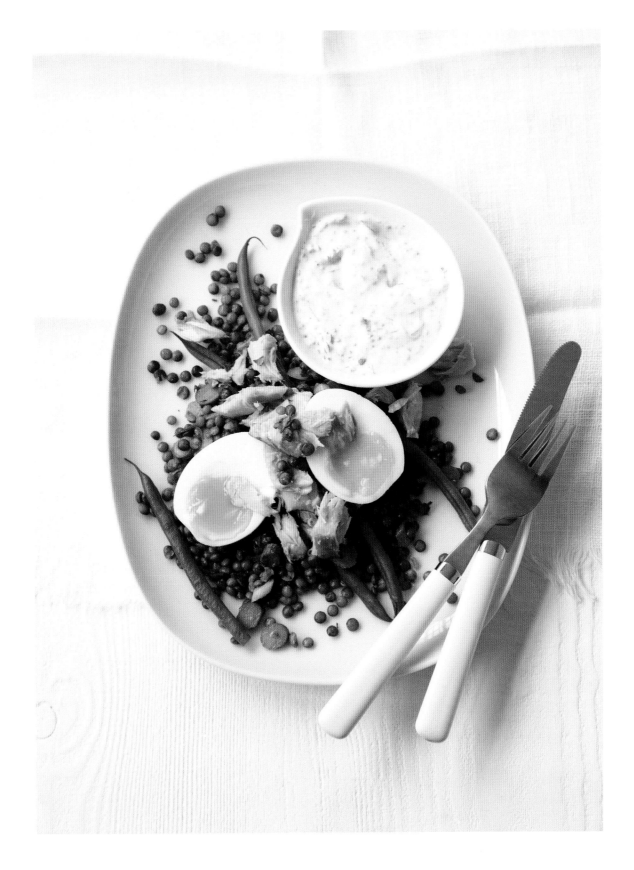

I came across *My New Roots*, Sarah Britton's fabulous food blog, while surfing the internet for lentil inspiration. I could hardly bypass a recipe with the title 'The Best Lentil Salad, Ever'. It lived up to expectations and has had many reincarnations since.

This lentil salad tastes all the better for a bit of resting and will keep for a couple of days in the fridge. Add fresh leaves, vegetables, cheese or whatever else takes your fancy at the last minute.

SPICED LENTIL SALAD

Serves 6–8

500 g/1 lb 2 oz/generous 2½ cups Puy lentils, rinsed

1 red onion, finely diced

150 g/5½ oz/scant 1 cup currants, sultanas or other dried fruit, diced to lentil size

4 heaped tbsp capers, rinsed, diced if large

FOR THE VINAIGRETTE

6 tbsp extra-virgin olive oil

4 tbsp apple cider vinegar

1 tbsp maple syrup

1 tbsp Dijon mustard

2 tsp salt

2 tsp pepper

1 tsp ground cumin

½ tsp ground turmeric

½ tsp ground coriander

½ tsp ground cardamom

¼ tsp cayenne pepper

¼ tsp ground cloves

¼ tsp freshly grated nutmeg

¼ tsp ground cinnamon

Put the lentils in a saucepan and cover with about 5 cm/2 in of cold water. Bring to the boil and then simmer until tender, but still with a bit of bite; this can take anything from 15 to 25 minutes.

Meanwhile, place all the vinaigrette ingredients in a jar and give it a good shake.

Once cooked, drain the lentils and rinse briefly with a little cold water to stop them overcooking and turning soggy.

While still just warm, combine the lentils with the onion, dried fruit, capers and vinaigrette.

HOW ABOUT?

... additions: Sarah suggests any of the following: rocket, parsley, coriander, basil, walnuts, goat's cheese, bean sprouts or seasonal vegetables.

... cheating! If the lengthy list of spices fills you with horror then, for a more predictable flavour, just add a good tablespoon of your favourite curry powder.

A stunning combination of colours and flavours. I love to vary the salad with the seasons, adding some grilled radicchio in the colder months and punchy pink radishes in the summer.

Do try to get around to sprouting some beans and radish seeds (see p.20) for this salad – they really do add an extra dimension.

CHICKEN, BEETROOT, AVOCADO AND SPICED LENTIL SALAD

Serves 4

1 ripe avocado
juice of 1 lemon
½ x spiced lentil salad (see p.opposite)
2 chicken breasts, poached (see p.250) and ripped into small pieces
300 g/10½ oz beetroot, roasted (see p.50) and chopped into
    rough chunks
large handful of sprouting beans, lentils, chickpeas and
    ideally some sprouted radish seeds
large handful of flat-leaf parsley, roughly chopped
salt and pepper
extra-virgin olive oil

Slice the avocado in half, twisting one side off to reveal the stone. Now, very carefully, tap the stone with a small sharp knife, which should lodge itself firmly; holding the avocado in one hand, turn the stone with the knife to remove the stone. Tap the knife sideways on your board and the stone will come off. Alternatively, use a spoon: it's just not quite so efficient. Cut the avocado halves in half again, peel and slice the flesh. Squeeze the lemon juice over the avocado to prevent it oxidizing and browning.

Spoon the lentil salad onto a wide serving plate. Scatter over the chicken, avocado, beetroot, your sprouted pulses and radish seeds and the parsley.

Season with a little salt and plenty of black pepper and give the salad a light drizzle of olive oil. Don't be tempted to toss the salad, or you will end up with a pink mushy mess.

HOW ABOUT?

... frying about 4 slices of streaky bacon until crisp and crumbling over the top.
... replacing the chicken with some goat's cheese for a vegetarian version.
... adding a bit of crunch with a handful of toasted nuts or seeds.

The mackerel/grapefruit pairing leapt out of a magazine when I was at the hairdresser's. The super-healthy salad article promised me a waspish waistline in a matter of weeks along with increased powers of concentration. I'm still waiting. Health issues aside, the combination is divine, especially with a bit of avocado thrown in.

SMOKED MACKEREL, GRAPEFRUIT AND LENTIL SALAD

Serves 4

2 grapefruits, preferably pink

2 ripe avocados

small bunch of watercress, washed and stalks removed

½ x spiced lentil salad (see p.124)

4 fillets of smoked mackerel, skin removed

2 tbsp toasted pumpkin seeds

pepper

Using a small serrated knife, slice off the top and bottom of the grapefruit and then cut away all the skin and pith. It's sometimes quite depressing as the grapefruit ends up half the size. Holding the grapefruit over a bowl to catch the juice, saw the knife carefully back and forth along the membrane that separates the segments until you reach the centre, turn the knife so you have effectively cut a V shape and out will drop the segment. Continue until you have removed all the flesh. Set the segments aside separately from the juice.

Slice the avocados (if in doubt, see the previous recipe) and stir gently in the bowl of grapefruit juice so that it doesn't oxidize and brown.

Add about half of the grapefruit, avocado and watercress to the lentil salad and flake in some of the mackerel. Fold rather than stir the salad very gently so that everything stays intact.

Place the salad in a wide bowl, or on individual plates, and scatter with the remaining ingredients including the grapefruit juice. Taste; it's unlikely that you'll need any more salt as the fish will be salty, but plenty of black pepper will really lift the flavour.

HOW ABOUT?

... using smoked trout, eel or prawns instead of the mackerel. There are some incredible smokehouses around the British coast; you'll often find their wares at farmer's markets or in good delis.

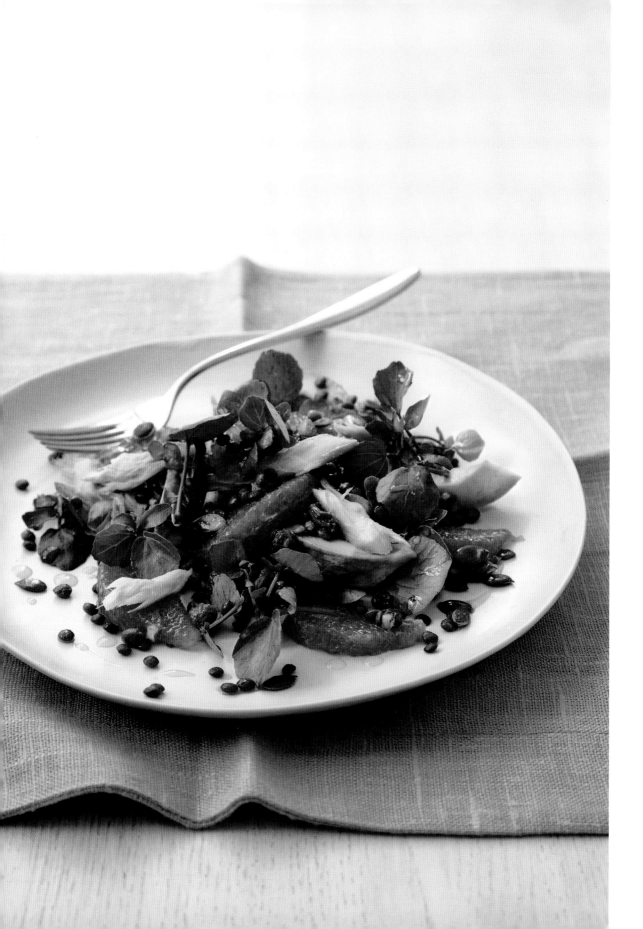

Oh, I know, all this superfood business is a bit of a cliché, but honestly you will have good reason to feel healthy and rather self-righteous after this salad. Most of these ingredients are vying for pole position in the world superfood ratings.

Quinoa is a complete protein (containing all the essential amino acids), it's gluten free and loaded with iron, phosphorus, magnesium and fibre. Pomegranates are packed with iron and fibre as well as vitamins A, C and E. Oranges are well known for their incredible burst of vitamin C but also contain loads of potassium, selenium and folic acid. Spinach is packed with vitamins A, E and K, folic acid and manganese. And then we come to the sprouts themselves: the vitamins, minerals and protein are said to increase substantially as the pulse bursts into life. In short, the salad is a nutritional powerhouse loaded with goodness and antioxidants. Eat this way regularly and it's widely believed that you will reduce the risk of obesity, diabetes, cancer, heart disease, Alzheimer's and Parkinson's. You'll also up the odds on becoming a centenarian supermodel, too.

SPROUTING BEAN AND QUINOA SALAD

Serves 4

200 g/7 oz/generous 1 cup quinoa, well rinsed

4 tbsp extra-virgin olive oil

2 tbsp red wine vinegar

salt and pepper

200 g/7 oz sprouting beans, bought or home-grown (see p.20)

½ red onion, diced

3–4 large sprigs of dill, stalks removed, roughly chopped

10 mint leaves, ripped up roughly

100 g/3½ oz baby spinach

1 pomegranate, seeds and juice but no pithy membrane

3 oranges, cut into segments

200 g/7 oz feta cheese, crumbled

Boil the quinoa in about 300 ml/10 fl oz/1¼ cups of water for about 15 minutes, until the grain has swelled up and you can see a Saturn-like ring around it. Drain off any excess moisture. While still warm, add the oil, vinegar and salt and pepper to taste. Set aside to cool.

Now toss the sprouting beans together with the onion, dill, mint, spinach, pomegranate and orange. Spoon out about a quarter of the mixture to use as a garnish, and then carefully tumble in the quinoa and half of the feta. Taste and balance the flavours with salt, pepper, vinegar and extra-virgin olive oil.

Serve, topped with the remaining feta and the technicolor bean mixture.

HOW ABOUT?

... using pearl barley, wheat berries, spelt or couscous instead of the quinoa (see Perfect Partners, p.18).

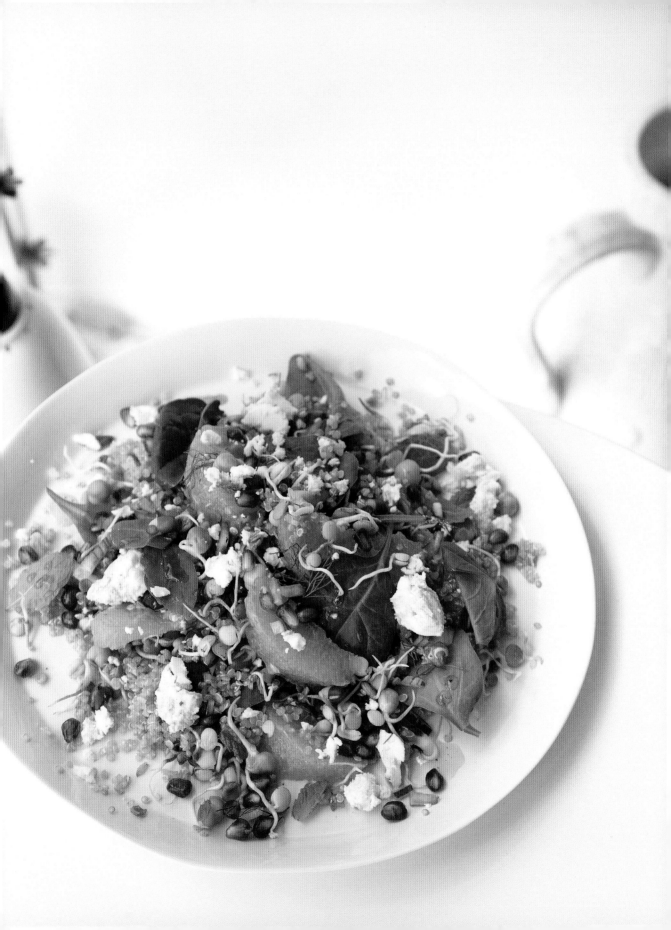

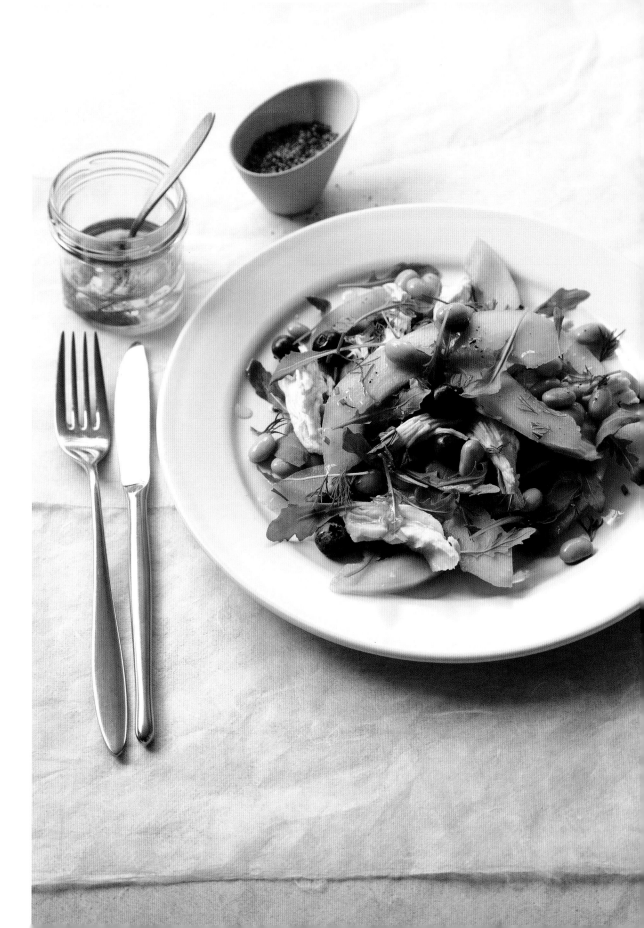

A heatwave salad. This incredibly refreshing and nutritious combination came together on one of those rare, searing-hot summer days. I love melon in its savoury incarnations – with prosciutto, or as a chilled soup – and thought about my melon baller, lurking redundantly in the kitchen drawer.

As well as being loaded with valuable antioxidants (apparently particularly good for keeping the memory up to scratch), the blueberries make a stunning contrast to the bright-green soya beans.

EDAMAME, MELON AND BLUEBERRY SALAD WITH POACHED CHICKEN

Serves 4

200 g/7 oz green soya beans, fresh or frozen

3 tbsp white wine vinegar, moscatel if possible

5 tbsp extra-virgin olive oil

about 2 tbsp finely diced shallot

salt and pepper

1 medium galia, cantaloupe, or any other sweet, ripe melon, diced, sliced or balled

100 g/3½ oz blueberries

100 g/3½ oz rocket (arugula)

½ tbsp finely chopped chives

5 sprigs of dill, stalks removed and fronds roughly chopped

10 mint leaves, finely chopped

2 chicken breasts, skin removed and poached (see p.250)

Bring some water to the boil and dunk the soya beans (don't worry if they haven't thawed) into the pan for about 3 minutes. Drain and rinse briefly with a little cold water so that they don't carry on cooking.

Tip the beans, still slightly warm, into a serving bowl. Add the vinegar, oil, shallot and some salt and pepper so that the flavours begin to marry. Leave to cool.

Once the beans are cool, tumble in the melon, blueberries, rocket and herbs.

Rip up or slice the chicken, season, then toss it in the salad. Taste; you may need more oil and vinegar and plenty of coarsely ground black pepper.

HOW ABOUT?

... sprinkling some crisped *jamón* or prosciutto (see p.250) over the salad.
... introducing some fresh, mild goat's cheese instead of, or as well as, the chicken.
... topping with a handful of sprouted baby leaves such as radish or broccoli (see p.20).

This salad comes from the Bertinet Kitchen in Bath, where I teach. We serve it alongside cured meats, cheese, pots of goodies such as tapenade and chickpea purée (and some fabulous bread of course – we're talking French baker extraordinaire); the perfect lunch.

The antithesis of the 1970s' stodgy bean salad, this is fresh, zippy and packed with vitamins. There's another bonus too: it takes about 5 minutes to prepare.

BEAN AND TOMATO SALAD WITH GINGER, CHILLI AND HERBS

Serves 4

2 shallots, finely sliced

4-cm/1½-inch piece of fresh ginger, finely diced

1–2 red or green chillies (see p.248), very finely diced

4 tomatoes, quartered

handful of fresh basil, coriander (cilantro) or any other herb,
    roughly chopped

2 x 400 g/14 oz cans of mixed beans
    or 500 g/1 lb 2 oz home-cooked beans

juice of ½ lemon or lime

1 tbsp red wine vinegar

extra-virgin olive oil

salt and pepper

Place all the ingredients in a large bowl, toss everything together, taste and balance the salt, pepper, acidity and oil.

HOW ABOUT?

... adding some chickpeas too. In fact, the more types of bean or pea the better, for both colour and texture.

... using spring onions instead of the more subtle shallots. Or you could tame some sliced red onion by soaking it in wine vinegar for 20 minutes, but do avoid using brown onions or your salad will come back to haunt you later in the day like the pickled onion in a ploughman's lunch.

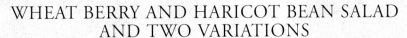

WHEAT BERRY AND HARICOT BEAN SALAD
AND TWO VARIATIONS

This versatile and healthy combination makes an ideal light lunch but is equally good alongside some soft sheep or goat's cheese, seared tuna or grilled meat. Wheat berries (whole wheat kernels) are increasingly available in health food shops and supermarkets, and you'll also find them in Turkish or Middle Eastern stores. You could substitute other whole grains such as spelt or pearl barley. Soaking overnight will not only speed up the cooking time but will also make them easier to digest. The basic recipe is followed by two distinctly different dressing options.

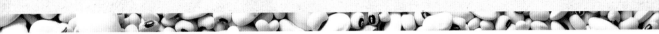

I love to use tiny Spanish *arrocina* beans but you can use any haricot, flageolet or whatever else takes your fancy.

WHEAT BERRY AND HARICOT BEAN SALAD

Serves 4

100 g/3½ oz wheat berries (preferably soaked overnight)

3 garlic cloves, peeled and left whole

salt and pepper

2 tbsp finely diced shallot

4 tbsp extra-virgin olive oil

juice of ½ lemon

250 g/9 oz home-cooked haricot (navy) beans
    or 1 x 400 g/14 oz can of haricot beans

large handful of parsley, coarsely chopped

Rinse the wheat berries thoroughly, place them in a saucepan and cover with plenty of cold water. Add the garlic and ½ teaspoon salt, bring to the boil and then reduce to a simmer. Cook the kernels until they are plump but still quite chewy, which will take between 45 minutes and 1¼ hours – or up to 2 hours if you haven't got round to soaking them. Drain, dig out the garlic and set aside.

Squash the garlic to a paste and mix it with the shallot, most of the oil, lemon juice, salt and pepper. Mix the dressing with the wheat berries while they are still warm. Stir in the beans and the parsley.

The salad is delicious just as it is. Taste and season if necessary. If you're going for one of the next two serving options, then taste and season later.

A feisty combination. Go easy on the harissa until you know how hot it is.

WHEAT BERRY AND BEAN SALAD WITH CAPERS, PRESERVED LEMON AND BLACK OLIVES

Serves 4

1 preserved lemon

wheat berry and haricot bean salad (see left)

3 tbsp capers, rinsed

3–4 tbsp pitted black Kalamata or Niçoise olives

1–2 tbsp harissa (see p.245)

large handful of fresh coriander (cilantro), roughly chopped

2 tbsp roasted almonds

Slice the lemon into quarters, remove the flesh, rinse and then slice the skin into fine needles.

Stir everything carefully into the salad, then taste and balance with more oil, lemon juice, salt or harissa.

HOW ABOUT?

... tossing in some leftover cold chicken or upping the game with some chargrilled squid.

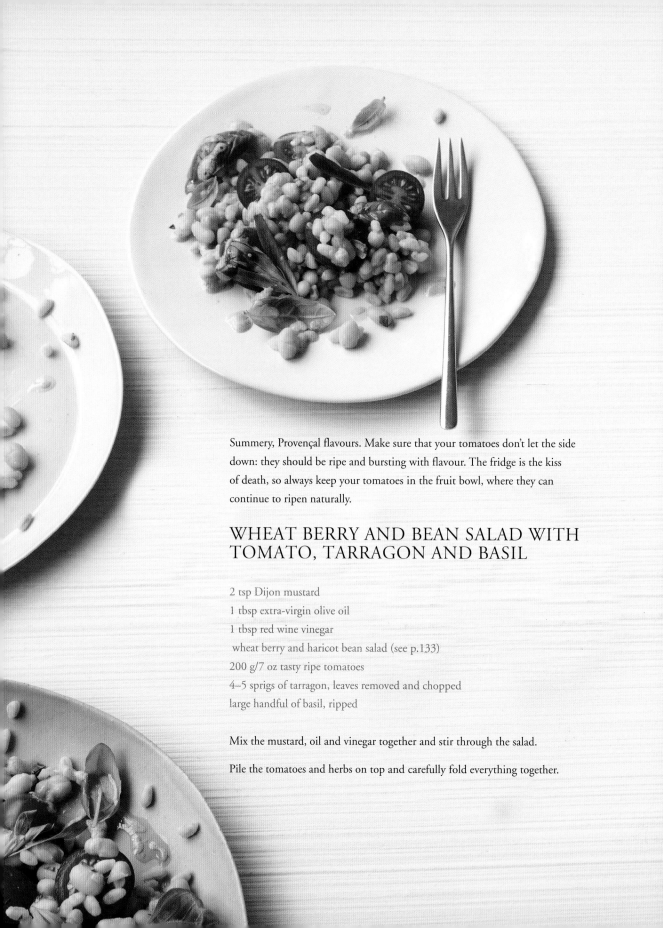

Summery, Provençal flavours. Make sure that your tomatoes don't let the side down: they should be ripe and bursting with flavour. The fridge is the kiss of death, so always keep your tomatoes in the fruit bowl, where they can continue to ripen naturally.

WHEAT BERRY AND BEAN SALAD WITH TOMATO, TARRAGON AND BASIL

2 tsp Dijon mustard
1 tbsp extra-virgin olive oil
1 tbsp red wine vinegar
 wheat berry and haricot bean salad (see p.133)
200 g/7 oz tasty ripe tomatoes
4–5 sprigs of tarragon, leaves removed and chopped
large handful of basil, ripped

Mix the mustard, oil and vinegar together and stir through the salad.

Pile the tomatoes and herbs on top and carefully fold everything together.

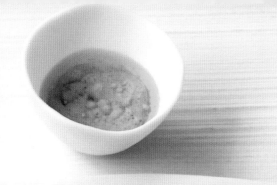

HOW ABOUT?

... serving this as a summer side with
roast chicken or poached salmon,
or throwing some ripe goat's cheese
into the mix.

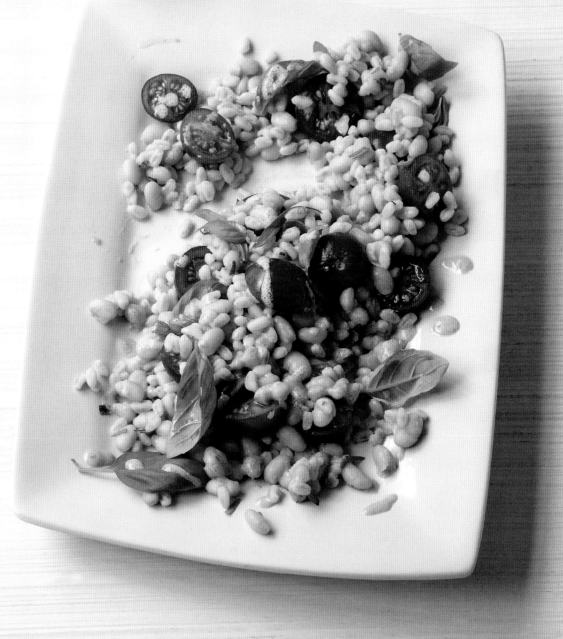

You can begin preparing this salad while cooking an evening meal. Double up the cauliflower and greens, eat half of them hot with your supper and the remains can reinvent themselves as tomorrow's lunch.

BUTTER BEAN AND WILD RICE SALAD WITH STEAMED GREENS AND ROASTED CAULIFLOWER

Serves 2

1 small cauliflower, divided into small florets

juice of 1 lemon

1–2 tsp curry powder or your choice of spice

1 red onion

2 tbsp olive oil

100 g/3½ oz/⅔ cup wild rice

150 g/5½ oz green beans, topped and halved

100 g/3½ oz fresh spinach, well washed

250 g/9 oz home-cooked butter beans (large lima beans) or 1 x 400 g/14 oz can of butter beans

FOR THE DRESSING

100 ml/3½ fl oz/7 tbsp extra-virgin olive oil

4 tbsp balsamic cider vinegar – or cider vinegar and 1 tbsp maple syrup

salt and pepper

Preheat the oven to 200°C/400°F/Gas mark 6.

Rinse the cauliflower and then toss it in the lemon juice. Place the florets in a roasting pan and sprinkle with the curry powder.

Peel the onion and chop into six, with each chunk held together by its root. Add the onion to the cauliflower and sprinkle with the olive oil. Roast in the oven for about 20–30 minutes, turning everything once until nicely golden and beginning to caramelize.

Rinse the rice and then place it in a pan (ideally the base of a tiered steamer) of cold water with a pinch of salt, bring to the boil and then cover and simmer for about 45 minutes, until tender and the grains begin to split. Drain.

Now to steam your veg. I cook mine in a steamer over the rice, but you may prefer to use a separate pan. Steam the beans for a couple of minutes, then refresh in cold water and drain well. Next, steam the spinach until it just collapses and drain well.

Combine all the ingredients for the dressing. While the roast vegetables are still warm, combine them with the rice, green vegetables and butter beans. Add the dressing and mix gently. Taste and balance the seasoning and set aside for the flavours to mingle and marry.

The recipe opposite can be used as a blueprint for any bean and rice salad, using similar quantities of each basic ingredient: beans, rice, roast vegetables and green vegetables. The soft roast onion and juicy spinach mean that the salad remains really moist.

Making up your own lunch box can not only save a fortune but it will most likely provide a much healthier, tastier and more varied option than the works canteen or local sandwich shop. The combination of beans and wholegrain rice provides a great balance of nutrients and slow-release energy to keep you going through the day.

This salad would also be great as part of a buffet spread or fabulous alongside roast chicken or a piece of fish. But for me, it's super selling point is the portability factor, there's nothing to wilt or spoil. The beans actually improve with a few hours' resting, so a night in the lunch box gives you a mature salad rather than an unappetizing soggy sandwich.

PERFECT PACKED LUNCH:
BEAN AND RICE SALAD

Here are a few combinations to try:

- red Camargue rice, haricot beans, roasted leeks, roasted courgettes, roasted peppers, steamed spinach and beans, plus a mustardy vinaigrette.

- brown rice, chickpeas, roasted red onions, parsnips, carrots with a good pinch of ras al hanout or ground cumin, steamed spinach and beans, plus a fresh lemon, honey and olive oil dressing.

- brown rice, mung beans, spring onions, roasted pumpkin, steamed mangetout and pak choy or spinach, sesame seeds, plus an orange juice, grated ginger, tamari, maple syrup and cold-pressed rapeseed oil dressing.

HOW ABOUT?

... sprinkling over a few hazelnuts, almonds, peanuts, cashews or walnuts.
... throwing in sunflower, pumpkin or sesame seeds.
... harvesting some sprouting beans (see p.20) and adding those too.
... adding crumbled cheese, such as feta.
... adding leftovers such as cold chicken or salmon.

This refreshing Cretan salad comes from Rosemary Barron. Her book, *Flavours of Greece*, was an absolute godsend when I cooked on a yacht in the Greek islands and I still dip into it regularly, 20 years later. Rosemary uses dried black-eyed peas, as any Greek cook would, but you could of course substitute canned if you are in a hurry.

BLACK-EYED PEAS WITH CORIANDER AND CAPERS

Serves 4 as a light lunch or side dish, 8 as *meze*

225 g/8 oz/generous 1 cup dried black-eyed peas, soaked for at least 2–3 hours

1 tbsp honey

3 tbsp red wine vinegar

salt and pepper

½ tbsp ground coriander

5 tbsp extra-virgin olive oil

3 tbsp capers, rinsed and roughly chopped if large

4 tbsp finely chopped parsley

TO SERVE

large handful of coriander (cilantro) leaves, coarsely chopped

1 small red onion, sliced into wafer-thin rings

225 g/8 oz Greek-style yogurt

Put the peas in a large saucepan, cover with plenty of cold water and bring to the boil. Drain and rinse out the pan. Return the peas to the pan, add cold water to cover by about 7 cm/3 in and bring up to the boil again. Turn down the heat and simmer for about 20–30 minutes, until tender (take care not to overcook). Drain in a colander and leave to dry off.

Meanwhile, in a large bowl, mix the honey, vinegar, salt, pepper and ground coriander. Gradually whisk in the olive oil, and then gently stir in the peas, capers and parsley. Taste and balance the flavours with more vinegar, oil, salt or pepper.

Carefully fold in the coriander leaves and serve the salad in a wide dish, scattered with the onion slices and accompanied by a bowl of yogurt.

HOW ABOUT?

... firing up the barbecue and serving the salad alongside some grilled halloumi cheese or lamb kebabs (you could first marinate the lamb with grated onion, lemon juice, olive oil and oregano for a few hours).

A traditional Tuscan dish that requires little more effort than opening a couple of cans. The recipe was a favourite of mine when I worked on an Italian racing boat. The idea was to spend as little time in the galley as possible while keeping all those strapping sailors happy and well nourished.

TUNA AND CANNELLINI BEAN SALAD
TONNO E FAGIOLI IN INSALATA

Serves 4

1 red onion, sliced very thinly

3 tbsp red wine vinegar

6 tbsp extra-virgin olive oil

salt and pepper

2 x 400 g/14 oz cans of cannellini beans
   or 500 g/1 lb 2 oz home-cooked cannellini beans

2 tbsp chopped flat-leaf parsley

200 g/7 oz canned tuna in olive oil, drained

Put the onion in a small bowl with the vinegar and stir it around; the vinegar makes the onion more mellow and digestible. Pour over the olive oil and add a pinch of salt. Leave the onions to sit for at least 10 minutes.

Tip the beans into a serving bowl, season with plenty of salt and freshly ground black pepper and add most of the onion slices, oil and vinegar. Stir in the parsley and lastly the tuna.

Taste and season, top with the remaining onion slices and serve with good, rustic bread.

HOW ABOUT?

... Tuscans look away! I love the simplicity of the salad in its virgin state but also like to ring the changes by adding any of the following: chopped celery, roasted peppers, semi-dried tomatoes (see p.249), diced chilli, capers, artichokes in oil, basil and marjoram.

Soya, mung and adzuki are the three great beans of the East. Soya has been consumed for thousands of years as tofu and in its fermented incarnations such as soy sauce and tempeh. Mung beans are most commonly eaten as bean sprouts, adding their crisp texture to salads and stir-fries, but here we enjoy them cooked. The adzuki bean is sometimes prepared with rice but most likely to end up as a sweet, red bean paste used for cakes and desserts. Combining the whole beans in a salad is a very unorthodox concept: let's call it East meets West.

Mung and adzuki require no soaking and cook quickly, so I'd never bother with canned (you can though if you're really up against it).

ASIAN-STYLE THREE -BEAN SALAD

Serves 4

100 g/3½ oz dried adzuki beans or 200 g/7 oz cooked beans

100 g/3½ oz dried mung beans or 200 g/7 oz cooked beans

250 g/9 oz edamame, fresh or frozen

2 spring onions (scallions), finely sliced

2 red peppers, finely diced

1 daikon (mooli/Japanese radish), peeled and
  finely diced (optional)

FOR THE DRESSING

2 tbsp white miso paste

2 tbsp grated fresh ginger

2 tbsp Japanese soy sauce

2 tbsp mirin (or white wine vinegar and 1 tsp sugar)

4 tbsp rapeseed or other vegetable oil

1–2 tbsp sesame oil

salt and pepper

Rinse the dried beans, and in separate pans, cover them with plenty of cold water and bring to the boil. Skim off any foamy scum and then turn down to a simmer. The beans will take anything from 20 minutes to 1 hour, depending on their age. They should be tender but still holding together well, or your salad will be a sludge. Drain the beans and set aside to cool.

Plunge the edamame into salted boiling water, or steam them for about 3 minutes. Drain and rinse with cold water to stop them cooking further.

Mix together all the dressing ingredients with a good pinch of salt and plenty of black pepper. Taste: you may need more salt, pepper, vinegar or even a pinch of sugar.

Place all the beans in a bowl with the spring onions, red peppers and daikon, if using (do try it, the texture is fabulous). Pour over the dressing and tumble everything together, taking care not to mash up the beans. If possible, leave for about 20 minutes for the flavours to marry and soak into the beans before serving.

HOW ABOUT?

... adding some mangetout, green beans, poached chicken, seared rare beef, marinated tofu (see p.199) or cooked prawns.

... combining with glass noodles (see p.111).

... using the dressing for any Asian-inspired salad.

... finishing up the leftover miso paste in soup (see p.95).

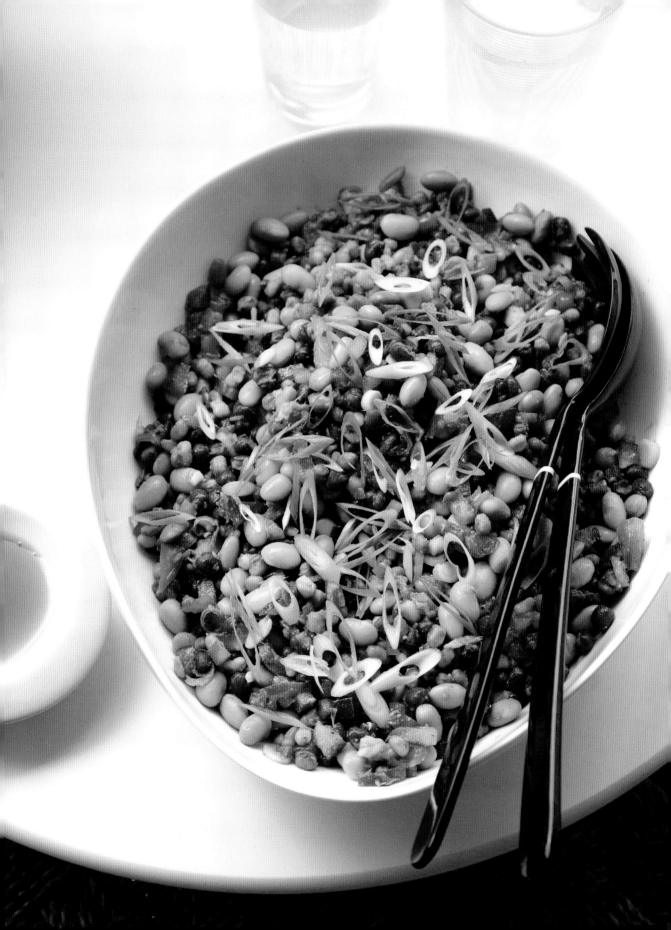

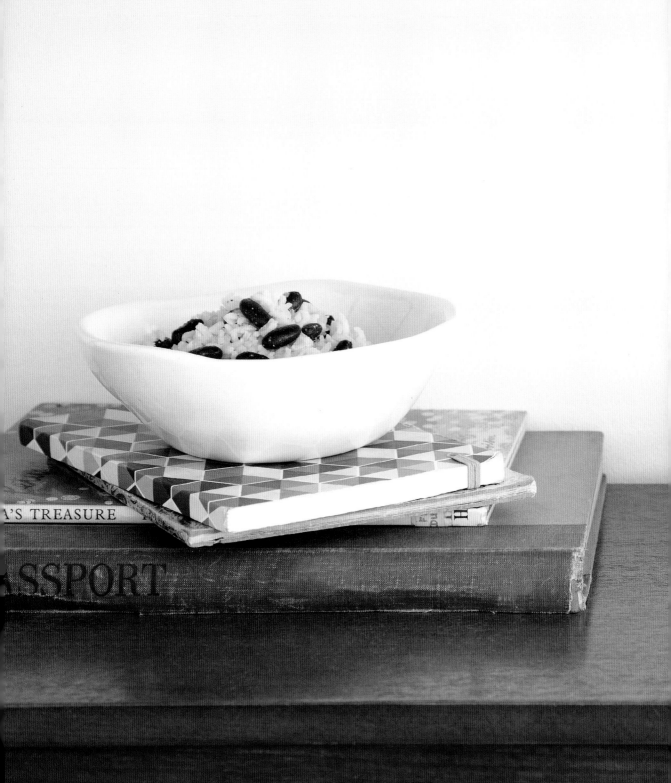

SIDES

Mashed, braised, spiced or fried, legumes offer so many options. Many of these dishes could also be eaten as main courses. Dals are a perfect example: in India, they are a staple meal with rice or bread – a very good one, too.

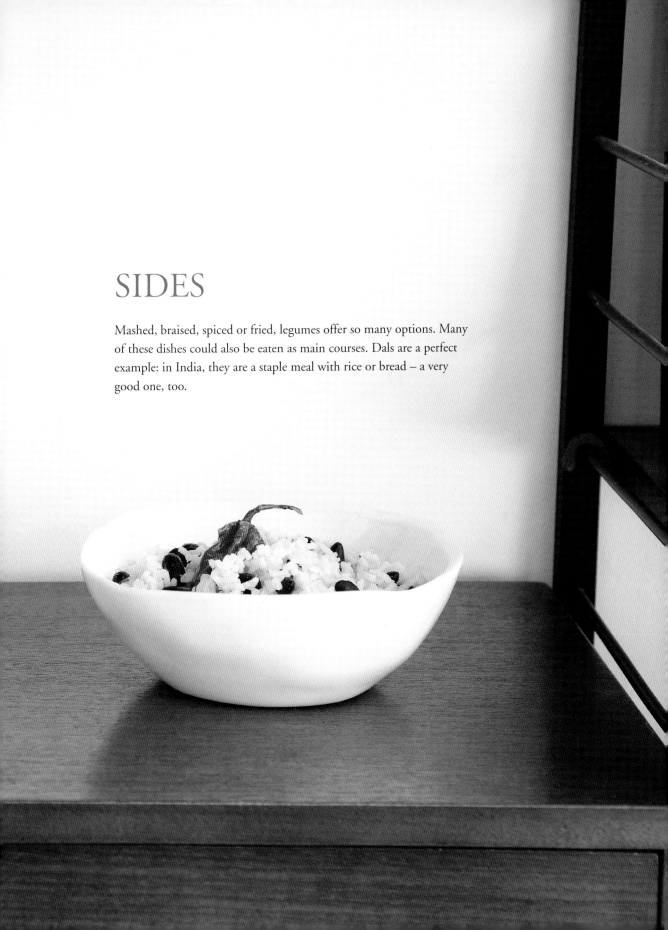

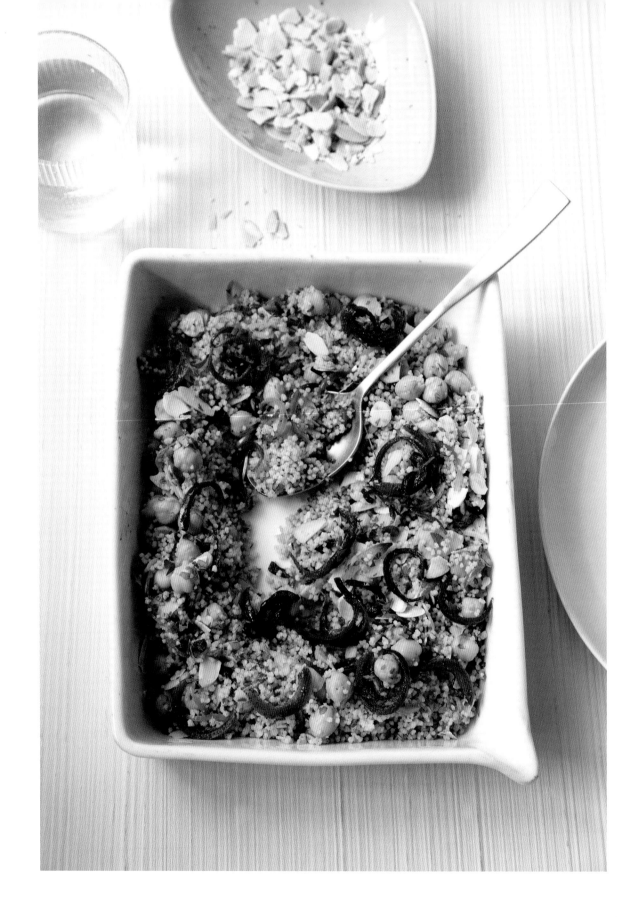

Great served warm alongside a tagine or some simple grilled food, and equally delicious cold. So double up the quantity and devour the next day with roast aubergine, pomegranate seeds and yogurt.

Couscous is quick, versatile and can be highly nutritious, too. It's worth looking out for the wholegrain spelt variety or barley couscous (for those with gluten intolerance). They are higher in fibre and have a lovely nutty flavour.

Ras al hanout is a blend of Moroccan spices and a convenient way of adding some North African magic to a dish without investing in dozens of different spices. There is no standard recipe; some blends contain up to 100 ingredients.

CHICKPEAS WITH COUSCOUS AND ALMONDS

Serves 4

2 tbsp olive oil

2 red onions, finely sliced

2 tsp ras al hanout – or use ½ tsp each of ground cumin, coriander, cayenne and cinnamon

200 g/7 oz/scant 1¼ cups couscous

300 ml/10 fl oz/1¼ cups boiling vegetable or chicken stock (vegetable bouillon or a vegetable stock cube will do)

4 tbsp extra virgin olive oil

250 g/9 oz home-cooked chickpeas (garbanzo beans) or 1 x 400g/14 oz can of chickpeas

large handful of fresh parsley, chopped

85 g/3 oz/scant 1 cup flaked (slivered) almonds, toasted

juice of 1 lemon

salt and pepper

Heat the olive oil in a pan and cook the onions gently until they are really soft, and then crack up the heat for a couple of minutes to brown a little. Stir in the spices.

Put the couscous in a large bowl and pour over the boiling stock. Cover with a plate and leave for about 5 minutes, until the stock is absorbed. Add the extra-virgin olive oil and fluff up the couscous with a fork. If it seems a little dry and granular still (this may well be the case if you are using a wholegrain version), just add a dash more boiling water and leave to swell again.

Fork in most of the fried onions, the chickpeas, parsley, some of the almonds and the lemon juice.

Taste and season with salt, pepper and more lemon juice or extra-virgin olive oil, if required.

Tip the couscous into a large mound on a platter or in a shallow bowl. Top with the remaining almonds and onions and serve warm or cold.

HOW ABOUT?

... adding fresh coriander, the chopped skin of 1 preserved lemon and some green olives for a sharper flavour.

... piling in some dried fruit such as chopped figs, sultanas, apricots or dates.

... stirring in a couple of spoonfuls of harissa (see p.245).

The Catalans love their chickpeas. They play a part in the traditional Christmas dish of *escudella i carn d'olla*, a slow-cooked brothy pot of meat and poultry. This dish is much quicker to throw together, especially when you can pick up some freshly cooked chickpeas from the market, corner shop or even the butcher's as they do in Catalonia. Home-cooked chickpeas or even a couple of cans will work a treat too.

Often served with salt cod, these are simply delicious alongside most fish, poultry or pork. I'm also very happy to dive into these as a light meal with a bit of good bread.

CATALAN CHICKPEAS WITH SPINACH
CIGRONS AMB ESPINACS

Serves 4 as a side, 2 as a main

6 tbsp olive oil

2 onions, diced

4 ripe tomatoes, peeled and diced

100 g/3½ oz lardons, pancetta or bacon (smoked or unsmoked), diced

3 garlic cloves, finely chopped

300 ml/10 fl oz/1¼ cups chicken stock, vegetable stock or chickpea cooking water

250 g/9 oz home-cooked chickpeas (garbanzo beans)
    or 1 x 400 g/14 oz can of chickpeas

250 g/9 oz fresh spinach, washed and trimmed of any tough stalks

salt and pepper

3 tbsp extra-virgin olive oil

Heat the oil in a large, heavy-bottomed frying pan or sauté pan and cook the onions gently for about 15 minutes, until they are really soft and golden.

Add the tomatoes, bacon and garlic, and cook until the mixture is thick and jammy.

Tip the stock into the pan, bring it to the boil and reduce by about a half before adding the chickpeas. Simmer for about 10 minutes (I like to leave my chickpeas at this stage to absorb the flavours for a while and then reheat).

Just before serving, add the spinach to the hot chickpeas: it needs only about a minute to wilt. Season with salt and pepper and drizzle with the extra-virgin olive oil.

HOW ABOUT?

... stirring in a handful of sultanas at the same time as the chickpeas.
... substituting the lardons with 200 g/7 oz of sliced chorizo for a one-pot supper.

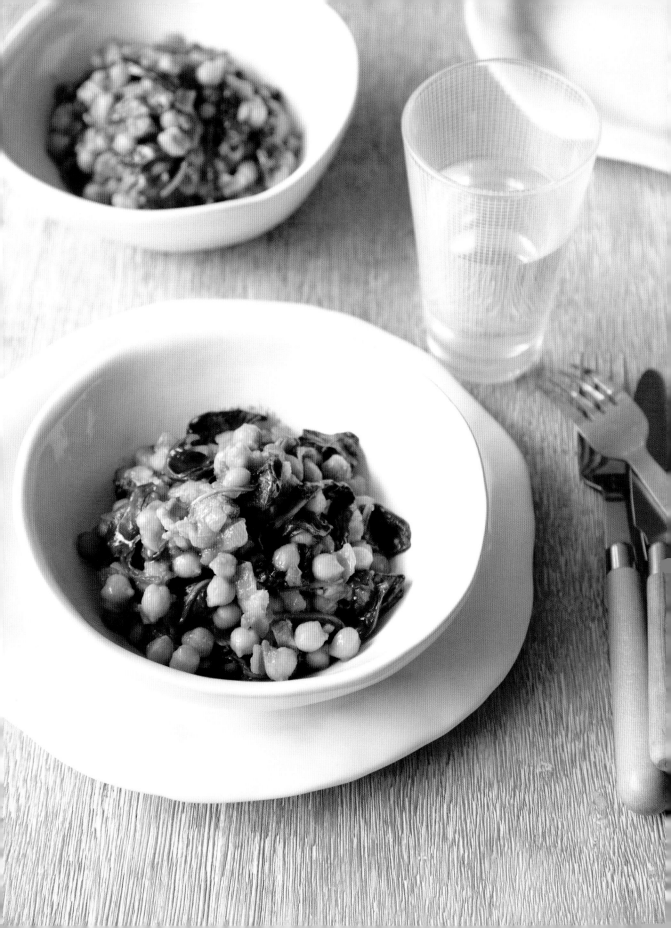

By August, Italian markets are stacked with wooden crates of fresh borlotti and cannellini beans. Every region has its own particular way of cooking them, which, being Italy, is of course quite simply the only way.

The Tuscans have an old nickname, *mangia fagioli*, or 'bean-eaters', historically a derogatory term since it implied that they were too poor to eat meat. Nowadays the traditional *fagioli all'uccelletto* is one of Florence's most celebrated dishes. *Uccelletti* are songbirds and the beans are supposedly prepared in a similar way to the tiny birds that are shot during the crazy Italian hunting season. (Just don't make the potentially fatal mistake of going for an autumnal stroll, I can assure you that it's a terrifying experience; you may never get back to your beans.)

TUSCAN CANNELLINI WITH TOMATO AND SAGE
FAGIOLI ALL'UCCELLETTO

Serves 6

500 g/1 lb 2 oz/generous 2½ cups dried cannellini beans, soaked overnight
(or, if you're very lucky, 500 g/1 lb 2 oz fresh podded cannellini beans)
2 sprigs of sage
salt and pepper
5 tbsp extra-virgin olive oil
3 garlic cloves, halved
8 ripe tomatoes, peeled and chopped

Place the drained (or fresh) beans in a pan, and cover by 5 cm/2 in of water. Throw in a sprig of sage, bring the water to the boil for 5 minutes, and then reduce to a simmer and cook until the beans are tender (anything between 30 minutes for fresh and 1½ hours for dried). Top up the water if the beans begin to emerge from the surface, but keep in mind that the beans should be juicy but not too soupy. Add some salt as the beans begin to soften.

Meanwhile, heat the oil very gently with the garlic and remaining sage. The idea is to infuse the garlic and sage flavours, but not lose the wonderful flavour of the extra-virgin olive oil. Stir in the tomatoes and simmer gently for a few minutes.

Add the tomatoes and sage to the beans, season with salt and pepper, cover and heat gently for about 15 minutes.

Serve with grilled meats, sausages or alone on a large slice of bruschetta.

HOW ABOUT?

... cheating: skip the bean cooking and use canned cannellini and drained canned tomatoes. This will definitely benefit from a few hours' resting, for the beans to absorb the juices.

... placing the beans in ramekins, cracking over an egg and baking in a hot oven (200°C/400°F/Gas mark 6). Add a dash of olive oil and a sprinkle of black pepper and salt to serve.

This is an almost instant supper option that goes brilliantly with any kind of stew or ragout or, for vegetarians, a ratatouille or a Sicilian sweet and sour caponata. You can of course use home-cooked chickpeas – you may even have some stashed away in the freezer for such occasions.

CHICKPEA MASH

Serves 4

3 x 400 g/14 oz cans of chickpeas (garbanzo beans)
    or about 750 g/1 lb 10 oz home-cooked chickpeas
salt
3 garlic cloves
5 tbsp extra-virgin olive oil
salt and pepper
juice of 1 lemon

Put the chickpeas in a pan, cover with salted water and bring to the boil (if you are using freshly cooked chickpeas, you can use some of their cooking water here). Toss in the garlic now if you prefer a more subtle garlic flavour; otherwise you can add raw garlic when you mash the chickpeas.

Once heated through, drain the chickpeas. Remove the garlic and crush it to a paste, then add it to the chickpeas (or add raw crushed garlic). Add the olive oil and mash the chickpeas using a potato masher, hand-held blender or, for a silky-smooth result, a food processor. Taste and season well with salt, pepper and lemon juice. If the mash seems too firm, then add a little stock, water or even a bit of liquid from the stew or vegetable dish you are about to eat it with.

HOW ABOUT?

... spicing it up with a teaspoon of ground cumin, ras el hanout, harissa paste, chilli or smoked paprika, or zipping it up with lime juice or tamarind paste (see p.247) instead of the lemon.
... adding chopped fresh chives, parsley, coriander or basil, or any herb that will marry well with your meal.
... a spot of indulgence: a few tablespoons of Greek yogurt, crème fraîche or melted butter would be delicious.

Good enough to eat on sourdough toast with a sprinkling of herbs or hot chilli.

CHICKPEA MASH WITH CARAMELIZED ONIONS

Serves 4
2 tbsp olive oil
2 onions, finely sliced
chickpea mash (see left)

Heat the olive oil in a frying pan over a low-medium heat and cook the onions for about 10 minutes while you prepare the chickpea mash. I find that the onions become especially sweet and soft if I start the process with a lid on and then take it off for the last few minutes. The onions should be deep gold by the time you have finished.

Tip half of the onion mixture in with the chickpeas as you mash. Taste and adjust the seasoning. Sprinkle the remaining onions over the top.

The familiar Provençal combination of aubergines, courgettes, peppers and tomatoes is given the Middle Eastern treatment in this traditional Turkish dish. The recipe calls for root vegetables too, so it's a great opportunity to use up any random bits in the vegetable basket. Especially good with lamb.

TURKISH ROAST VEGETABLES WITH CHICKPEAS
TURLU TURLU

Serves 6

1 aubergine (eggplant), cut into long fingers

1 red pepper, deseeded and cut into strips

2 small red onions, cut into quarters

2 potatoes, cubed

2 carrots, cut in half lengthwise

2 other roots, such as parsnip, beetroot or turnip,
    cut into chunks

1 tsp coriander seeds, crushed

good pinch of ground cinnamon

1 tsp chilli flakes (mild Aleppo chilli flakes are good)

2 tbsp extra-virgin olive oil

salt and pepper

2 courgettes (zucchini), cut into 2.5-cm/1-inch thick slices

handful of flat-leaf parsley, chopped

handful of coriander (cilantro), roughly chopped

FOR THE TOMATO SAUCE

2 tbsp olive oil

1 onion, finely diced

4 garlic cloves, crushed

400 g/14 oz can of chopped tomatoes

250 g/9 oz home-cooked chickpeas (garbanzo beans)
    or 1 x 400g/14 oz can of chickpeas

1 tsp honey (optional)

Preheat the oven to 200°C/400°F/Gas mark 6.

Toss all the vegetables (except the courgettes) with the spices and extra-virgin olive oil in a large roasting pan, season with salt and place in the oven. After 20 minutes, turn the vegetables and roast for a further 20 minutes. Turn again and add the courgettes for a final 10 minutes.

Meanwhile make the sauce. Heat the oil in a saucepan and cook the onion until soft and golden. Add the garlic and stir until fragrant, then throw in the tomatoes. Stir, add the chickpeas, and then season well with salt, pepper and honey if you like.

Combine the sauce with the roasted vegetables and serve sprinkled with plenty of fresh parsley and coriander.

HOW ABOUT?

... adding fennel, green beans or pumpkin to the roast vegetables.

... serving with bulgur, wheat berries or rice and Greek yogurt as a vegetarian main.

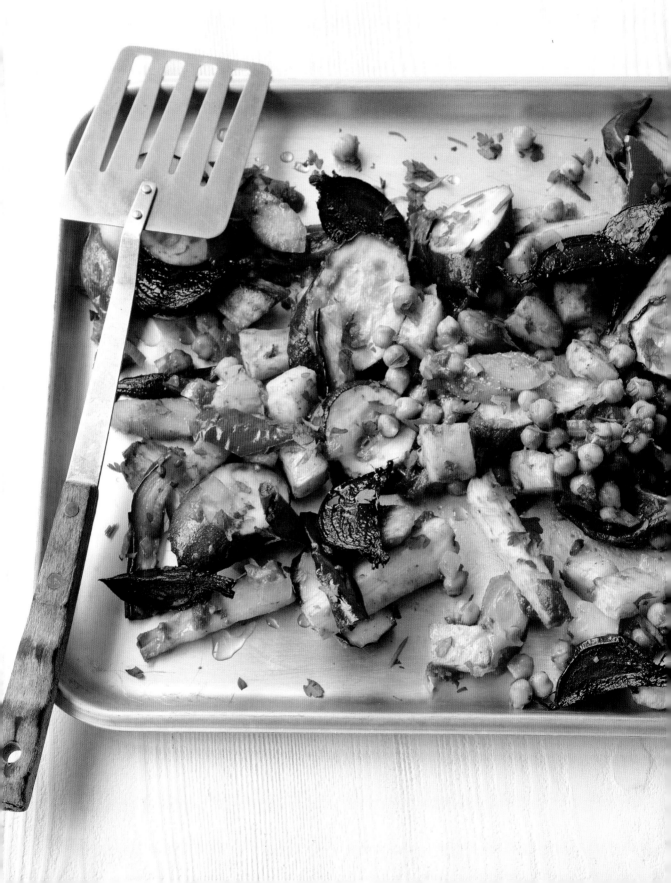

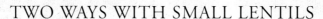

TWO WAYS WITH SMALL LENTILS

Tiny Puy lentils, black belugas, Spanish *pardinas*, Umbrian or Castelluccio lentils all have one thing in common: they hold together well and thus make wonderful side dishes when you don't want the mushier consistency of bigger green and brown lentils. Do make sure that the lentils are properly cooked: they should be intact but really juicy and tender, otherwise they seem rather mean and mealy.
Feel free to interchange the tiny lentils in these recipes.

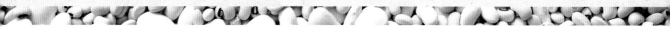

'As a separate vegetable dish this is hard to beat, especially in winter when there are no fresh green vegetables', said Elizabeth David of parsley buttered lentils in her seminal *French Provincial Cooking*. Fifty years on and the supermarkets are laden with tempting displays of unseasonal baby greens. Ignore them, and embrace the cold weather with these superbly simple lentils.

PUY LENTILS WITH PARSLEY BUTTER

Serves 4
250 g/9 oz/1¼ cups Puy lentils, rinsed
bouquet garni
150 ml/5 fl oz/⅔ cup chicken, veal or beef stock
50 g/1¾ oz/4 tbsp unsalted butter
large handful of fresh parsley, very finely chopped
lemon juice
salt and pepper

Put the lentils in a large pan, cover with at least 5 cm/2 in of cold water, bring to the boil and then simmer until tender. (I add a bouquet garni of celery, parsley, thyme and bay for an extra layer of flavour, but Elizabeth David did not, so don't worry if you don't have the celery or even some of the herbs.)

Drain the lentils and then return to the pan with the stock and cook for a further 5–10 minutes, until the stock is absorbed.

Stir in the butter and parsley, season to taste with lemon juice, salt and pepper and serve piping hot.

A wonderful accompaniment to game, sausages and oily fish such as sardines. I could happily tuck into these lentils on a slice of toast for lunch.

WINE-BRAISED CASTELLUCCIO LENTILS

Serves 4
2 tbsp olive oil
1 onion, diced
4 slices unsmoked streaky bacon, chopped finely (optional)
3 garlic cloves, crushed
250 g/9 oz/1¼ cups Castelluccio lentils or other small, firm lentils, rinsed
bouquet garni
400 ml/14 fl oz/scant 1¾ cups red wine
500 ml/18 fl oz/2 cups chicken stock
salt and pepper

Heat the oil in a large saucepan. Cook the onion and bacon until the bacon fat has begun to render and the onion is soft. Stir in the garlic and, when fragrant, tip in the lentils and stir to coat in the oil. Add the bouquet garni, wine and just enough stock to cover the lentils by about 5 cm/2 in. Bring up to a simmer and cook for about 30 minutes, until really juicy and tender. Add more stock, a ladle at a time, if the lentils seem dry, but remember you are not making soup and you don't want to strain away any of the tasty juices. Remove the bouquet garni, taste and season before serving.

HOW ABOUT?

... using canned chopped tomatoes in place of the stock.
... adding a couple of tablespoons of Dijon mustard, particularly if serving with sausage or game.

Red lentils add texture and body to a simple sweet potato purée. The secret is the zappy seasoning: plenty of chilli, lime juice, soy sauce and maple syrup. This is a really good accompaniment to the Sunday roast alongside more traditional greens and roast potatoes. Add a dash more lime and the tart mash makes a great backdrop for some freshly grilled mackerel.

RED LENTIL AND SWEET POTATO MASH

Serves 4

2 tbsp olive oil

2 onions, diced

1–2 fresh red chillies, deseeded if you like (see p.248), sliced

2 orange-fleshed sweet potatoes, peeled and roughly diced

300 g/10½ oz/1½ cups red lentils, rinsed

about 1 litre/1¾ pints/4 cups water

juice of 1–2 limes

1–2 tbsp tamari soy sauce

1 tbsp maple syrup or palm sugar

large handful of fresh coriander (cilantro), roughly chopped

Heat the oil in a large saucepan and cook the onions gently until soft. Turn up the heat and let them begin to colour before adding the chilli and the sweet potato. Stir to coat the potato in the oil.

Add the lentils and about three-quarters of the water and bring up to a simmer. Cover and cook for 15–20 minutes, until the potato and lentils are tender. The mixture will splutter and spit as it thickens. You will need to be fairly attentive for the last 10 minutes, stirring regularly and adding just enough water to make a mash (and not a soup).

Using a potato masher, hand-held blender or food processor, work until you reach a good smooth consistency.

Seasoning is crucial, so taste and add lime juice, tamari, maple syrup or sugar until you are really happy with the flavour. Stir in the coriander and serve.

HOW ABOUT?

... using any leftover mash in a toasted wrap for a quick lunch. Spread a thick layer of the purée on one half of the wrap, fold over to make a half moon. Toast in a dry frying pan until crisp on both sides and heated right through. Serve with a green salad.

DAL

Dal makes a wonderful side dish alongside a curry or a stand-alone simple family supper. You can adjust the tarka, or tempering (see right), to keep everyone happy, from a toddler to a fire-eating *phal* fanatic. One of the ultimate comfort foods, dal is extraordinarily cheap and easy to prepare, it is also extremely nutritious and can be flavoured in a myriad of ways. No wonder then that it is a staple right across the Indian subcontinent, where, combined with roti or rice, it provides invaluable protein. It is often thought of as a lentil dish, but a great variety of skinned, split and even whole pulses are used, depending on the country or region. Most common are masoor dal (red lentils), moong dal (skinned and split mung beans) and chana dal (skinned and split chickpeas), but other legumes such as urad dal (split black urad beans), toor dal (split pigeon peas) and even rajma dal (red kidney beans) can go in too.

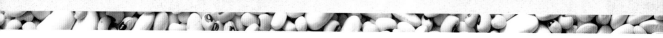

What gives this dal its character is commonly known as the tarka or the tempering, a mixture of spices and aromatics, and possibly onions, shallots or garlic, that is thrown over the dal just before serving.

TARKA DAL

Serves 8 as a side dish, 4 as a main with flatbread or rice

400 g/14 oz/2 cups moong dal, masoor dal,
    or a mixture of both

1.2 litres/2 pints/5 cups water

5-cm/2-inch piece of fresh ginger, chopped

3 garlic cloves, finely chopped

1 tsp ground turmeric

½–1 tsp salt

2 tbsp roughly chopped fresh coriander (cilantro)

squeeze of lemon juice (optional)

FOR THE TARKA

2 generous tbsp ghee, butter or vegetable oil

1 red onion, sliced

3–4 fresh green chillies, sliced

Wash the dal thoroughly and check for any tiny stones. Place them in a large saucepan with the water. Bring them to the boil and skim away any frothy scum.

Throw in the ginger, garlic and turmeric and simmer, with lid ajar, on the lowest heat possible for about 1½ hours. (A ridged griddle pan can help to diffuse the heat if you have a particularly fierce gas hob, just put your saucepan on top.) Stir from time to time and add more water if the dal is getting very thick.

When the lentils have collapsed, taste and season with salt. Add more water if you like a soupy consistency; I prefer mine to be more like a loose porridge.

For the tarka, heat the ghee, butter or oil in a small pan. (I would go for the luscious creaminess of ghee or butter every time.) Add the onion and cook until golden. Add the chillies and stir for a moment or two over a high heat.

Tip the tarka over the dal, stir it in along with a squeeze of lemon juice and then sprinkle with coriander.

HOW ABOUT?

... stirring in a handful of spinach leaves just before adding the tarka.

... adding tamarind paste (see p.247), lime juice or even a pinch of *amchur* (an intriguingly sharp powder made from dried green mango) instead of the lemon. Or leave out the sharp element for a more mellow dal that would work alongside a zippy curry or pickle.

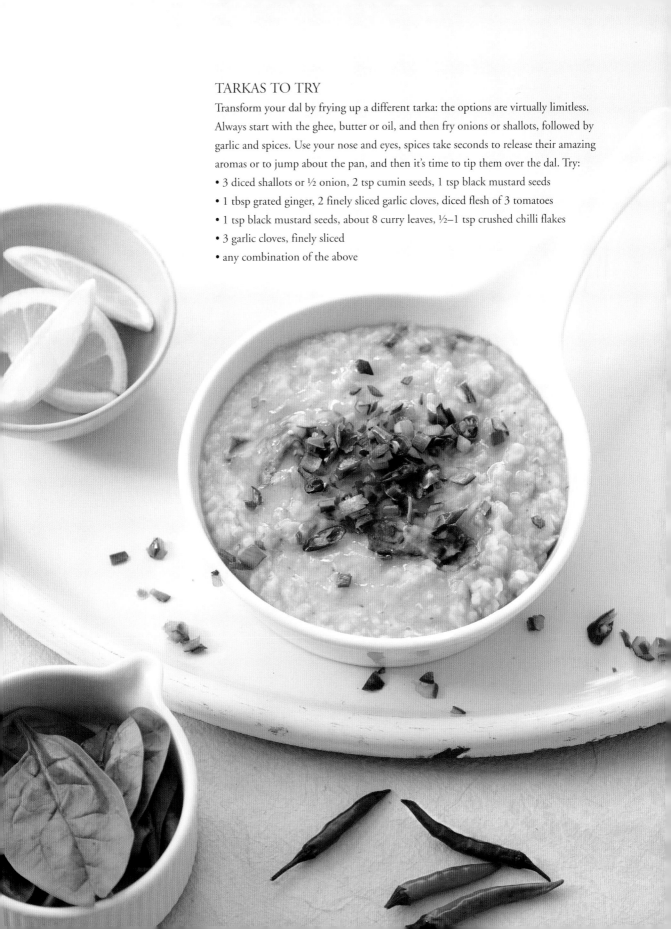

TARKAS TO TRY

Transform your dal by frying up a different tarka: the options are virtually limitless.
Always start with the ghee, butter or oil, and then fry onions or shallots, followed by
garlic and spices. Use your nose and eyes, spices take seconds to release their amazing
aromas or to jump about the pan, and then it's time to tip them over the dal. Try:

- 3 diced shallots or ½ onion, 2 tsp cumin seeds, 1 tsp black mustard seeds
- 1 tbsp grated ginger, 2 finely sliced garlic cloves, diced flesh of 3 tomatoes
- 1 tsp black mustard seeds, about 8 curry leaves, ½–1 tsp crushed chilli flakes
- 3 garlic cloves, finely sliced
- any combination of the above

A special occasion dal, served in restaurants all over northern India. Indulgence is what the dish is all about, so we are piling in the butter and cream. There are plenty of healthier dals to choose from; this one's a high days and holidays recipe. Delicious alongside a curry spread, but also a meal in itself with some naan bread.

Track down the little black urad dal (which are in fact beans, not lentils) in Asian shops or online. You will need to begin soaking them 10 hours in advance.

BUTTERED DAL
DAL MAKAHNI

Serves 6–8 as a side dish, 4 as a main with rice or flatbread

150 g/5½ oz/¾ cup whole urad dal (black gram), well picked over, rinsed and soaked overnight

85 g/3 oz/generous ⅓ cup dried red kidney beans, soaked overnight

½ tsp ground turmeric

2 green chillies, deseeded if wished (p.248), chopped finely

3 garlic cloves, crushed

2.5-cm/1-inch piece of fresh ginger, finely chopped

FOR THE TARKA

1 tbsp ghee or unsalted butter

½ onion, finely diced

2 garlic cloves, crushed

1 tsp ground cumin

2 tbsp tomato purée

salt

TO FINISH

100 g/3½ oz/7 tbsp unsalted butter

2–3 tbsp double (heavy) cream

1 tsp garam masala (see p.247)

handful of fresh coriander (cilantro), roughly chopped

Drain the urad dal and kidney beans and place them in a large saucepan with the turmeric, chillies, garlic and ginger. Cover with about 2 cm/about 1 inch of cold water and bring to the boil. Cover and bubble away for 10 minutes before lowering the heat to a gentle simmer. The beans will take anything from 1 to 1½ hours to become soft and tender. Check them regularly and top up the pan with water when necessary (the beans should only just be covered).

Once the beans are cooked, purée about a third of them. I find it easiest to do this with a hand-held blender in the pan. It's traditionally done with the back of a ladle and plenty of elbow grease (a potato masher would do the trick).

For the tarka, melt the ghee in a small frying pan and cook the onion until golden. Add the garlic and cumin, and once you're enveloped in wonderful smells, add the tomato purée. Stir the tarka into the beans along with a good sprinkling of salt and cook over a really low heat for about 10 minutes.

The dal will taste pretty good right now and you could just serve it with a dollop of yogurt, but it isn't dal makahni. If you're going for the real thing, stir in the butter, cream and a good teaspoon of garam masala. Taste and add more salt or chilli to balance. Sprinkle with fresh coriander and serve.

HOW ABOUT?

… using a pressure cooker up to the point of adding the tarka: it really does speed things up.

… sprinkling finely sliced fresh ginger and chilli as a garnish.

… cheating: add canned red kidney beans once the urad dal is ready.

… adding a handful of soaked chana dal (split chickpeas) right at the start, for extra texture and flavour.

Mushy peas are a northern English staple that usually accompany a traditional pie or fish and chips. They are sometimes referred to as Yorkshire caviar (the locals apparently have a rather tight-fisted reputation). Mushy pea fans are, quite rightly, appalled at the notion of a fresh or frozen pea purée being served up in their place; dried marrowfat peas are the only choice.

Bicarbonate of soda does leach out some of the nutrients from the peas, but without it you can be cooking away for hours, especially if your water is hard, and still end up with bullets. The bicarb helps retain the bright colour too.

MUSHY PEAS

Serves 4
250 g/9 oz/1¼ cups dried marrowfat peas
2 tsp bicarbonate of soda (baking soda)
1 tsp salt
knob of butter
large pinch of sugar (optional)
malt vinegar, to serve

Place the marrowfat peas and bicarbonate of soda in a large bowl and cover with plenty of water (they will swell up and double in size). Leave to soak for 12 hours.

Drain and rinse the peas and then place them in a large saucepan and cover with cold water. Bring to the boil and then simmer gently for anything between 40 minutes and 1½ hours, until tender and mushy.

Season with salt to taste, and I can't resist a bit of butter. A touch of sweetness is delicious too, so perhaps a pinch or two of sugar. Serve with some malt vinegar on the table. This is not the moment for your aged balsamic, this is British to the core.

HOW ABOUT?

… using split green peas instead: you can forego the bicarbonate and the texture will be more porridgey. Delicious, but not quite mushy peas.

A virtually instant accompaniment to stews or simple grills; quick, nutritious, endlessly versatile and, above all, very tasty. What more could you ask for?

The recipe comes from Clara at Notting Hill's legendary shop Books for Cooks, where I teach from time to time. The fabulous smells of bread, buttery cakes and aromatic stews waft among the shelves every morning as recipes are tested from the books and served up for lunch. Clara finds these simple, speedy beans are a great way to feed a crowd. They're incredibly popular, and make an interesting alternative to mashed potatoes.

CREAMY WHITE BEAN MASH

Serves 2–4
1 x 400 g/14 oz can or 300 g/10½ oz home-cooked
    cannellini or butter beans (large lima beans)
100 ml/3½ fl oz/7 tbsp double (heavy) cream
salt and pepper
extra-virgin olive oil

Heat the beans with a few tablespoons of water, or your own bean cooking liquid.

Stir in the cream and some salt and pepper and then mash to a rough texture or alternatively purée with a hand-held blender until smooth. Add more of the bean liquid if necessary.

Taste and adjust the seasoning, and add a little extra-virgin olive oil to taste.

HOW ABOUT?

… adding horseradish, Dijon or grainy mustard, grated Parmesan or finely chopped herbs. A favourite combination is butter bean mash with grainy mustard, tarragon and chives, served alongside roast chicken and steamed greens.

A fabulous way to tart up home-cooked or canned beans. Braised beans make a great accompaniment to roasts, barbecues or grilled meat and fish. They are good enough to go solo too, mopped up with a chunk of good crusty bread. The combinations are endless.

BRAISED BEANS
THE BASIC RECIPE

Serves 4 as a side

500 g/1 lb 2 oz home-cooked
    or 2 x 400 g/14 oz cans of beans
100 ml/3½ fl oz/7 tbsp extra-virgin olive oil
150 ml/5 fl oz/⅔ cup dry white wine
150 ml/5 fl oz/⅔ cup chicken, vegetable stock or
    bean water (if you have cooked your own)
4 garlic cloves, crushed
salt and pepper

Preheat the oven to 180°C/350°F/Gas mark 4. Put the beans in a shallow ovenproof dish and pour over the olive oil, wine and enough stock or bean water to just cover the beans. Stir in the garlic, a little salt and pepper and any other herbs or seasonings. Cover the dish with foil and place in the oven.

After about 30 minutes, take a look at the beans. Season with salt and pepper, give them a stir, check there is enough liquid and return to the oven without the foil. Cook for a further 20 minutes, until the liquid has reduced a little.

Taste and season with salt and pepper and serve hot or at room temperature.

To top it all
Transform your braised beans into a gratin with a crispy breadcrumb, cheese and herb crust.

4 tbsp dried breadcrumbs
2 tbsp extra-virgin olive oil
2 tbsp very finely grated Parmesan cheese
2 tbsp very finely chopped fresh herbs such as basil, parsley
    or marjoram (unless the braised beans are already herby)

Combine all the ingredients in a bowl and sprinkle over the beans for the last 20 minutes of cooking.

The combination of flageolets and rosemary screams for lamb, but would also be delicious with goat's cheese.

BRAISED FLAGEOLETS WITH SUN-DRIED TOMATOES AND ROSEMARY

braised beans (see left) made with flageolet beans
8 sun-dried tomatoes, finely sliced
4 small sprigs of thyme, leaves removed
2 sprigs of rosemary, leaves removed and very finely chopped

Add the sun-dried tomatoes and herbs along with the garlic.

The tiny, round *arrocina* beans from northern Spain would be heaven if you can find them, but any haricot will be good. The fennel and orange work beautifully with duck; you could also serve these beans with white-fleshed fish.

BRAISED HARICOTS WITH FENNEL AND ORANGE

braised beans (see left) made with haricot (navy) beans
2 bulbs of fennel
2 tsp fennel seeds, roasted and crushed
zest and juice of ½ orange
2 tbsp chopped flat-leaf parsley

First trim the fennel. Chop off the frondy tops and set aside for the garnish. Remove the tough outer layer and then chop the bulb into quarters.

Follow the braised bean recipe, adding the fennel and fennel seeds to the beans along with the garlic.

Before serving, check that the fennel is tender. Stir in the orange zest and juice, parsley, any chopped fennel fronds, and season with salt and pepper.

HOW ABOUT?

... stirring some baby spinach leaves into the beans as soon as they come out of the oven, they will add a lovely freshness.

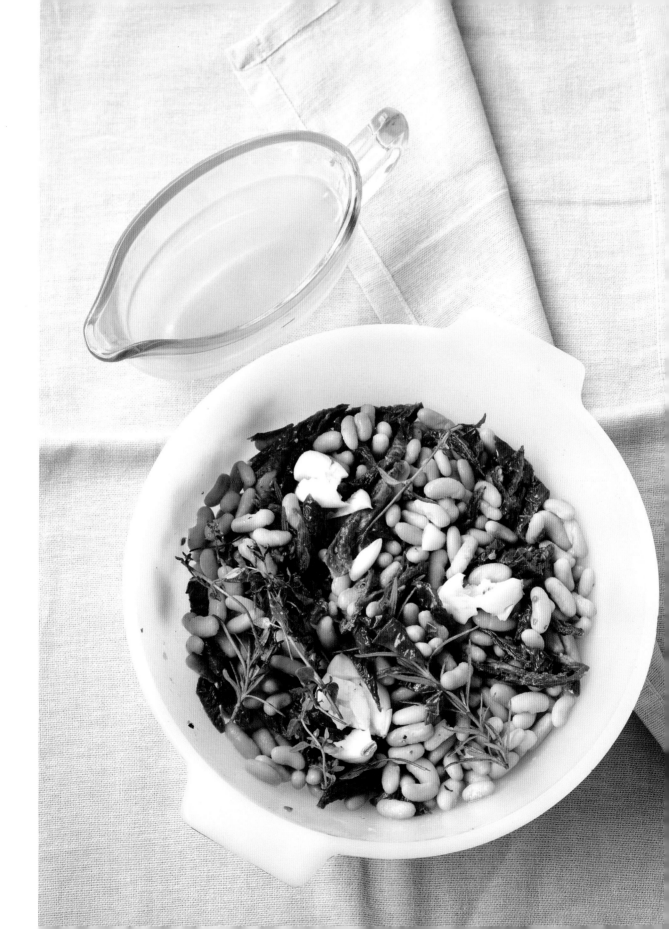

Black-eyed peas and wild greens are a classic Greek combination. Locals forage for leaves such as purslane, dandelion, dock, chard, wild fennel and even thistles. Back at home, a good selection of greens and plenty of fennel gives this dish its wonderful, if not totally authentic, flavour.

Black-eyed peas cook relatively quickly, especially when pre-boiled as here, and the beans (they are actually beans rather than peas) really do benefit from cooking with all the aromatic vegetables. Hence this is a cook-from-scratch rather than open-the-can recipe.

Try these beans served alongside simply cooked fish or pork.

GREEK BLACK-EYED PEAS WITH FENNEL AND GREENS

Serves 6–8

250 g/9 oz/1¼ cups dried black-eyed peas, rinsed

3 tbsp olive oil

2 onions, finely diced

2 carrots, diced

1 bulb of fennel, halved, cored and really finely sliced

4 garlic cloves, crushed

1 tsp fennel seeds, lightly bruised

2 tsp sweet Aleppo chilli flakes or ½ tsp hot chilli flakes

1 bay leaf

salt and pepper

300 g/10½ oz mixed greens such as Swiss chard, kale, spinach or beetroot leaves

3 tbsp tomato purée

juice of 1 lemon

Place the beans in a saucepan, add enough water to cover by about 5 cm/2 in. Bring to the boil and boil for 5 minutes and then remove the pan from the heat.

Meanwhile, heat the oil in a large saucepan and add the onions, carrots and fennel. Stir over a medium heat until they begin to colour and then add the garlic, fennel seeds, chilli flakes and bay leaf. As soon as you can smell the garlic, turn down the heat, give the pan a good stir and cover with a tight-fitting lid. Cook very gently for about 15 minutes, taking care that the garlic does not catch or burn.

Drain the beans and then add them to the vegetables, adding enough water to cover by about 5 cm/2 in. Cover and simmer gently for anything between 30 minutes and 1 hour, checking from time to time whether you need to top up the water. The beans should be moist but not too soupy by the time they are tender. (You can drain away some of the broth if they seem too wet.) Add a large pinch of salt.

When the beans are just ready, add the greens and the tomato purée to the pan. Cook until the greens have wilted and then taste and adjust the seasoning with salt, pepper and lemon juice.

HOW ABOUT?

… putting on your rubber gloves and gathering some young nettle leaves in the springtime. Cook for about 4–5 minutes instead of, or along with, your other greens.

BEANS DOWN MEXICO WAY

Beans are a staple in Mexican cooking; rarely does a day go by without a bowl of beans. The classics are black beans and pinto beans, but stroll into a Mexican market and there will be dozens of varieties to choose from, with evocative names such as Flor de Mayo, Sangre de Toro and Vaquita Roja. A green herb called epazote, or Jesuit's tea, is often added to the beans. It reputedly reduces flatulence, but is also thrown in for extra flavour. Mexican stockists will have some; try online.

Cook up a large pot and use in dips, soups, quesadillas (see p.62), burritos (see p.196), refried or drunken beans (p.162), or just tuck into a bowl of them by themselves. You can freeze some too. As you can see, you may as well cook for more than just one meal.

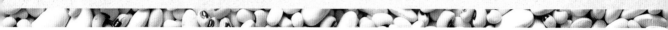

Pork lard will give these beans their authentic flavour, but we're not talking about the white block of over-processed grease that you find in the supermarket. Many butchers sell good lard, or you could even buy a piece of pork back fat and render it yourself. Just chop up the fat, place in an ovenproof dish with a few tablespoons of water and pop it in a medium oven (about 180°C/350°F/Gas mark 4) for up to an hour, until the fat has melted. If pork fat doesn't float your boat, then just use olive oil instead.

Soak your beans overnight (Mexicans don't, but I find the soaked beans cook more quickly and evenly).

POT OF BEANS
FRIJOLES DE LA OLLA

Serves 8

2 tbsp lard (see above) or olive oil

2 onions, diced

2 garlic cloves, bruised

500 g/1 lb 2 oz/generous 2½ cups dried black turtle beans, pinto beans or any other Mexican bean, soaked overnight

2 tsp dried epazote (optional)

1–2 tsp salt

Melt the lard in a large pot over a medium heat, then add the onions and cook until they start to soften. Toss in the garlic and stir until really fragrant. Tip in the beans and enough cold water to cover them by about 2–3 cm/1 inch. Sprinkle in the epazote.

Boil for 5 minutes, then reduce the heat to a barely wobbling simmer. Cook for anything between 1 and 2 hours, depending on the age of your beans. You'll need to check occasionally; the beans must be covered by water and do give them a stir to make sure they're not sticking.

Once the beans are soft, season to taste: they need plenty of salt.

HOW ABOUT?

... serving as part of a Mexican spread, alongside dips, salsas, enchiladas, a feisty beef stew or even a fried egg.

... giving the beans a starring role. Top with diced red onion and chopped coriander and squeeze over some lime juice.

Liven up your frijoles with a good dousing of beer.

DRUNKEN BEANS
FRIJOLES BORRACHOS

Serves 8

½ tbsp pork lard or olive oil

1 onion, diced

4 rashers streaky bacon, chopped

2 garlic cloves, crushed

3–4 fresh red or green chillies (see p.248), deseeded and
    sliced finely

4 or 5 ripe tomatoes, diced,
    or 200 g/7 oz canned chopped tomatoes

1 bottle of Mexican lager

500 g/1 lb 2 oz cooked frijoles (see p.161)
    or 2 x 400 g/14 oz cans of pinto or black beans

salt and pepper

fresh coriander (cilantro), chopped

Melt the lard/heat the oil in a large sauté pan or saucepan
and cook the onion and the bacon. Once the onions
are golden, throw in the garlic and chillies. Cook for
3–4 minutes and then add the tomatoes and stir over the
heat. Tip in the beer and bring to the boil.

Add the beans and enough of their cooking liquid
(or stock if using canned beans) to just cover the beans.
Simmer gently for about 20 minutes so that the juices
reduce and thicken.

Season with salt and pepper to taste and sprinkle
with coriander.

HOW ABOUT?

... adding some chopped mushrooms instead of, or as well
as, the bacon.

Oddly, a refried bean is not refried at all, just a cooked
bean that's fried. So it's up to you whether your beans come
from the *olla* (see p.161) or the can. If using home-cooked
beans, you will have the wonderful bean broth, but a few
tablespoons of vegetable or chicken stock work very well
too. Brilliant with all manner of Mexicana.

REFRIED BEANS
REFRITOS

Serves 4

1–2 tbsp lard or 2 tbsp olive oil

1 onion, diced

1 tsp ground cumin

good pinch of chilli powder

250 g/9 oz home-cooked or 1 x 400 g/14 oz can of pinto
    or black beans

salt

Heat the lard in a large frying pan and cook the onion until
it begins to colour.

Add the cumin, chilli, beans and a couple of tablespoons of
their cooking liquid (or stock if using canned beans). Now
mash with a flat-ended wooden spoon or potato masher as
the beans cook and the stock evaporates. Add more liquid,
a tablespoon at a time, as the pan becomes dry and the
beans begin to stick.

After about 15 minutes, your beans should be thick, almost
smooth and quite dark. Season with salt to taste.

HOW ABOUT?

... spreading a layer of refritos in a chicken and avocado
sandwich.

... serving on toast with diced tomato and crumbled mild
cheese such as Wensleydale.

... stirring in some chipotle paste (see p.248) for a bit of
smoky heat.

Super speedy and infinitely flexible, here's the way to magic up a bowl of tasty beans at a moment's notice. Equally happy alongside a fillet steak or an after-school fish finger.

The technique is borrowed from the Mexican kitchen but the recipe is really down to what you have in the cupboard.

QUICK SUPPER BEANS

Serves 4–6

2 tbsp olive oil

1 onion, roughly chopped

2 x 400 g/14 oz cans of any cooked beans

or about 500 g/1 lb 2 oz home-cooked beans

2 garlic cloves, crushed (optional)

salt and pepper

2–3 tbsp extra-virgin olive oil

Heat the olive oil in a large pan and cook the onion until golden. Add half of the beans and really squash them around with the back of a wooden spoon, allowing them to catch and colour in places.

Stir in the remaining beans and the garlic, and cook until everything is heated through and smells fabulous.

Season with salt and pepper to taste and add a couple of tablespoons of extra-virgin oil to add richness.

Now's the time to get creative (see right), but remember that just a couple of additions will work better than ten.

HOW ABOUT?

... adding finely chopped parsley, basil, tarragon, chives, rosemary, sage or thyme.

... throwing in some grated Parmesan, pecorino or lemon zest.

... tarting things up with capers, olives, anchovies or sun-blush tomatoes.

... zipping it up with lemon juice, verjuice, balsamic or wine vinegar.

... spicing it up with roasted cumin seeds, smoked paprika, sweet chilli flakes or ras al hanout.

The Jamaican Sunday side dish of rice and peas is made with beans rather than peas. Originally it was made with pigeon peas or cow peas (both of which are actually beans), but nowadays many people use red kidney beans.

The dish pops up all over the Caribbean and makes a great accompaniment to jerk chicken or any barbecued meats. So light the barbie and dream about steel drums, rum punch and flambée bananas.

JAMAICAN RICE AND PEAS

Serves 4–6

2 tbsp vegetable oil

1 onion, finely diced

2 garlic cloves, crushed

1 tsp grated fresh ginger

300 g/10½ oz/generous 1½ cups long-grain rice

salt

400 ml/14 fl oz/scant 1¾ cups canned coconut milk

400 ml/14 fl oz/scant 1¾ cups chicken stock, vegetable stock or water

1 tsp dried thyme

250 g/9 oz home-cooked or 1 x 400 g/14 oz can of pigeon peas,
    black-eyed peas or red kidney beans

1 Scotch bonnet chilli, left whole but spiked in a few places

Heat the oil in a large sauté pan or saucepan and cook the onion until soft and beginning to caramelize.

Stir in the garlic, ginger, rice and a good pinch of salt, and as soon as everything is fragrant, tip in the coconut milk and the stock or water.

Add the thyme and the beans, give the pot just one stir (otherwise the rice will become sticky) and then pop the Scotch bonnet on the top. The chilli is there to infuse the rice with flavour rather than heat, and is removed later.

Bring the liquid to a simmer and cover. Cook for about 15–20 minutes, until the rice has swollen and the liquid disappeared. Leave to rest, covered, for 10 minutes, then remove the chilli and fluff up the rice with a fork before serving.

HOW ABOUT?

... making a jerk marinade for chicken, pork or even goat. Purée (in a blender or food processor) 2–3 Scotch bonnet chillies, 6 spring onions, 1 tbsp dried thyme, 1 tbsp brown sugar, 3 tbsp soy sauce and 5 tbsp lime juice. Grind and add 10 allspice berries and 10 black peppercorns.

... serving with some dried banana chips scattered over.

... another great rice and bean combination: adzuki beans, brown rice and roasted cashews. Soften the onion and add brown rice along with twice its volume of water and a pinch of salt. Cover and boil until tender. Stir in cooked adzuki beans and a handful of roasted cashews. Season with tamari and sprinkle with fresh coriander.

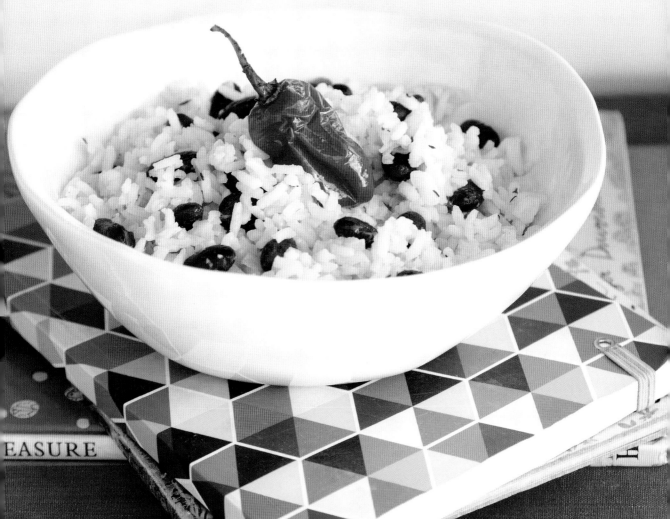

These greens are spectacularly good and have such a depth of savoury *umami* flavour that I could happily dive into a pile with some boiled white rice and call it a day. However, the combination of this stir-fry with roast belly pork, Chinese-style pork spare ribs or the more authentic *cha siu* (sticky sweet roast pork), if you happen to live near Chinatown, is out of this world. You could stir in some marinated and fried tofu (see p.199) for a delicious vegetarian alternative.

STIR-FRIED GREENS WITH FERMENTED BLACK BEANS

Serves 4 as a side dish
250 g/9 oz pak choi (bok choy), spring greens, purple sprouting broccoli
2 tbsp vegetable oil
2 garlic cloves, sliced
1 tbsp grated fresh ginger
1–2 fresh red chillies, sliced finely, seeds in or out (see p.248)
1 tbsp fermented black beans, rinsed and drained
1–2 tsp light soy sauce
1 tsp sugar (optional)

Quarter the pak choi, slice the spring greens or trim and divide the purple sprouting broccoli. Bring a pan of water to the boil and cook the vegetables for a couple of minutes, until just tender. Refresh in cold water and then drain.

Heat the oil in a wok or large pan. Stir-fry the garlic, ginger and chilli until you're enveloped in wonderful smells – a matter of seconds, as you must not burn the garlic.

Throw in the black beans and greens and stir-fry over a high heat for a couple of minutes, adding a tablespoon of water if the pan gets dry. Taste and season with soy sauce and sugar if needed. Serve at once.

HOW ABOUT?

... using sliced courgettes or runner beans, whole green beans, broccoli florets or a medley of any of the suggested vegetables.
... adding finely sliced fillet steak for the last minute in the wok.

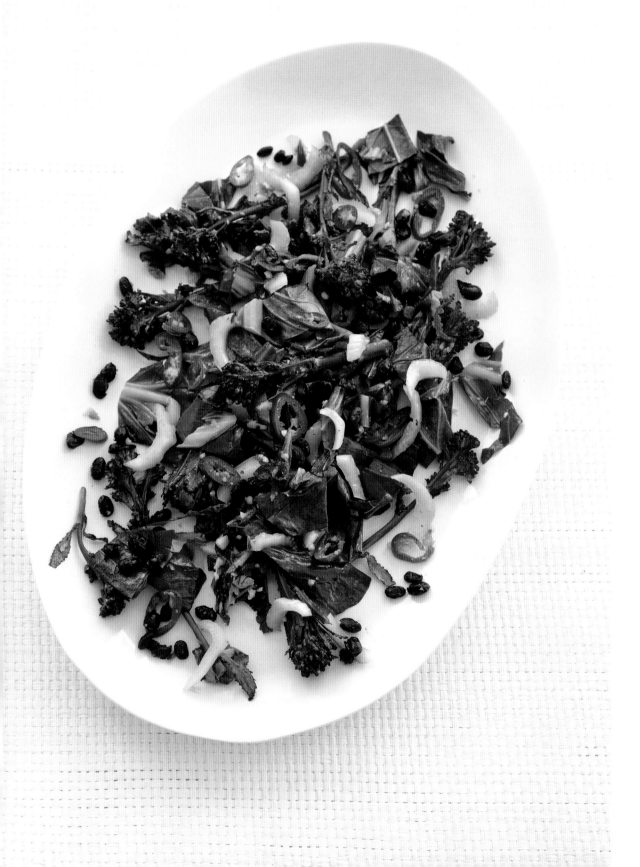

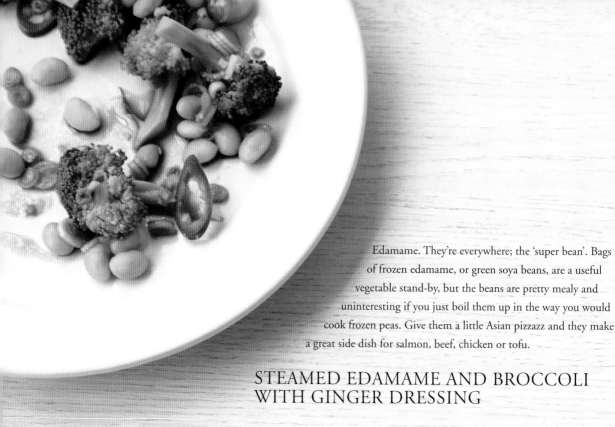

Edamame. They're everywhere; the 'super bean'. Bags of frozen edamame, or green soya beans, are a useful vegetable stand-by, but the beans are pretty mealy and uninteresting if you just boil them up in the way you would cook frozen peas. Give them a little Asian pizzazz and they make a great side dish for salmon, beef, chicken or tofu.

STEAMED EDAMAME AND BROCCOLI WITH GINGER DRESSING

Serves 4
450 g/1 lb broccoli, broken into small florets
300 g/10½ oz podded edamame beans, fresh or frozen

FOR THE DRESSING
1-cm/½-inch piece of fresh ginger, diced
1–2 fresh red chillies, sliced or diced
3 spring onions (scallions), finely sliced
1 tsp grated palm sugar, jaggery or demerara sugar
juice of 1 lime
2 tsp tamari soy sauce
2 tsp sesame oil

HOW ABOUT?

... green beans, sugarsnap peas or courgettes instead of/as well as the broccoli.
... making a meal of it, with glass noodles (see p.257), a few roasted cashews or peanuts, some tofu or cooked prawns.

Mix together the dressing ingredients and taste. Now 'exercise its extremities', as my food-obsessed friend Jerry would say, adjusting the salty, sour, sweet and hot flavours until perfectly balanced.

Steam the broccoli and beans separately until tender and cooked. Timings will vary depending on the size of your florets and whether your edamame are frozen or fresh, but around 5 minutes.

Toss the hot vegetables in the dressing and serve immediately. Alternatively, dunk your cooked vegetables into iced water to cool and keep their colour, and serve as a salad, with the dressing.

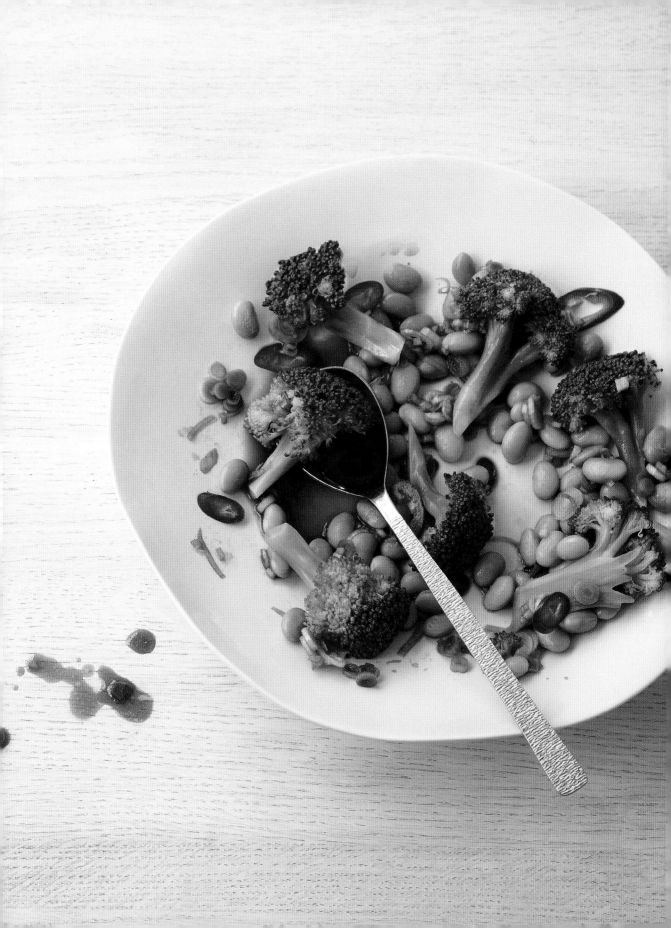

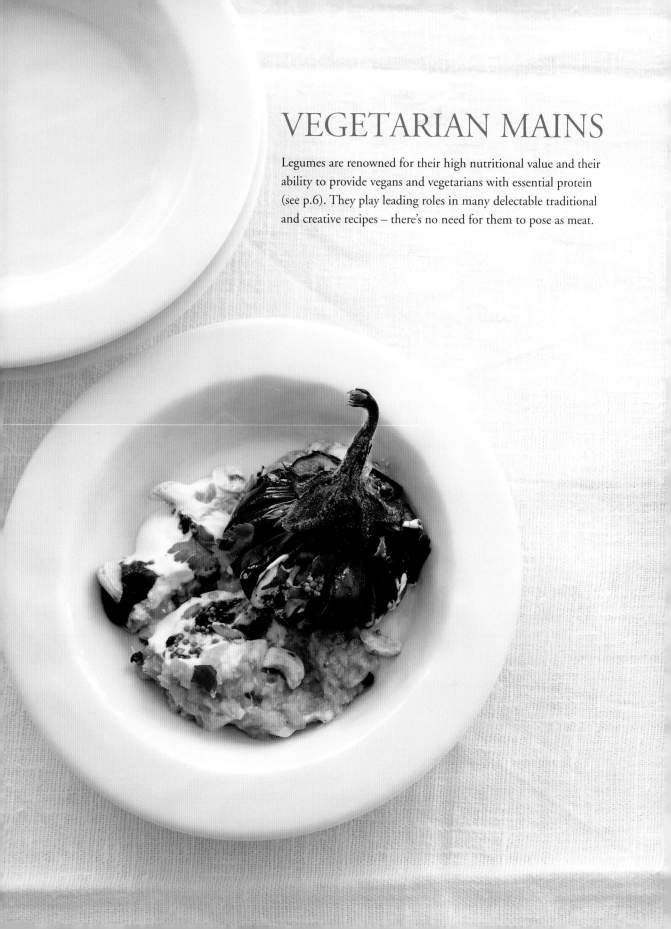

VEGETARIAN MAINS

Legumes are renowned for their high nutritional value and their ability to provide vegans and vegetarians with essential protein (see p.6). They play leading roles in many delectable traditional and creative recipes – there's no need for them to pose as meat.

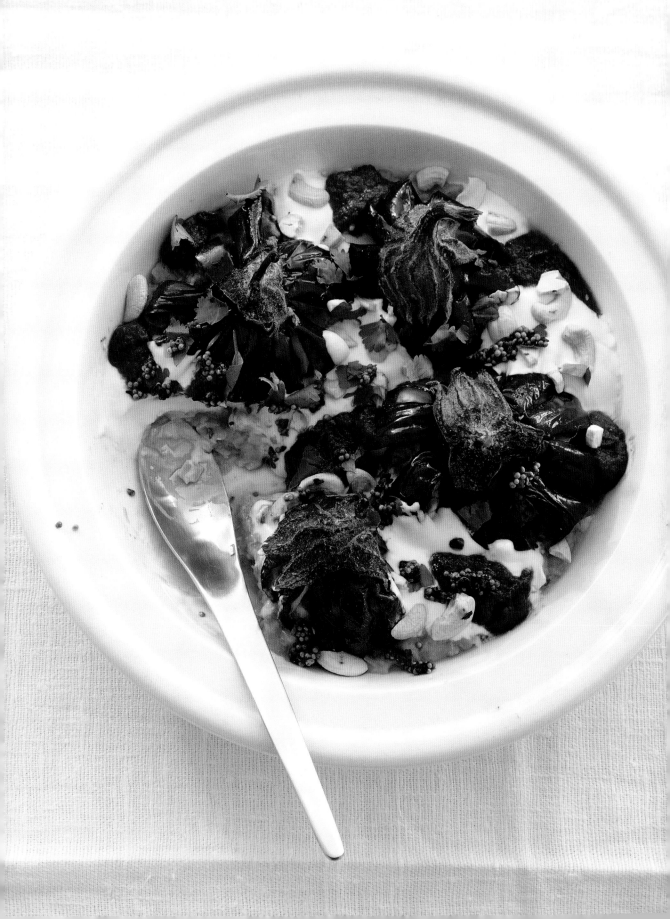

Seven is considered a lucky and magical number by many cultures: in the Muslim world, the Koran speaks of seven heavens and seven earths. Hence the vegetable tagine of Morocco with its traditional seven vegetables.

It's difficult not to become slightly obsessive about the vegetable tally here, so just count the onions, garlic and tomatoes as base flavours if it seems that you're coming in on the high side. After all, this is a great opportunity to empty the vegetable box or fridge drawer.

SEVEN-VEGETABLE TAGINE

Serves 4–6

2 tbsp olive oil

2 onions, finely diced

2 garlic cloves, crushed

2.5-cm/1-inch piece of fresh ginger, finely diced

1 fresh red chilli, deseeded and very finely diced

1 tsp sweet paprika

1 tsp cumin

1 cinnamon stick

2 carrots, cut into large chunks

1 small butternut squash, cut into large dice

500 g/1 lb 2 oz turnip, cut into large dice

1 red pepper, sliced

1 bulb of fennel, trimmed and sliced

400g/14 oz can of chopped tomatoes

1 x 400 g/14 oz can of chickpeas (garbanzo beans)
   or 250 g/9 oz home-cooked chickpeas

handful of dried apricots, chopped roughly

3 courgettes (zucchini), cut into large chunks

1 tbsp chopped fresh parsley

1 tbsp chopped fresh coriander (cilantro)

juice of 1 lemon

salt and pepper

Heat the oil in a large saucepan over a medium heat and cook the onion until soft. Toss in the garlic, ginger, chilli and spices, and keep stirring over the heat until you hit by the heady smells.

Now add the carrots, squash, turnip, red pepper and fennel, stirring everything together. Tip in the tomatoes and enough water to cover the vegetables and then simmer until the root vegetables are just tender. Throw in the chickpeas, apricots and courgettes, and simmer for a few minutes.

Stir in the herbs, taste and balance with lemon juice, salt and pepper. Serve hot, with couscous and harissa.

HOW ABOUT?

... straining off some of the finished tagine liquid and using it to soak couscous or, less orthodox, some quinoa (see p.128) to serve alongside the vegetables.

... serving with flatbreads, yogurt and harissa (see p.245).

... using other vegetables such as parsnips, sweet potato, green beans, broad beans, according to the season.

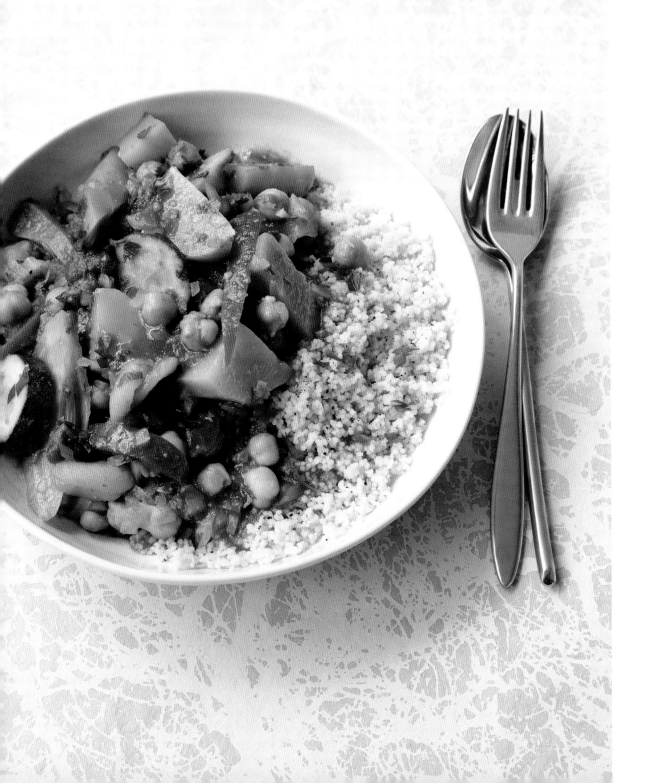

Today's recipes often call for all sorts of weird and wonderful ingredients destined to languish in the back of the cupboard until they reach their 'best before' date. You might consider this sweet-and-sour pomegranate molasses to be one of them. Think again. The syrup makes a fabulous Middle Eastern dressing with a touch of lemon juice and plenty of olive oil, and can be brushed on roasting chicken, duck or lamb for a glorious glaze, is fantastically refreshing when mixed with chilled fizzy water and seems to keep *ad infinitum*. Naturally sweet root vegetables and chickpeas make a great combination with the yogurt, but it's the pomegranate molasses and spices that lift this dish onto another plain.

ROASTED ROOTS WITH CHICKPEAS

Serves 4

400 g/14 oz carrots, preferably small ones, halved if large

3 parsnips, quartered lengthwise, woody core removed

4 tbsp olive oil

salt and pepper

300 g/10½ oz beetroot, peeled and cut into quarters
   or bite-sized chunks

250 g/9 oz home-cooked chickpeas (garbanzo beans)
   or 1 x 400g/14 oz can of chickpeas

4 tbsp pomegranate molasses

1 tsp caraway seeds

1 tsp cumin seeds

½ tsp chilli flakes or milder Aleppo chilli flakes

juice of 1 lemon

extra-virgin olive oil

large handful of flat-leaf parsley, coriander (cilantro)
   or a mixture of both, chopped

250 g/9 oz Greek-style yogurt

Preheat the oven to 200°C/400°F/Gas mark 6.

Toss the carrots and parsnips in a large roasting pan with 2 tablespoons of the olive oil and a little salt. If the pan is large enough, use a small corner for the beetroot and toss that in the remaining oil; otherwise you will require a separate pan. Try not to toss the beetroot with the other vegetables at any stage, otherwise your entire dish will turn a rather unappetizing, lurid pink.

Roast the vegetables for about 15 minutes, then add the chickpeas. Turn the vegetables carefully and roll the chickpeas around to pick up any oil in the pan.

Roast for a further 10 minutes, then tip over the molasses and scatter with the spices. Turn the vegetables in the sticky syrup and roast for a further 5–10 minutes, until just tender, but not soft, and starting to brown. Season well with salt, a bit more chilli or pepper, some lemon juice and a dash of extra-virgin olive oil.

Pile the vegetables on a large platter and scatter with the herbs. Serve hot or warm, with a bowl of yogurt to spoon out at the table.

HOW ABOUT?

... adding pumpkin, sweet potato or celeriac to the mix.

... piling the roots and chickpeas on top of some cooked wheat berries, barley or spelt (see p.18) for a really nutritious hearty meal.

... serving this as a side dish with lamb or chicken.

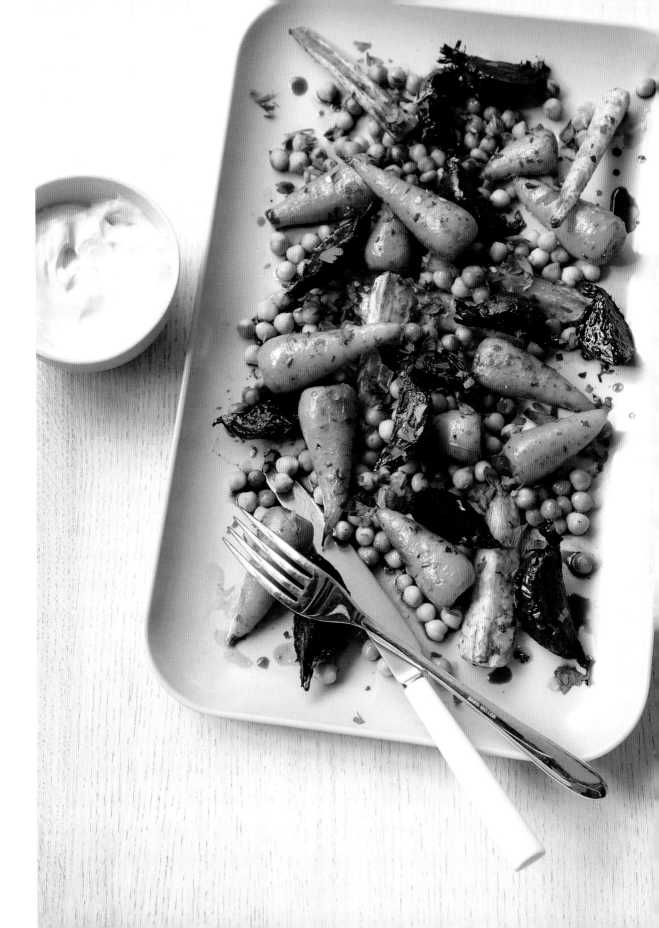

There are many traditional Italian pasta and chickpea combinations – this isn't one of them! I gleaned the idea from a cookbook by Denis Cotter (of the acclaimed vegetarian Cafe Paradiso in Cork) on a recent trip to Ireland. I adore the simplicity and freshness of this dish, especially teamed with a fabulous pasta like the long, ripple-edged ribbons of *mafalda*, but any good-quality long pasta will work well.

PASTA WITH CHICKPEAS AND LEMON

Serves 4

500 g/1 lb 2 oz *mafalda* or other long, dried pasta

salt

5 tbsp extra-virgin olive oil

2 garlic cloves, halved

250 g/9 oz home-cooked chickpeas (garbanzo beans)
    or 1 x 400 g/14 oz can of chickpeas

grated zest of 2 unwaxed lemons

juice of 1 lemon

large bunch of flat-leaf parsley, very roughly chopped

salt and pepper

100 g/3½ oz Parmesan cheese, grated

Cook the pasta in a really big pot of well-salted boiling water until *al dente*. Check the cooking time on the packet and begin tasting about 2 minutes before the time is up. Overcooked pasta is inexcusable, especially when the sauce is so simple to put together.

Meanwhile, pour the olive oil into a saucepan and add the garlic, chickpeas, lemon zest and juice, parsley and some salt and cracked black pepper. Heat the oil very gently for a couple of minutes and then set aside and leave to infuse. Search out and remove the garlic (you could add crushed garlic and leave it in if you're a garlic fiend).

Drain the pasta, reserving a few tablespoons of the cooking water. Toss the pasta and sauce together, adding about half of the Parmesan. Taste and add more salt, pepper, lemon juice or extra-virgin olive oil until beautifully balanced. If the ~~pasta~~ sauce seems too dry, you may want to add some of the reserved pasta water or chickpea cooking water.

Serve at once, with Parmesan and extra-virgin olive oil on the table.

HOW ABOUT?

… zipping this up with some chilli flakes, adding a few halved cherry tomatoes and substituting aged pecorino for the Parmesan.

… adding 3 tablespoons of double cream, a large handful of baby spinach and a few thyme leaves to the sauce.

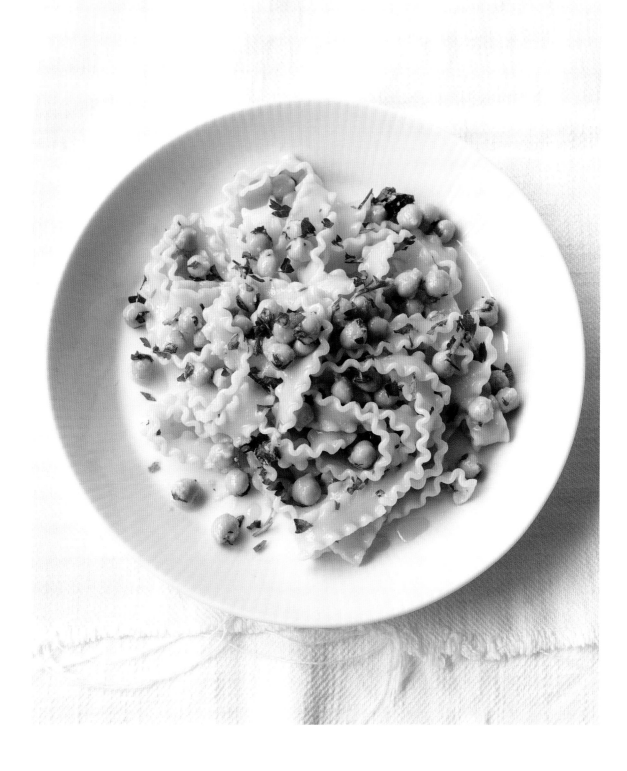

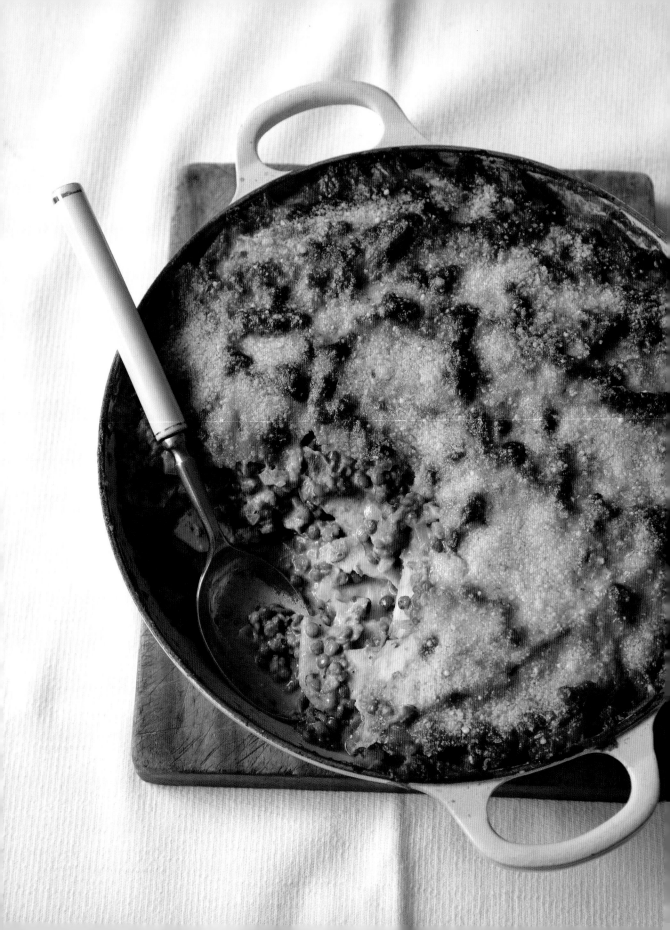

I've been cooking this recipe for years, but I can't remember where it came from, so thank you to whoever dreamt it up, it's inspired. The nutty celeriac has a wonderful texture and the creamy tomato sauce lends the lentils a touch of luxury. Serve with a big green salad and some really good bread.

CELERIAC AND LENTIL GRATIN

Serves 4–6

2 tbsp olive oil

1 onion, finely diced

4 garlic cloves, crushed

2 x 400 g/14 oz cans of chopped tomatoes

300 g/10½ oz/1½ cups Castelluccio lentils, rinsed

salt and pepper

large handful of parsley, roughly chopped

225 ml/8 fl oz double (heavy) cream

1 celeriac, about 1 kg/2¼ lb, peeled, quartered and finely sliced

zest and juice of ½ lemon

100 g/3½ oz Parmesan cheese, grated

Preheat the oven to 190°C/375°F/Gas mark 5.

Heat the oil in a large saucepan and cook the onion gently until soft and beginning to turn golden. Add the garlic and stir until its wonderful smell wafts up from the pan. Tip in the tomatoes and simmer for about 10 minutes.

Meanwhile, put the lentils in a pan, cover with about 5 cm/2 in of water and simmer for about 20 minutes, until just soft and creamy rather than *al dente*. Drain if necessary, and then season well with salt and pepper. Stir in the parsley and 3 tablespoons of the cream.

Add the celeriac to the tomato sauce, cover and cook for about 15 minutes or until tender. At first, there will not appear to be enough tomato sauce, but the celeriac will release plenty of moisture as it cooks. When the celeriac is tender, add the remaining cream, the lemon zest and juice, and season with salt and plenty of black pepper to taste.

Layer the celeriac and tomato mixture alternately with the lentils in a large, shallow ovenproof dish, finishing with a layer of celeriac. Sprinkle with the grated Parmesan and bake for about 30 minutes, until nicely browned on the top.

This can be prepared ahead and even frozen. Thaw before baking for an extra 10–15 minutes, covering with foil if the top begins to get too dark.

HOW ABOUT?

... using any whole brown or green lentil for the dish. Not red lentils though, as they will collapse into a mush.

So here it is in all its splendour, the quintessential veggie recipe. Just like the bean burgers, lentil rissoles and three-bean salads of old, some pretty dubious variations of this loaf have been churned out over the decades. This is the version to silence all the doubters out there. It comes from the *Avoca Café Cookbook*.

The Irish company Avoca is nowadays as well known for its award-winning cafés as for the stunning handwoven rugs and throws that originally made it famous. This nut loaf has been on the menu since the word go and apparently there's public outcry every time they threaten to drop it. You'll understand why.

The loaf will keep for up to 5 days in the fridge; ideal for a buffet spread or for healthy suppers, picnics and packed lunches.

LENTIL AND NUT LOAF

Serves 8–10

50 g/1¾ oz/5 tbsp Puy lentils, rinsed

300 g/10½ oz/1½ cups red lentils, rinsed

50 g/1¾ oz/4 tbsp unsalted butter

1 large onion, diced

3 carrots, diced

1 large red pepper, diced

3 celery stalks, diced

½–1 fresh red or green chilli (see p.248), deseeded and finely diced

2 heaped tsp ground cumin

75 g/2¾ oz fresh breadcrumbs

150 g/5½ oz Cheddar cheese, grated

75 g/2¾ oz roasted nuts, such as pistachios, hazelnuts or peanuts, chopped

6 eggs

salt and pepper

sunflower, pumpkin or other seeds for sprinkling (optional)

Preheat the oven to 160°C/325°F/Gas mark 3. Line the base and sides of a 900 g/2 lb loaf tin (or 2 smaller tins if you prefer) with greaseproof paper.

Put the lentils in a bowl, pour boiling water over them, and leave to soak for 20 minutes. (The original recipe says to cook them, but after a couple of decades of practice, the Avoca team are happy just to soak.)

Melt the butter in a large saucepan and throw in all the vegetables, the chilli and cumin. Cover the pan and cook gently for about 5 minutes, no longer or the vegetables will lose their colour.

Drain the lentils and place in a large bowl. Tip in the vegetables along with the breadcrumbs, cheese, nuts and eggs. Mix everything together thoroughly and then taste. Season well; this loaf is all about flavour. Spoon the mixture into the prepared tin(s) and sprinkle with seeds, if you like. Bake for 45–55 minutes, until firm (smaller loaves will be more like 40–45 minutes).

To serve hot, leave to stand for 5–10 minutes before slicing. Alternatively, turn out and leave to cool, then cut into slices to eat cold, or to warm up when you want them. Serve with a tasty chutney and salad.

Ful medames is not just the national dish of Egypt, it's hugely popular from Sudan right up through the Middle East to Syria. The beans are often eaten at breakfast time, particularly during the Ramadan fast, when a plate of *fuls* can just about keep you going until nightfall.

The favas, or *fuls* as they are known, vary from tiny plump beans the size of your little fingernail to much larger, flatter varieties. It just depends where you are: the Egyptians like a small bean while the Syrians favour the large. Whatever the size, make sure you cook them really well or they can seem a bit leathery. The recipe varies hugely through the region; garlic, lemon juice and oil are essential but then you may add cumin, tahini, parsley or coriander, a tomato or pepper sauce.

MIDDLE-EASTERN FAVA BEANS
FUL MEDAMES

Serves 4

500 g/ 1 lb 2 oz home-cooked whole fava beans
    or 3 x 400 g/14 oz cans of *ful* beans (cooked fava beans)
salt and pepper
2 garlic cloves, crushed
150 ml/5 fl oz/⅔ cup extra-virgin olive oil
juice of 1–2 lemons
1–2 tsp cumin seeds, roasted and ground
pitta bread to serve

GARNISHES – ANY OF THE FOLLOWING:

fresh tomatoes, diced
sliced spring onions (scallions) or, more traditionally,
    wedges of white onion
handful of rocket (arugula)
fresh coriander (cilantro) or parsley, roughly chopped
hard-boiled eggs
black olives
Aleppo or Urfa chilli flakes (see p.248)
tahini
extra-virgin olive oil

Heat the beans with plenty of seasoning. If using cans, just tip their liquid into the saucepan with them. If you've cooked your own beans, make sure that they are really tender and almost mushy.

Drain off some of the liquid, leaving behind just a few tablespoons with the beans. Stir in the garlic, olive oil, lemon juice and cumin to taste. Spoon into bowls and serve.

This simple combination makes a wonderfully sustaining dish scooped up with flatbread, but you can turn it into a feast with a selection of the garnishes set out in small bowls so that everyone can help themselves. Everyone loves to get stuck in, making up their own magical combination.

HOW ABOUT?

.. throwing a handful of red lentils in with the beans if you're cooking from scratch: they will thicken up the sauce.
... mashing up about a third of the beans once cooked to give the dish a creamy texture.
... adding a few chickpeas too, as they do in Lebanon.
... cooking a double quantity of favas and freezing some for your next brunch gathering.

Small, egg-shaped aubergines are often available in Indian grocers and are worth seeking out for this dish. They look beautiful, opened out like paper lanterns. If you can't get them, the larger common aubergine will taste just as good.

I fell in love with this dish at a restaurant in Kochi (formerly known as Cochin), the ancient hub of the Indian spice trade. I asked an extremely courteous waiter how the aubergines were cooked and was, to my surprise, immediately ushered into the hottest hell-fire of a kitchen that I have ever experienced. I emerged about 10 minutes later feeling, and quite possibly looking, as if I had been in the tandoor itself, but most importantly I had scrawled down the recipe.

KERALAN AUBERGINES WITH LENTILS, CASHEW AND TAMARIND

Serves 4

3 large or 8–12 baby, egg-shaped aubergines (eggplants)

1 tbsp vegetable oil, plus extra for brushing

2 onions, finely diced

5 garlic cloves, crushed

5-cm/2-in piece of fresh ginger, diced

2 tsp dried chilli flakes

100 g/3½ oz/½ cup red split lentils (masoor dal), rinsed

½ tsp cumin seeds, roasted and ground

salt

3 tbsp yogurt

3–4 tbsp tamarind paste (see p.247)

handful of coriander (cilantro) leaves

3 tbsp cashew nuts, roasted

ON THE TOP (OPTIONAL)

2 tbsp ghee or clarified butter

1 tbsp mustard seeds

4 dried chillies

Preheat the oven to 200°C/400°F/Gas mark 6. Prick the aubergines once or twice, brush with a little oil, and roast in the oven until they are soft (about 30 minutes for regular aubergines, 15 minutes for the egg-sized ones). Cool for a few minutes.

Meanwhile, heat the vegetable oil in a large frying pan and cook the onions until translucent. Add the garlic, ginger and chilli flakes and, once you are enveloped by the wafts of garlic, tip in the lentils and enough water to cover by 5 cm/2 in. Simmer the lentils for about 20 minutes, until they are soft and creamy, topping up the water if necessary. Stir in the cumin and season with salt to taste.

Cut large aubergines lengthwise into quarters. For egg-shaped aubergines, hold them by their stalks and make vertical slashes at regular intervals, leaving the base and top intact. Push down on the stalk, and the skin will open up like a Chinese lantern. Add the aubergines to the lentils, pushing them down halfway so that they're not totally engulfed. You can prepare the dish to this stage and reheat later.

Dollop over the yogurt and tamarind. Don't stir it in, the idea is to get bursts of different flavours. Sprinkle with coriander and cashews. The topping is optional but it really is the icing on the cake. Just before serving, melt the ghee, and heat the mustard seeds and chillies until they sizzle and pop. Tip over the aubergines and eat at once with Indian flatbreads or rice.

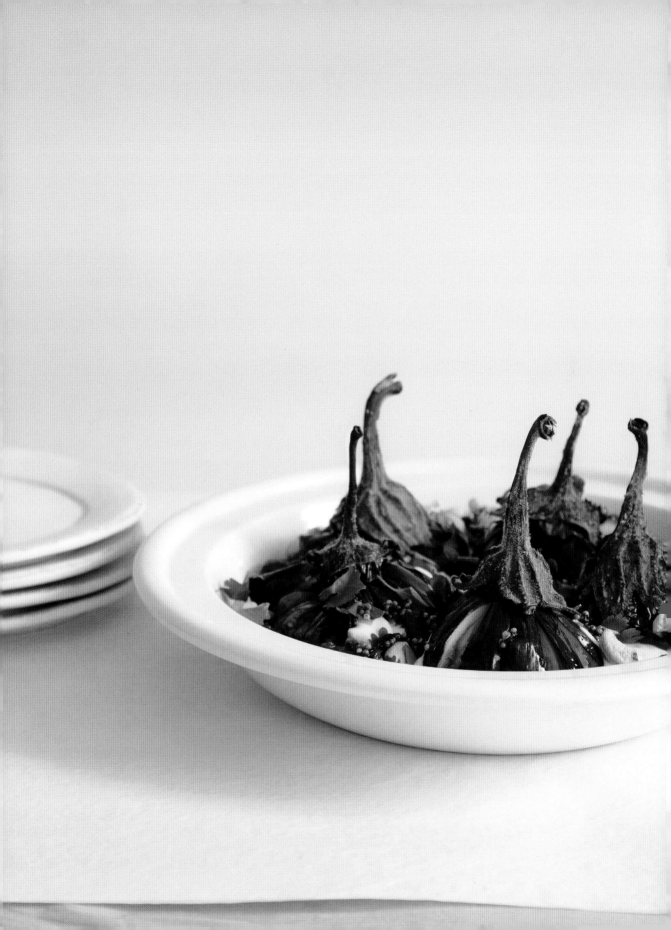

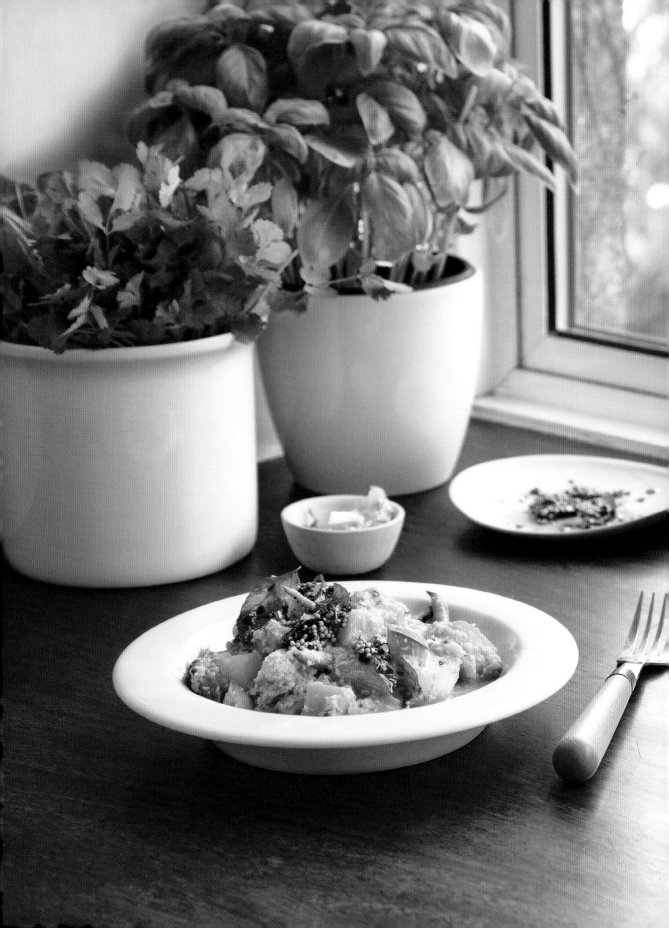

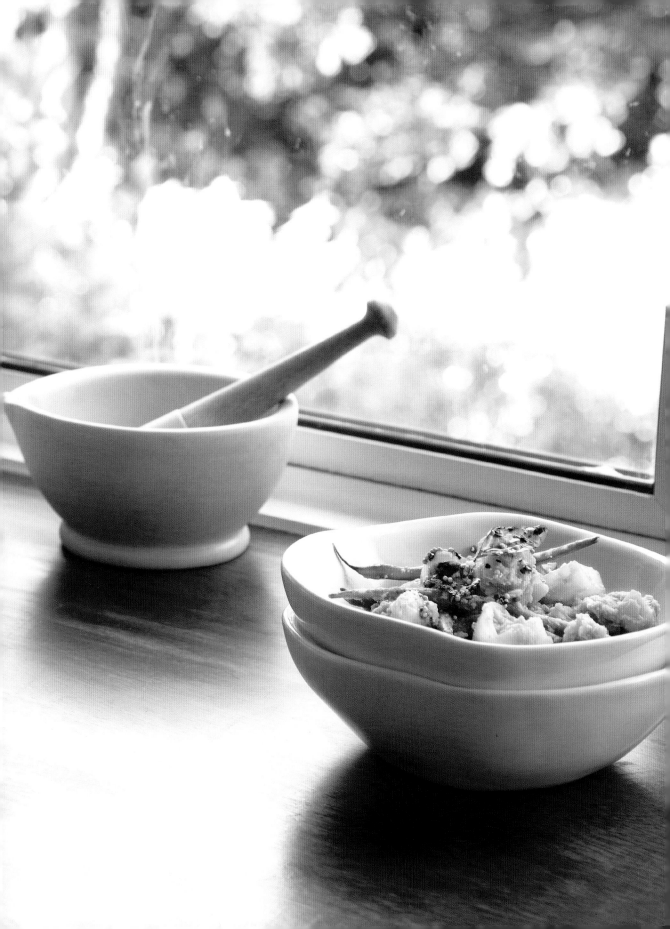

Sambar is a southern Indian staple. It's essentially a dal cooked with whatever vegetables are in season. You might be able to track down exotica such as snake beans, okra, bottle gourd or white radish, but more readily available potato, tomato, pumpkin and aubergine are authentic too.

Traditional sambar has a loose, almost soup-like consistency and is served alongside rice, dosa or flatbreads. I like to make mine a little thicker. Toor/toovar dal (split pigeon peas) are the pulse of choice, but you could use any of the split lentils, peas or beans for an unorthodox but tasty result. *Illustrated on pp.184–185.*

SOUTHERN INDIAN VEGETABLES WITH DAL
SAMBAR

Serves 4

100 g/3½ oz toor dal (or other split lentils), rinsed

1 tsp ground turmeric

2 onions, each cut into 8 wedges

small potatoes, cubed

2 tomatoes, quartered

1 aubergine (eggplant), diced

100 g/3½ oz pumpkin, diced

handful of green beans, topped but not tailed

3–4 tbsp tamarind paste (see p.247)

salt

FOR THE SPICE PASTE

1 tbsp vegetable oil

3 shallots, diced

100 g/3½ oz freshly grated or desiccated coconut
(unsweetened please!)

2 tsp coriander seeds

1 tsp cumin seeds

2 dried chillies

FOR THE TARKA

1 tbsp ghee or vegetable oil

1 tsp black mustard seeds

10–15 fresh or frozen curry leaves

1 tsp dried chilli flakes

Put the lentils in a large pan with the turmeric and cover with 600 ml/1 pint of water. Simmer, covered, for about 45 minutes or until the lentils are soft. Add the onions, potatoes, tomatoes, aubergine and pumpkin, and cook until tender.

Meanwhile, make the spice paste. Heat the oil in a small frying pan and cook the shallots until soft. Add the coconut, coriander, cumin and chillies. As soon as the mixture is aromatic and golden, remove it from the heat. Grind to a fine paste using a pestle and mortar, a spice grinder or small food processor.

Stir the green beans, tamarind and spice paste into the lentils, and cook until the beans are tender. Add more water if you like the traditional, soupier consistency.

Using the frying pan (no need to wash it), make the tarka, or tempering. Heat the ghee and cook the mustard seeds until they begin to splutter, then add the curry leaves and chilli, stir once and then tip over the sambar.

These chickpeas predate the partitioning of India by hundreds of years and they are traditional on both sides of the Punjab region that straddles the Indian/ Pakistani border. Great with flatbreads, rice, as a side dish, with yogurt, chutney. The curry improves over a couple of days, too.

I've given a recipe for garam masala (see p.247) that I'd love you to use, but let's not get too sniffy about shop-bought masalas. If you only use spices once in a while, then a jar of ready-mixed masala makes more sense than a dozen pots of stale spice. I recently discovered an ingenious product from Bart Spices with the whole masala spices packed together in their own little spice mill. If you want to be truly authentic, you could track down a chana masala spice mix to use instead of the garam masala.

PUNJABI CHICKPEA CURRY
CHANA MASALA

Serves 4

3 tbsp vegetable oil

2 tsp cumin seeds

2 onions, diced

4 garlic cloves, crushed

2.5-cm/1-inch piece of fresh ginger, finely diced or grated

2–3 green chillies, slit lengthwise, or deseeded and diced if feeling a little cautious (see p.248)

½–1 tsp chilli powder

1 tsp ground turmeric

1 tsp ground coriander

400 g/14 oz can of chopped tomatoes (or about 6 tomatoes, peeled, deseeded and chopped)

500 g/1 lb 2 oz home-cooked chickpeas (garbanzo beans) or 2 x 400 g/14 oz cans of chickpeas, drained

1 tsp garam masala

handful of fresh coriander (cilantro), chopped roughly

½–1 tbsp *amchur* (sour green mango powder) or juice of ½–1 lemon

salt

4 tbsp Greek-style yogurt, to serve

Heat the oil in a large pan, add the cumin seeds and cook over a medium heat until you are hit by their fabulous smell. Throw in the onions and cook until soft.

Add the garlic, ginger, chillies, chilli powder, turmeric and ground coriander. Stir over a medium heat, taking care not to burn the garlic.

Tip in the tomatoes, chickpeas and just enough water to give a loose sauce. Simmer for about 10 minutes, then add the garam masala and the fresh coriander. Taste and add the *amchur* or lemon juice, salt and perhaps a little more chilli to balance the flavours. Ideally, I like to leave this for a couple of hours before eating, allowing the flavours to develop.

Serve with a dollop of yogurt and some rice or flatbread. Do warn everyone to look out for the whole green chillies, if using, they can and have been mistaken for a green bean!

HOW ABOUT?

... adding some tea. If you are cooking your own chickpeas, some traditionalists like to darken them by adding tea leaves, tied in a muslin pouch, when they boil them; Darjeeling seems to be the number one choice. I even came across a recipe with a tea bag thrown in.

... throwing 2 diced aubergines into the pan before you add the cumin, and cooking until soft. You may need to add a little more oil, but don't overdo it. Raw aubergines soak up masses of oil but release it back into the pan once they soften and collapse.

Sprouting beans for cooking has been a revelation to me (see pp.20–21). Yes, you do have to be quite organized, but the nutty texture and taste of these beans is just fabulous. Moth beans are extraordinary: soak overnight and sprout for one day and these little powerhouses are ready to go. If you have trouble tracking down moth (matki) beans, then you could use sprouted mung beans or adzuki instead, although they will take a little longer to sprout. Begin 36 hours in advance or buy your sprouted beans. They're increasingly available in shops and supermarkets.

Matki usal is a staple on the streets of Mumbai and all over the Indian state of Maharashtra. The stir-fried beans make a cheap, nutritious and very tasty breakfast, snack or light lunch; they're often crammed into a '*pav*', a type of soft white bread roll, like a burger bun. I love to eat this with rice, chapatis, stuffed inside a pitta bread or as a side dish with a curry. Throw in a bit of chutney, pickle or raita (see p.246) and you have a real treat.

INDIAN STIR-FRIED SPROUTED BEANS
MATKI USAL

Serves 4

200 g/7 oz dried moth beans, soaked and sprouted (or sprouted adzuki or mung beans)

2–3 tbsp vegetable oil

handful of raw peanuts

1 tsp cumin seeds

1 tsp black mustard seeds

10 curry leaves

1 onion, diced

2.5-cm/1-inch piece of fresh ginger, finely chopped

2 garlic cloves, crushed

1 tsp garam masala, bought or home-blend (see p.247)

½ tsp chilli powder

1 tsp salt

1–2 tsp light brown sugar or jaggery

handful of fresh coriander (cilantro), chopped

1 lime, quartered

Rinse the sprouted beans and put them in a pan, cover them with plenty of cold water and boil for about 10 minutes, until tender.

Meanwhile, heat the oil in a karahi, wok or frying pan, and cook the peanuts for a couple of minutes, until golden and toasted. Scoop out the nuts and set aside.

In the same oil, heat the cumin and mustard seeds until they begin to hop about. Add the curry leaves and onion. Cook until the onion is soft and turning golden.

Now add the ginger, garlic, garam masala, chilli powder and salt. As soon as you smell the amazing spicy aromas, you can throw in the drained beans. Stir to coat in the spices and then add a slosh of water to prevent them from catching on the bottom of the pan. The amount of liquid is up to you. Some usal is quite wet, with a bit of soupy sauce to mop up, or you may prefer to leave it a little drier, as I do. Cook over a high heat for a couple of minutes, taste and then season with sugar (or jaggery) and salt.

Sprinkle with the peanuts and coriander and serve with a wedge of lime.

HOW ABOUT?

... replacing the garam masala with the more authentic Maharashtrian *goda masala* (there are plenty of versions available online).

... using slices of roasted coconut (available from health food shops) instead of the peanuts.

... adding 4 peeled and diced tomatoes at the same time as the garlic.

... stirring in some baby spinach leaves for the last few minutes of cooking.

Winter bean casseroles can sometimes seem rather worthy and stodgy. This Iranian/Afghani combination loaded with ginger, chilli and lime juice is anything but. It comes from Sally Butcher's magical book *Veggiestan*, an incredible collection of Middle Eastern vegetarian recipes, anecdotes, history and folklore.

We tend to associate mung beans with East Asian cooking, but they are widely used in the Middle East and India too.

MUNG BEAN CASSEROLE

Serves 6

1 tbsp ghee or vegetable oil

1 tsp fenugreek seeds

1 tsp cumin seeds

3 garlic cloves, crushed

2-cm/¾-inch piece of fresh ginger, finely chopped

1 Scotch bonnet or 4 green chillies

1 large onion, diced

2 red, yellow or green peppers, diced

2 potatoes, cut into 2–3-cm/1-inch cubes

1 tsp ground turmeric

350 g/12 oz/1½ cups dried mung beans

1 litre/1¾ pints/4 cups water or vegetable stock

500 g/1 lb 2 oz fresh spinach, roughly chopped

3 tomatoes, chopped into chunks

juice of 2 limes

salt

handful of fresh coriander (cilantro), chopped

onion wedges, to serve

Heat the ghee or oil in a large, heavy pan, add the fenugreek and cumin, and cook for a minute before adding the garlic, ginger, chilli, onion and peppers.

Once the onion is soft and translucent, throw in the potatoes and turmeric. Stir for a couple of minutes, then stir in the mung beans and the liquid. Bring to the boil and then simmer for about 45 minutes, or until the beans are tender.

Add the spinach and tomatoes, and let everything bubble away for another 10 minutes.

Squeeze in the lime juice, taste and season. Serve with a sprinkling of coriander and an onion wedge on the side. (The onion wedge is a typical Middle Eastern accompaniment, which is said to aid digestion.)

HOW ABOUT?

... adding other vegetables, such as carrots or pumpkin, along with the potatoes.

... should you require a truly fortifying feast, serve with rice.

Risotto should feature in any good cook's repertoire. Gone are the days when we were happy to throw yesterday's leftovers into the pot with some long-grain rice and call the resulting sludge a risotto.

The key is a good risotto rice (Carnaroli would be my preference), well-flavoured stock (I would usually plump for chicken stock but the pea pods do wonders here) and plenty of Parmesan cheese. A little patient stirring delivers a creamy base with an *al dente* bite that becomes a fabulous backdrop for whatever the allotment, veg box or grocer has to offer. Here it's summery green peas and beans, plenty of them, to give the risotto a light, fresh finish. You could use frozen beans, but fresh peas, please, as the pods give masses of flavour.

Usually eaten as a *primo piatto*, or first course, in Italy, risotto's more likely to appear as a main in my home.

FRESH PEA AND BROAD BEAN RISOTTO
RISOTTO CON PISELLI E BACCELLI

Serves 4–6

2 litres/3½ pints/2 quarts vegetable stock
1 kg/2¼ lb fresh peas in the pod, podded and pods set aside
salt and pepper
300 g/10½ oz frozen or fresh podded broad (fava) beans
150 g/5½ oz/generous ½ cup unsalted butter
2 onions, finely diced

300 g/10½ oz/1½ cups risotto rice (preferably Carnaroli)
150 ml/5 fl oz/⅔ cup dry white wine
large handful of flat-leaf parsley, chopped
small handful of basil, ripped
100 g/3½ oz Parmesan cheese, grated

Bring the stock to the boil and add the pea pods and a pinch of salt. Simmer for about 15 minutes, then strain the stock or lift the pods out with a slotted spoon. For an even more intense pea flavour, you can purée the pods with some of the stock and then push the mush through a sieve to add to the risotto with the peas later. (If you have a mouli for legumes then here is the time to use it.)

Place the stock over a medium heat to keep hot.

Blanch or steam the peas and broad beans for 4–5 minutes, until tender, drain and set aside. Slip at least half of the broad beans out of their skins if you have the time.

Heat about half of the butter in a large, heavy-bottomed pan and cook the onions gently until soft but not coloured.

Stir in the rice and coat with all the buttery juices for a couple of minutes.

Tip in the wine and then add a ladleful of hot stock, stirring continuously (a square-ended wooden spoon will prevent sticking). When the stock is absorbed, add more stock, a ladleful at a time.

HOW ABOUT?

... throwing in some asparagus too (any tough stalks will enhance the stock).
... adding a beaten egg to any leftovers and shallow-frying them in a cake the next day. Individual cakes served with an Italian-style tomato salsa (see p.244) and a few salad leaves make an elegant starter.
... stirring in some baby spinach leaves or rocket to wilt at the last moment

After 15–20 minutes, the rice will be cooked but still have a little firm centre; you'll need to sample a grain or two. You may not need all the stock, or you may need to add a little more hot water from the kettle. The risotto should be quite fluid, as it will continue to cook and set as you serve it.

Stir in the remaining butter, the peas, pea mush (if you have some), beans, herbs and half of the Parmesan. Taste and season with salt and freshly ground black pepper. Serve immediately, with the remaining Parmesan alongside.

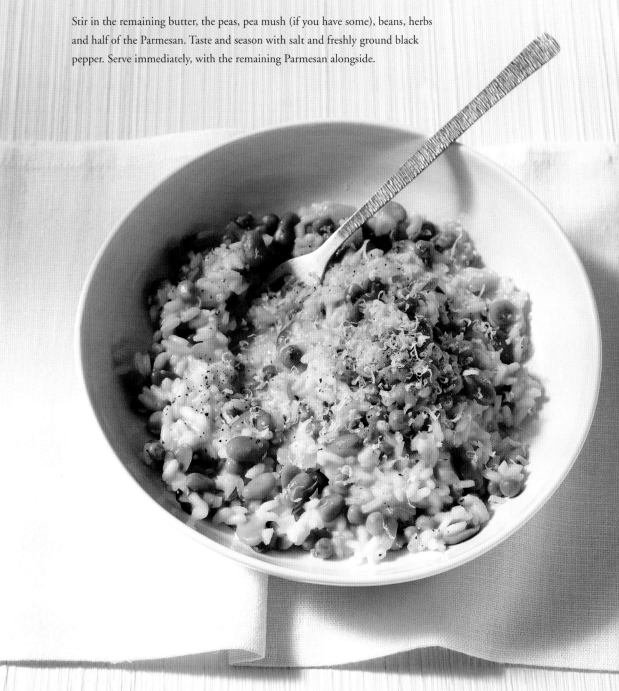

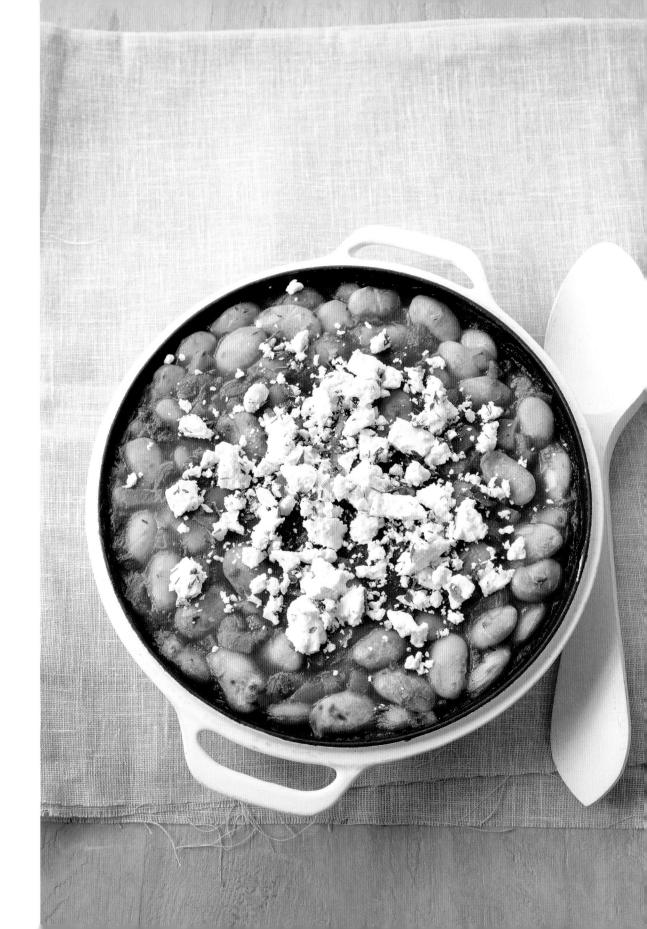

Try seeking out the signature supersize Greek *gigantes* beans for this if you have a local Greek grocer's or an especially well-stocked deli, or try online. If you can't find the traditional 'elephant' beans, then any butter beans are wonderful.

The beans make a great main course topped with feta cheese and served with crusty bread and a green salad. *Gigantes plaki* (literally 'baked giants') are also sometimes served alongside fish or meat.

GREEK BAKED BUTTER BEANS WITH FETA
GIGANTES PLAKI

Serves 6

3 tbsp olive oil

1 large onion, roughly diced

2 carrots, diced

2 large celery stalks, diced

3 garlic cloves, crushed

400 g/14 oz can of chopped tomatoes

2 tbsp tomato purée

3 bay leaves

½ tsp dried chilli flakes

salt

½ tsp dried oregano

large bunch of parsley, roughly chopped

3 sprigs of dill, stems removed, roughly chopped

½ tbsp brown sugar or honey

1 tbsp red wine vinegar

1 kg/2¼ lb home-cooked *gigantes* or large butter beans (lima beans) or 4 x 400 g/14 oz cans of butter beans

200 g/7 oz feta cheese

Preheat the oven to 180°C/350°F/Gas mark 4.

Heat the oil in a large pan and cook the onion, carrots and celery gently until they soften and begin to colour.

Add the garlic, stir until fragrant, then tip in the tomatoes, tomato purée, bay leaves and pepper flakes. Season with a good pinch of salt, add the oregano, most of the parsley and dill, and bubble away for about 10 minutes.

Taste, keeping in mind that you are will be adding a large quantity of beans that require plenty of acidity and savoury seasoning. Balance the sauce, adding a little sugar and vinegar.

Add the beans. Now all the soakers and simmerers among you can feel rather smug as you can add enough of the nutrient-rich bean cooking water to just cover the beans. Otherwise use tap water. Tip the beans into a wide, ovenproof dish – I use a Spanish terracotta *cazuela* – and place in the oven for about 1 hour.

After 30 minutes, check that the beans still have plenty of liquid around them; the juices will have thickened, but you don't want the beans to dry out. The top needs to become a bit crispy and crunchy while the beans wallow in delicious juices.

Crumble the feta into a bowl and tumble it around with the remaining parsley and dill. Sprinkle the cheese over the beans and serve hot or warm.

HOW ABOUT?

... adding some smoked lardons or pancetta when you cook the onion, for an extra layer of flavour.

I can't get enough of San Francisco-based Heidi Swanson's recipes; her blog *101 Cookbooks* is truly inspiring. While Heidi is a vegetarian crusader for natural wholefoods, her food never seems remotely 'worthy'. This dish evolved out of the White Beans and Cabbage recipe from her book *Super Natural Every Day*.

FLAGEOLETS WITH KALE AND CRISPED POTATOES

Serves 4

3 tbsp olive oil

1 large potato, cut into 2-cm/¾-inch dice

salt and pepper

1 small red onion, finely sliced

250 g/9 oz home-cooked flageolets or 1 x 400 g/14 oz can of flageolet beans

2 garlic cloves, finely chopped

200 g/7 oz kale, well washed, tough stalks removed, sliced into ribbons

juice of ½ –1 lemon

5 tbsp grated Parmesan cheese

Heat the olive oil in a large frying pan (with a lid) over a medium-high heat. Toss in the potato dice and a pinch of salt. Cover the pan and cook for a few minutes, then carefully turn the potatoes. Continue until the potatoes are golden, crisp and cooked through.

Add the onion and beans to the pan, and carry on cooking, with the lid off. Leave the beans to brown and catch a little on the bottom of the pan. You will want to stir – don't!

After a couple of minutes, when the onion has softened and the beans have a few golden, crusty flecks, stir in the garlic and the kale. Reduce the heat slightly and cover the pan.

The kale will take about 3 minutes to wilt, and then you are ready to taste and season. Add salt and plenty of coarsely ground black pepper, lemon juice and a good sprinkling of Parmesan, and serve.

HOW ABOUT?

... kale out of season? Try Heidi's suggestion of white cabbage, or perhaps shredded spring greens or Brussels sprouts.

... removing the casing from 3 good pork sausages and crumbling the meat into the pan along with the potatoes.

... using cannellini, haricots (navy beans) or butter beans (lima beans).

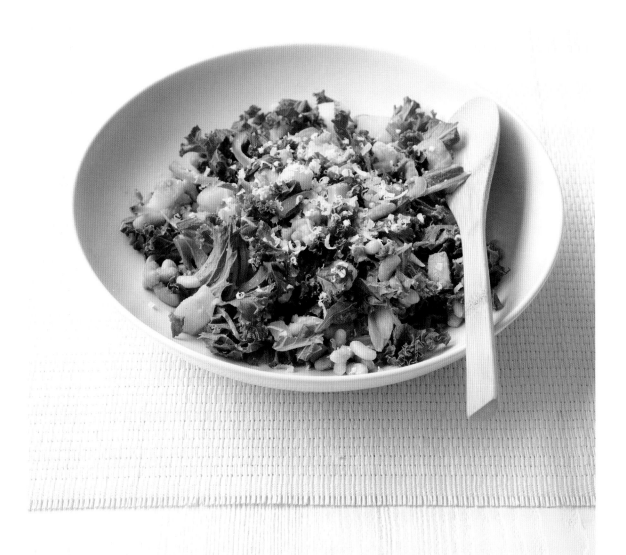

This is not so much a recipe as an amalgamation of recipes found elsewhere in this book. But I didn't want you to miss out – burritos are one of my favourite things to nosh into at lunchtime. They're simple to make at home, too.

BLACK BEAN BURRITOS

Serves 4

½ x *frijoles borrachos* (see p.162) or 1 x refried beans (see p.162)

4 wheat tortillas or wraps

guacamole (see p.243)

4 tbsp sour cream or crème fraîche

100 g/3½ oz Wensleydale or Cheddar cheese, grated

½ iceberg lettuce, finely shredded

EXTRAS

sliced jalapeño peppers, straight from the jar,

　　or finely diced chilli peppers, a dash of Tabasco sauce, salsa (see p.242)

　　or some smoky chipotle relish/chipotles in adobo

rare-cooked steak, sliced into ribbons,

　　or shredded chicken/turkey left over from the Sunday roast

a couple of tablespoons of cooked rice (brown if possible)

a sprinkling of grated dark chocolate

Warm the beans in a pan or microwave oven, and heat a heavy frying pan or, better still, a ridged griddle pan.

Place the tortillas in the pan one at a time to soften, warm through, and ideally get some attractive charring. You need only cook them on one side. Pile the tortillas up, wrapped in a tea towel to keep warm, until you are ready to fill your burritos.

Lay the tortillas, one at a time, on the work surface and imagine each one as a globe. If you are using *frijoles borrachos*, strain off any excess liquid, using a slotted spoon. Spoon a good helping of beans just below the equator, leaving a 5-cm/2-inch margin along the east and west edges. Add a couple of tablespoons of guacamole and a tablespoon of sour cream and then sprinkle with grated cheese and lettuce. Throw any extras in too.

Fold in the naked eastern and western margins of your tortilla, to cover the edges of the filling. Now take the south pole and fold it up to just cover the filling and roll the whole thing up towards the north pole. Turn the tortilla over and you should have something a little more rectangular-envelope than carpet-roll in shape. Dive in.

HOW ABOUT?

... having a DIY production line so that people can pile in their own favourite ingredients.

... using any leftover chilli (see pp.225, 230, 231 and opposite). Be sure not to flood the tortilla – use a slotted spoon to drain off any excess moisture.

... rolling up some simple bean burritos as above with just the sour cream (no guacamole, cheese or lettuce) and placing them in an ovenproof bowl. Add a spicy tomato sauce (see below) and tip it over the burritos. Sprinkle with cheese and more sour cream and bake in a hot oven (200°C/400°F/Gas mark 6) for 30 minutes – you've just made enchiladas!

... for a tomato sauce, you can use the chickpea and tomato sauce on p.208, omitting the chickpeas and adding oregano in the place of the cinnamon.

Bulgur wheat is an inspired addition to a meat-free chilli, giving fabulous texture while combining with the beans to create a complete protein. The idea comes from Mollie Katzen, the American doyenne of vegetarian food writing, whose *Moosewood Cookbook* has sold millions of copies.

The bean mix is up to you. If you are cooking from scratch, you probably won't get around to preparing three types, but you need about 800 g/1 lb 12 oz of cooked beans in total.

There's no point in making a small pot of chilli, it tastes even better after a couple of days in the fridge or you could freeze any leftovers.

THREE-BEAN CHILLI WITH BULGUR

Serves 6–8

6 tbsp olive oil

2 aubergines (eggplants), cut into large dice

2 onions, diced

4 garlic cloves, crushed

2.5-cm/1-inch piece of fresh ginger, finely diced

1 tbsp cumin seeds, roasted and ground (or ground cumin)

1–2 tbsp chilli powder

450 g/1 lb squash or pumpkin, peeled, deseeded and cut into large dice

2 x 400 g/14 oz cans of chopped tomatoes

300 ml/10 fl oz/1¼ cups vegetable stock or water

50 g/1¾ oz bulgur wheat

400 g/14 oz can of black turtle beans

400 g/14 oz can of red kidney beans

400 g/14 oz can of pinto beans

salt

Tabasco sauce or chopped fresh chill (optional)

juice of 1 lime

2 tbsp chopped fresh coriander (cilantro)

Heat 2 tablespoons of the oil in a large cast-iron casserole or heavy-bottomed saucepan, and cook half of the aubergine until really soft and translucent. Set aside and cook the remaining aubergine in the same way. Set aside.

Add the remaining 2 tablespoons of oil to the pan and cook the onions until golden.

Throw in the garlic, ginger, cumin and as much chilli as you dare, keeping in mind that heat is the very essence of this dish. Stir for a couple of minutes over the heat – the chilli will probably leave you gasping for breath – and then add the pumpkin and the cooked aubergine. Once the vegetables are well coated in the spicy juices, add the tomatoes and stock and then simmer for about 15 minutes.

Add the bulgur and the beans and leave to bubble away for about 10 minutes, until the wheat has plumped up and become tender. Taste and season with salt and more chilli (I'd opt for Tabasco or fresh chillies at this stage), if you were too cautious earlier on.

Add the lime juice and coriander just before serving.

HOW ABOUT?

... serving with warmed corn tortillas, sour cream and guacamole (see p.243).

... feeding a crowd with baked potatoes and grated Wensleydale or other mild cheese.

... adding some freshly steamed vegetables such as courgettes, green beans, broccoli or kale just before serving. (If you cook them with the beans, you will have a soggy mess when reheating leftovers.)

If you're a tempeh virgin, then let this be your first tantalizingly tasty experience. I love to serve this simply, with steamed greens and a few fine slices of red chilli thrown in. If you're feeling hungry, cook up a bit of rice, too.

The recipe is well travelled. It comes from the thoroughly inspiring Australian chef and food writer Jude Blereau's book *Coming Home to Eat... Wholefood for the Family*. I originally came across Jude, and the recipe, on *101 Cookbooks*, San Francisco-based Heidi Swanson's blog.

ORANGE PAN-GLAZED TEMPEH

Serves 4

1 tbsp grated fresh ginger

250 ml/9 fl oz/1 cup fresh orange juice

2 tsp tamari soy sauce

1½ tbsp mirin

2 tsp maple syrup

½ tsp ground coriander

2 garlic cloves, crushed

300 g/10½ oz tempeh

2 tbsp extra-virgin olive oil or, better still, unrefined coconut oil

large handful of coriander (cilantro) leaves

juice of ½ lime

Squeeze the juice from the grated ginger into a bowl. I find it easiest to pile up the ginger in the middle of a small square of muslin, gather up the edges and then twist the cloth into a tight ball until the juice runs out. Discard the pulp.

Add the orange juice to the bowl along with the tamari, mirin, maple syrup, ground coriander and garlic. Stir everything together and then set aside.

Chop up the tempeh into thin-ish, bite-sized slithers, triangles, fingers or whatever shape takes your fancy.

Heat the oil in a large frying pan until hot, but not smoking, and cook the tempeh for about 5 minutes on each side until golden.

Pour in the orange juice mixture and simmer for 10 minutes, until the sauce has reduced to a thick glaze. Turn the tempeh once as you simmer and spoon over the sauce from time to time.

Serve the tempeh drizzled with the sauce. Sprinkle with coriander leaves and a good squeeze of lime juice.

HOW ABOUT?

... serving with steamed or stir-fried tender-stem broccoli or any mixture of seasonal greens.

... replacing the tempeh with firm tofu. Pat the tofu dry with kitchen paper before you fry.

Most stir-fry recipes call for the tofu to be pre-fried, which stops the bean curd from breaking up. I think that marinating the tofu first is equally important to boost the flavour.

Here's an opportunity to pile up loads of fresh greens and enjoy a truly cleansing meal. I crave this type of food after the excesses of Christmas or whenever I'm feeling a bit fat and flat.

MY ULTIMATE TOFU STIR-FRY

Serves 4, with rice or noodles

FOR THE MARINATED TOFU

6 tbsp light soy sauce or tamari soy sauce

2 tbsp mirin, rice vinegar or, at a pinch,
    dry sherry

2 tsp sesame oil

2 garlic cloves, crushed

2.5-cm/1-inch piece of fresh ginger, grated

250 g/9 oz firm tofu, drained and cut
    into 2.5-cm/1-inch cubes

FOR THE STIR-FRY

4 tbsp sunflower, groundnut or rapeseed oil

5 spring onions (scallions), sliced finely

2 garlic cloves, chopped

2.5-cm/1-inch piece of fresh ginger, finely diced

2–3 green or red chillies (see p.248),
    very finely chopped

300 g/10½ oz firm green vegetables such as
    green beans, mangetout, snow peas, asparagus, broccoli
    or purple sprouting, chopped into bite-sized pieces

200 g/7 oz leafy greens, ideally pak choi (bok choy), but
    Swiss chard or spinach will work too, chopped if large
    and any tender stalks chopped and set aside

juice of 1 lime

2 tbsp toasted sesame seeds

Mix all the marinade ingredients together in a bowl, add the tofu and leave to marinate for at least 30 minutes.

Drain the tofu, reserving the marinade.

Heat the oil in a wok or large frying pan, and carefully cook the tofu cubes on all sides until golden. Stand back and turn with tongs, they may spit a bit. Drain on kitchen paper.

The rest is fast work. Stir-fry the spring onions, garlic, ginger, chilli, firm vegetables and any crisp stalks from your greens for a minute or so. Take great care not to burn the garlic, as soon as you can really smell it, toss in the greens with a good splash of water and keep stirring.

Once the greens have wilted, add the tofu and a couple of tablespoons of the leftover marinade, give it a stir and then squeeze over the lime juice. Taste. If the dish needs saltiness, add soy sauce, or if you want a bit more of the sweet–sour balance, then stir in a dash more mirin or rice vinegar.

Sprinkle with sesame seeds and serve at once, with noodles, white or brown rice.

HOW ABOUT?

... doubling the marinade and preparing some extra tofu for another occasion. It will keep in a resealable plastic bag in the fridge for a couple of weeks, so you have flavoursome tofu to hand.

... sprinkling over roasted peanuts or cashews in place of the sesame seeds.

... replacing some or all of the greens with mushrooms such as chestnut, enoki or shiitake.

... throwing in a few thawed green soya beans if you happen to have some in your freezer.

A vibrant, fresh and filling salad that I virtually lived on while backpacking around Indonesia and Malaysia many moons ago. Any combination of cabbage, pak choi, spring greens or carrot can be added to the mix. But where are the pulses? The bean sprouts, tofu (soya bean curd) and even the peanuts are actually legumes. It goes to show that legumes offer so much more than their hearty image suggests.

For convenience, I happily use peanut butter to make the sauce, but if you're a purist you could roast and grind some peanuts yourself.

INDONESIAN VEGETABLE SALAD WITH PEANUT SAUCE
GADO GADO

Serves 4 as a main, 8 as a starter

FOR THE PEANUT SAUCE

2 tbsp vegetable oil

30 g/1 oz shallots, finely diced

2 garlic cloves, finely chopped

2–3 fresh red chillies (see p.248), finely chopped

2 tsp grated fresh ginger

2 tbsp soy sauce

2 tsp palm sugar or brown sugar

5 heaped tbsp unsweetened, organic peanut butter
    or 5 tbsp ground, roasted (but not salted) peanuts

400 ml/14 fl oz canned coconut milk or water

juice of ½–1 lime or lemon or tamarind paste (see p.247)

FOR THE SALAD

250 g/9 oz new potatoes, quartered or halved

1 tsp ground turmeric

salt

3 eggs, boiled (see p.249)

½ small cauliflower, divided into florets

100 g/3½ oz green beans

100 g/3½ oz bean sprouts

½ cucumber, sliced thickly

½ cos or romaine lettuce, sliced

1–2 tbsp vegetable oil

100 g/3½ oz tofu, sliced into fingers and well drained
    (optional)

TO GARNISH

2 tbsp roughly chopped coriander (cilantro) leaves

large handful of prawn crackers

First, make the sauce. Heat the oil over a medium heat and cook the shallots until soft. Throw in the garlic, chillies and ginger, and cook for a minute or two. Add the soy sauce, sugar, peanut butter or ground peanuts, and stir around for a moment. Now add the coconut milk (which I strongly recommend) or water to the sauce and bring it to the boil, then simmer for about 15 minutes to thicken. Remove from the heat and add your citrus juice or tamarind. Taste. Add more soy, sugar, sour juice and chilli until you have a really fresh and feisty sauce. Set aside.

Boil the salad potatoes with the turmeric and a pinch of salt until tender. Drain.

Boil the eggs for 7 minutes and then plunge into cold water and shell.

Steam or blanch the cauliflower (about 5 minutes), the beans (3 minutes) and the bean sprouts (1–2 minutes) until just tender. Refresh in cold water and drain.

Brush a frying pan with vegetable oil and cook the tofu until golden on all sides.

HOW ABOUT?

... using fried tempeh instead of tofu, marinating it as in the previous recipe, or leaving the bean curd out altogether as many Javan cooks do.

... serving the components separately in bowls or on a platter, with the sauce on the side, and inviting guests to create their own combination.

... adding some chicken or beef kebabs (marinated in soy sauce, Tabasco, honey and ginger) and doubling up on the sauce.

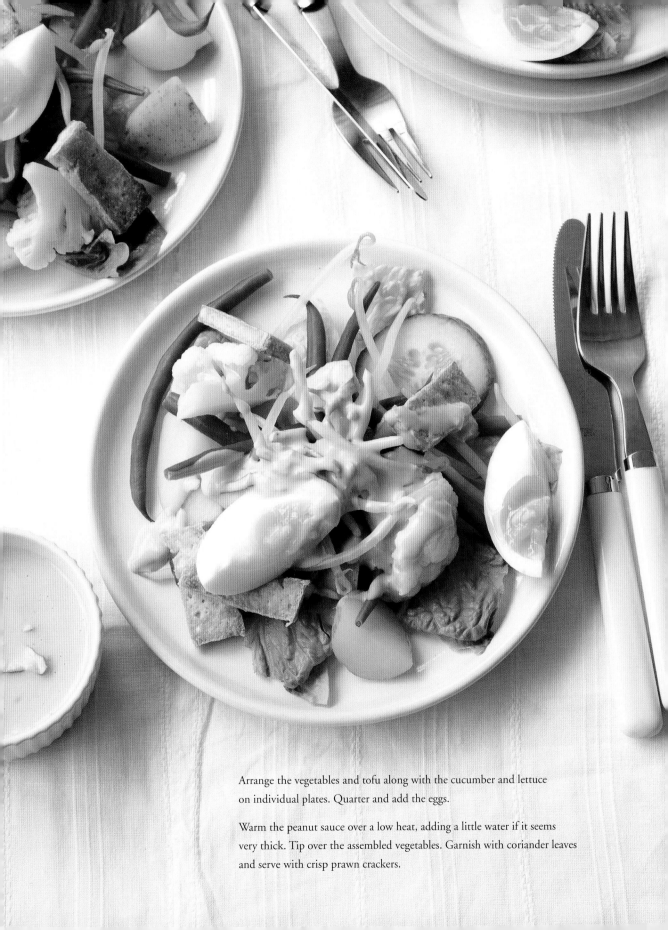

Arrange the vegetables and tofu along with the cucumber and lettuce
on individual plates. Quarter and add the eggs.

Warm the peanut sauce over a low heat, adding a little water if it seems
very thick. Tip over the assembled vegetables. Garnish with coriander leaves
and serve with crisp prawn crackers.

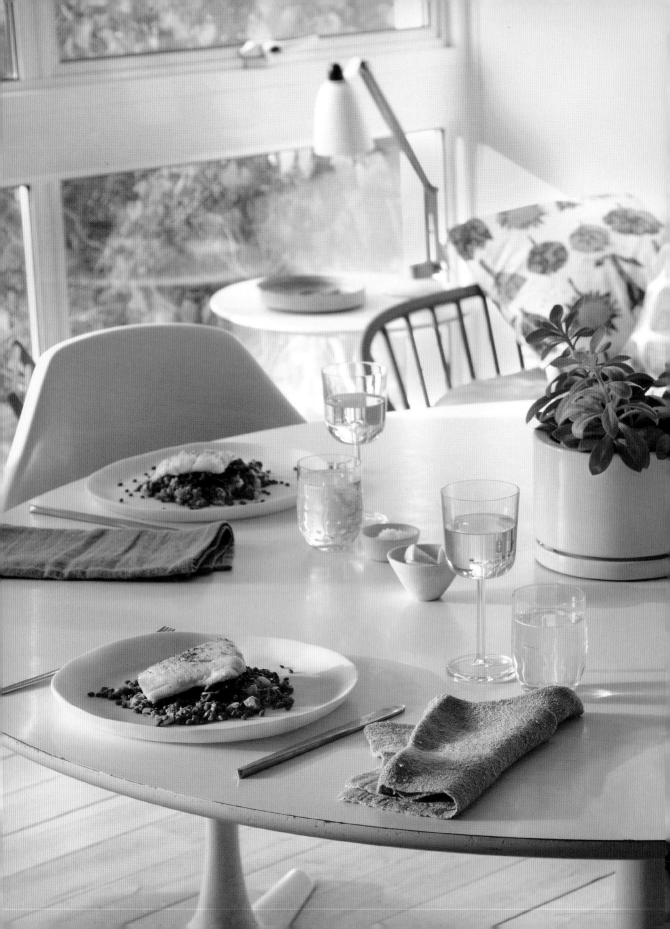

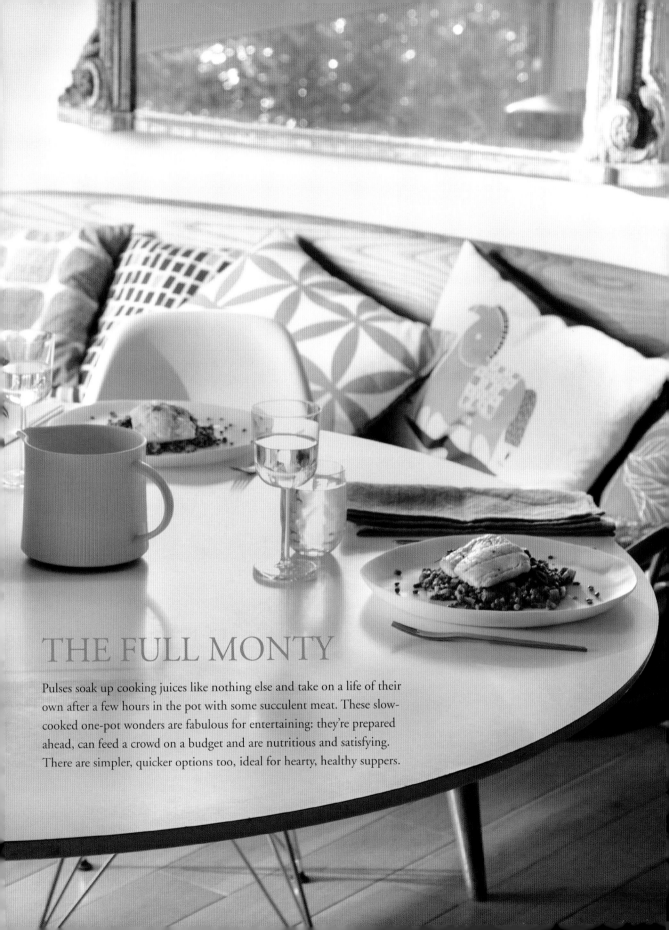

THE FULL MONTY

Pulses soak up cooking juices like nothing else and take on a life of their own after a few hours in the pot with some succulent meat. These slow-cooked one-pot wonders are fabulous for entertaining: they're prepared ahead, can feed a crowd on a budget and are nutritious and satisfying. There are simpler, quicker options too, ideal for hearty, healthy suppers.

You might like to garnish the top of this dish with a few whole, shell-on prawns, but don't underestimate the flavour you will get by making a stock with most of the heads. True seafood lovers suck and chew the heads with gusto, while most people just shove them to the side of the plate – it's a crime to see all that flavour go to waste.

SMOKY PRAWNS WITH CHICKPEAS AND AIOLI

Serves 4

16–24 shell-on raw prawns (shrimp)

4 tbsp olive oil

1 onion, diced

2 old-crop potatoes, diced and cooked
    until tender

500 g/1 lb 2 oz home-cooked or 2 x 400g/
    14 oz cans of chickpeas (garbanzo beans)

salt

1 tbsp hot smoked paprika

75 ml/2½ fl oz/5 tbsp dry white wine

200 g/7 oz cherry tomatoes, halved

2 tbsp roughly chopped flat-leaf parsley

TO SERVE

4 lemon slices

aioli (see p.242)

Remove the heads from the prawns and place them in a small saucepan with 1 tablespoon of the oil. The tails are up to you: shell-on will be messier to eat but give you juicier prawns, shell-off will be a more elegant dining experience (and the shells can join the heads in the pan).

Fry off the heads until they begin to turn pink and then add 3 tablespoons of water. Now you need to crush the heads to release all the fabulous flavour. You can use a mouli legumes, a potato masher and then push the juices through a sieve, or a potato ricer, which looks like a giant garlic press. Set aside the deep orange, prawny juices.

Heat 2 tablespoons of the oil in a large pan, ideally something you can put on the table, and cook the onion until soft. Add the diced potatoes, chickpeas, a pinch of salt and the prawn juices, and stir around carefully. Leave over a low heat.

Sprinkle the prawns with the paprika. Heat the remaining oil in your largest frying pan and throw in the prawns. As soon as you can really smell the paprika, it's time to add the wine and the tomatoes. Cook until the prawns are just firm and the flesh is opaque.

Tip the prawns, tomatoes and juices over the chickpeas, sprinkle with parsley, taste and season.

Serve with a slice of lemon and generous quantities of aioli. You can worry about the garlic later (Campari works wonders).

HOW ABOUT?

... replacing the prawns with squid or cuttlefish; just add a dash of fish stock instead of the prawn juice.

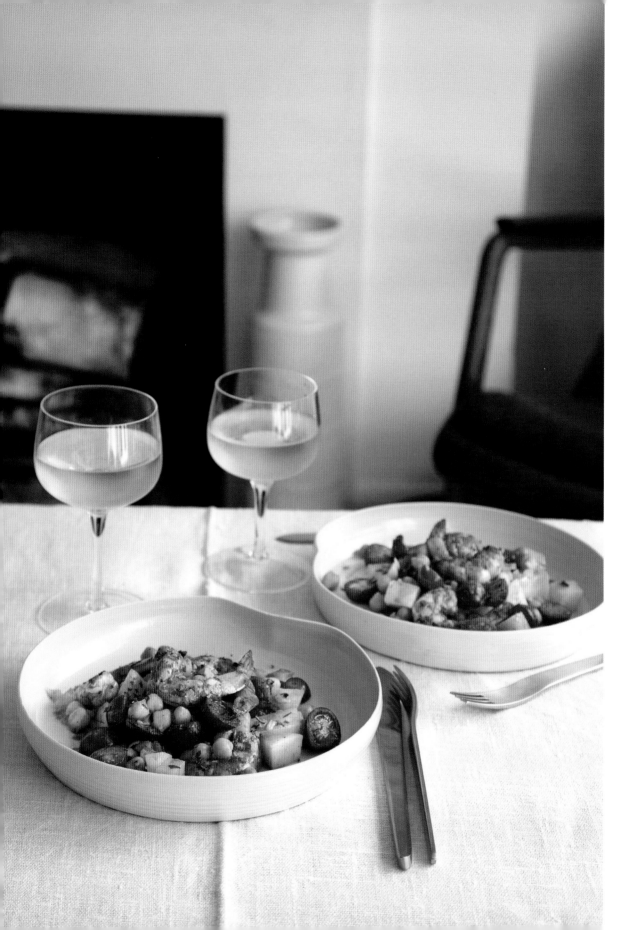

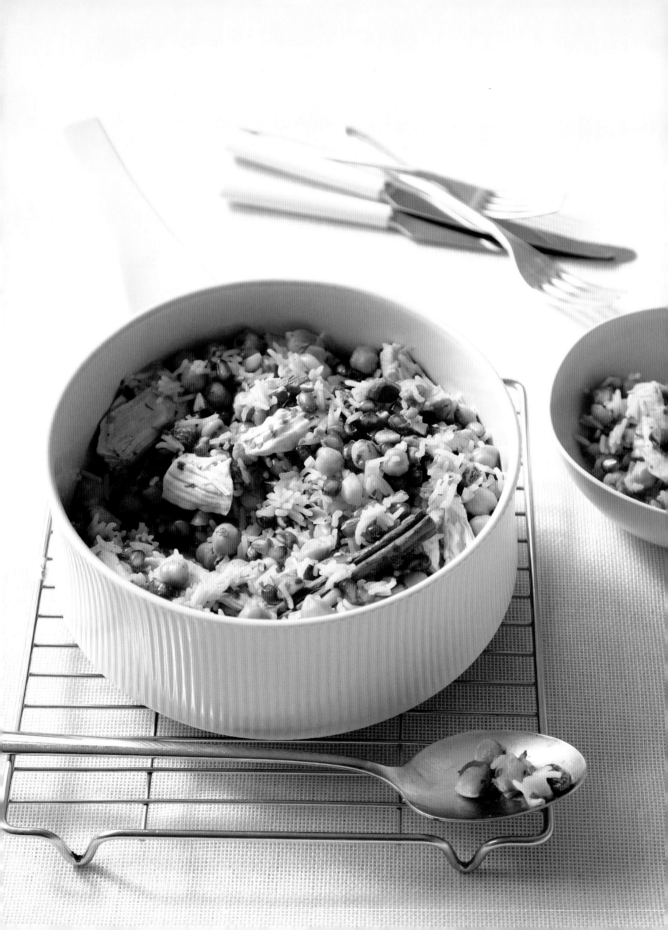

Pilafs are fantastically versatile one-pot dishes. I dreamt this up after Christmas a few years ago, faced with the inevitable leftover turkey. It's now a regular in my festive repertoire, using up both the last pickings from the carcass and the stock, too. The pistachios and pomegranates give the dish a bit of glamour, making it an easy entertaining option. Serve a fresh green salad alongside.

Pilafs provide endless possibilities. Once you have the basic quantities worked out, you'll find dozens of combinations. The subtle Middle Eastern spicing is crucial, as are the dried fruit and nuts.

TURKEY, CHICKPEA AND PISTACHIO PILAF

Serves 4–6

200 g/7 oz/generous 1 cup basmati rice, soaked in tepid water for 1 hour

12 saffron threads, ground with a pestle and mortar

300 ml/10 fl oz/1¼ cups turkey stock

50 g/1¾ oz/4 tbsp unsalted butter

2 onions, sliced

½ cinnamon stick

3 cardamom pods, bruised

500 g/1 lb 2 oz home-cooked or 2 x 400 g/14 oz cans of chickpeas
    (garbanzo beans)

50 g/1¾ oz sultanas (golden raisins)

salt and pepper

about 250 g/9 oz cooked turkey meat, shredded

100 g/3½ oz/generous ¾ cup lightly toasted pistachios, roughly chopped

large bunch of fresh parsley, chopped

seeds and juice of 1 pomegranate

juice of 1 lemon

Add a couple of tablespoons of stock to the saffron in the mortar.

Heat the butter in a large heavy pan (one that has a well-fitting lid), add the onions, cinnamon and cardamom, and cook until the onions are completely soft.

Drain the rice and add to the pan, turning it in the butter to cover. Add the chickpeas, sultanas, saffron stock, stock and a touch of salt and pepper.

Cover with a lid and boil for 5 minutes, reduce the heat and simmer for 5 more minutes, and then leave to rest (still covered) for at least 10 minutes.

Fork in the turkey, pistachios, parsley and about half of the pomegranate. Season to taste with salt, pepper and lemon juice. Sprinkle with the remaining pomegranate seeds, tip over the juice and serve at once.

HOW ABOUT?

... partridge or pheasant, dried fig and almond pilaf. Try this with orange juice instead of lemon.

... lamb, cumin, dried apricot, almond and fresh coriander pilaf.

... leftover chicken and whatever's in the cupboard pilaf – a great way of using up sultanas or pine nuts lurking in the bottom of the packet.

Chickpeas absorb the warm North African spices beautifully and will taste even better if made a day ahead. I like to make a double batch of the chickpeas in tomato sauce, using some with my meatballs and reheating the remainder with greens such as Swiss chard or spinach stirred in. Pile on plenty of fresh mint and parsley, serve with yogurt and flatbread, and you have a magnificent vegetarian lunch.

MOROCCAN CHICKPEAS AND MEATBALLS

Serves 4–6

FOR THE TOMATO AND CHICKPEA SAUCE

2 tbsp olive oil

1 onion, finely chopped

6 garlic cloves, finely chopped

½ tsp ground cinnamon

1 tsp cumin seeds, ground

1 tsp unsmoked paprika, hot or sweet

250 g/9 oz home-cooked or 1 x 400 g/14 oz can of
    chickpeas (garbanzo beans)

400 g/14 oz can of chopped tomatoes

1 tbsp honey

salt and pepper

FOR THE MEATBALLS

450 g/1 lb minced lamb

3 tbsp fresh breadcrumbs

1 onion, very finely chopped or grated

2 garlic cloves, crushed

handful of fresh coriander (cilantro), chopped

2 tsp cumin seeds, ground

1 tsp ground cinnamon

1 tsp salt

pinch of cayenne pepper

1 egg, beaten

2–3 tbsp olive oil for frying

2 tbsp chopped fresh coriander (cilantro), to serve

First make the tomato and chickpea sauce. Heat the oil in a large cast-iron pan or ovenproof sauté pan and cook the onion until just soft. Add the garlic and spices and stir until fragrant. Add the chickpeas and stir them around in the spicy oil, then add the tomatoes, honey, salt and pepper. Simmer for 20 minutes, stirring from time to time.

Meanwhile, mix all the meatball ingredients together with your hands. Form a little patty with a teaspoon of the mixture, heat some oil in a frying pan and cook the patty to check the seasoning. You may like to add more spices and/or salt.

Dip your hands into a bowl of cold water, which will stop the mixture from sticking, and roll the meat into walnut-sized balls.

Cook the meatballs over a medium-high heat until well browned and then pop them into the pan with the chickpeas. Simmer for about 15 minutes, sprinkle with fresh coriander and serve.

HOW ABOUT?

... **Italian style:** Substituting chilli flakes and rosemary for the chickpea spices. Making beef and pork meatballs (meat in equal quantities) and flavouring with lemon zest, grated Parmesan and parsley in place of the coriander, cumin and cinnamon.

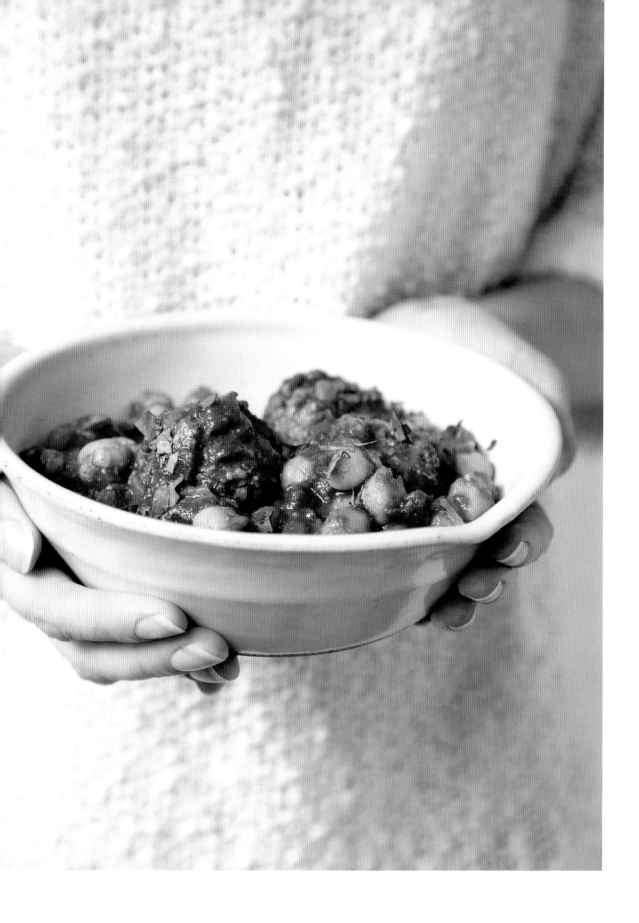

Chermoula is a fabulously aromatic and spicy marinade hailing from north-west Africa, traditionally used for fish, poultry and meat. Recipes vary across Morocco, Algeria and Tunisia, but the fresh coriander, garlic and lemon are constant.

I would recommend the juicy chicken leg or thigh for this dish (breast is much better suited to grilling and frying). The skin gives extra flavour, so don't be tempted to remove it unless you're really counting the calories.

MOROCCAN CHICKPEAS WITH CHERMOULA CHICKEN

Serves 4

6 chicken legs

Moroccan tomato and chickpea sauce (see p.208)

16 green olives, pitted

salt

parsley or coriander (cilantro) sprigs, to garnish

FOR THE CHERMOULA MARINADE

1 onion, roughly chopped

3 garlic cloves

4 tbsp olive oil

handful of flat-leaf parsley

handful of fresh coriander (cilantro)

1 tsp sweet paprika

1 tsp ground cumin

1 tsp ground coriander

½ tsp ground ginger

½ tsp cayenne pepper or chilli flakes

1–2 preserved lemons (depending on size)

Put all the chermoula ingredients except the lemon in a food processor and pulse to a slightly rough paste. You could do this by hand, but make sure that the herbs and onion are really fine: the end texture should resemble a chunky pesto.

Wash the preserved lemon, then cut it open to remove the salty flesh. Slice the skin finely. It smells like detergent and has a very strong flavour, so should be used judiciously. Genuine North African preserved lemons are tiny, with a fine skin, so you could use two of them, but otherwise one will be plenty.

Slash the chicken skin in a couple of places, put the legs in a bowl with the chermoula, and massage the paste into the flesh. Leave for a couple of hours if you have time.

Preheat the oven to 190°C/375°F/Gas mark 5.

Tip the tomato and chickpea sauce into a large oven-to-table dish, such as a terracotta *cazuela* or tagine base.

Remove the chicken from the marinade, wiping away any excess so that it doesn't burn. Stir the excess marinade into the chickpeas, along with the olives.

Lay the chicken on top of the chickpeas, sprinkle over a good pinch of salt and bake for 30–40 minutes. The chicken is ready once skin is crisp and the flesh is cooked through (insert a knife or skewer into the thickest part of the thigh and check that the juices run clear). Serve garnished with parsley or coriander.

HOW ABOUT?

... cooking the chermoula chicken on a baking sheet and serving with the chickpeas with couscous (see p.19) and harissa (see p.245).

... rubbing the chermoula over a butterflied leg of lamb. Leave overnight. Remove the excess marinade and stir it into the tomato and chickpeas, and roast the lamb on top.

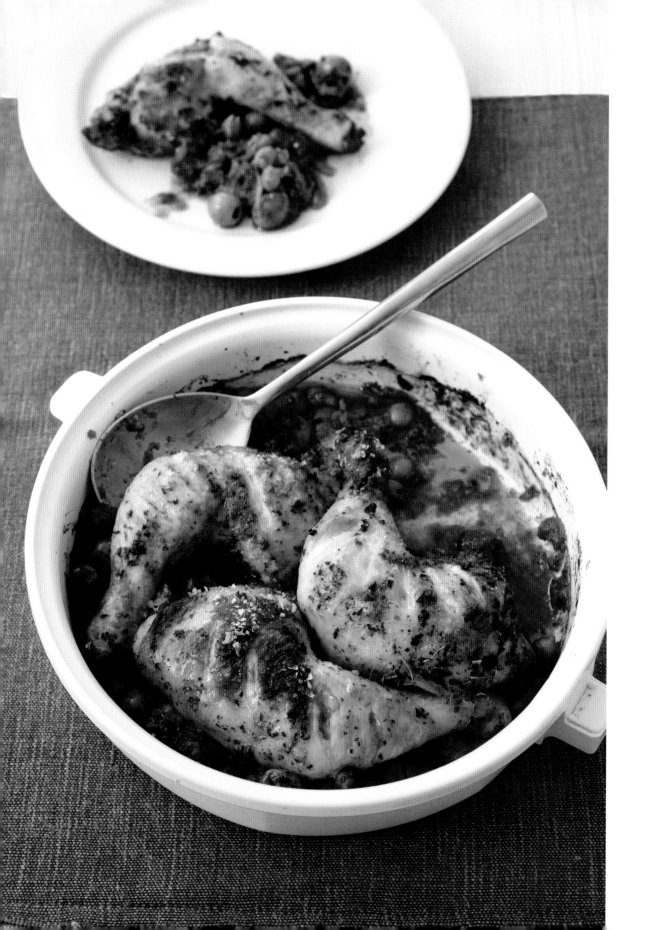

Smoked haddock has a great affinity with curry flavours, best known in kedgeree. I am happy to use a good-quality ready-made curry powder here, but of course you can mix up your own blend. Just make sure that your spices are not too old.

SMOKED HADDOCK, SPINACH AND CURRIED LENTILS

Serves 4

600 g/1 lb 5 oz smoked haddock fillet, skinned and boned

juice of 1 lemon

250 g/9 oz/1¼ cups small lentils such as pardina, Puy or Castelluccio, well rinsed

2 bay leaves

salt and pepper

100 g/3½ oz/7 tbsp unsalted butter

1 onion, diced

1 carrot, diced

2 garlic cloves, crushed

2-cm/¾-inch piece of fresh ginger, finely diced

2 stalks of lemongrass, outer leaves removed, very finely diced

1–2 tbsp medium curry powder

100 ml/3½ fl oz/7 tbsp double (heavy) cream

400 g/14 oz fresh spinach, washed

2 tbsp olive oil

2 tbsp roughly chopped fresh parsley or coriander (cilantro)

1 lemon, cut into wedges, to serve

Check over the fish, remove any bones and cut into 4 pieces. Squeeze over the lemon juice and place in the fridge.

Put the lentils in a large saucepan with the bay leaves and cover with about 5 cm/2 in of cold water. Bring to the boil, then simmer until tender, about 30–45 minutes. Keep an eye on them; they may need topping up with a little water. Drain off any excess water and season with a little salt and black pepper.

Heat half the butter in a saucepan and cook the onion and carrot until the onion is soft. Add the garlic, ginger and lemongrass. Stir for a minute or two, taking care not to burn the garlic, before adding the curry powder. Stir again and then tip in the cream. Pour the curry cream over the lentils, give them a good stir, taste and season well. These lentils can be prepared well in advance and gently reheated.

Cook the spinach in another pan. There will probably be enough moisture from washing the leaves. Cover with a well-fitting lid and cook over a medium heat until the spinach has collapsed. Drain, squeeze well (I love to drink the juice) and season. Too much washing up? Just add the raw spinach to the hot lentils and allow to wilt. A little wetter, not quite as pretty, but hey ho.

Heat the oil and the remaining butter in a large frying pan and pan-fry the haddock until cooked through and beginning to flake – a matter of minutes on each side, depending on the thickness of the fish.

Place a mound of lentils on each plate, then a spoonful of spinach and crown with the fish. Sprinkle with parsley or coriander and serve with a wedge of lemon.

HOW ABOUT?

... serving this with a poached egg (see p.249) on top.

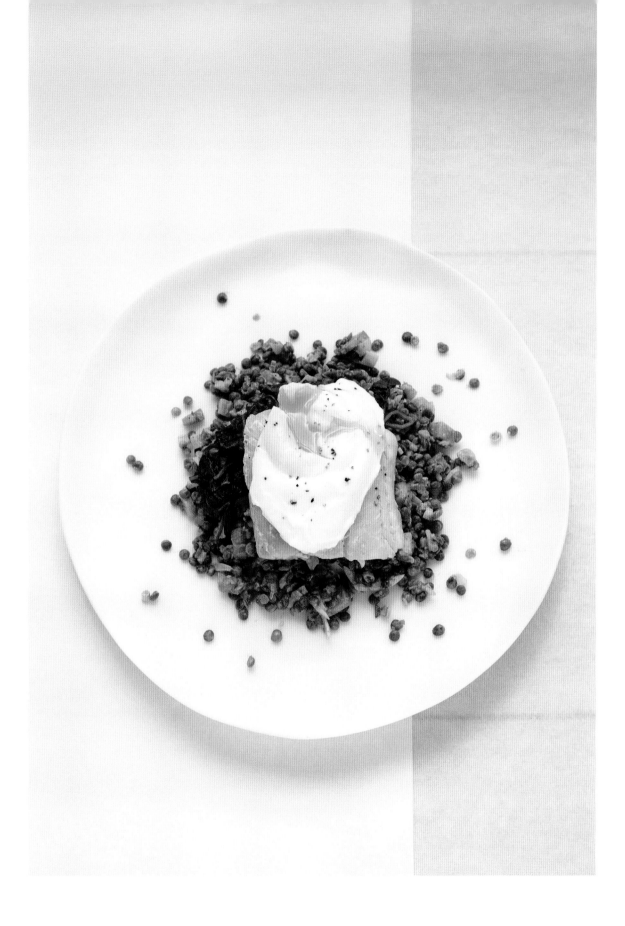

Pheasant can become rather dry if you roast it traditionally, but cooked in the pot with all the vegetables and wine it stays juicy and tender. The lentils soak up the gamey flavours and the brandy-plumped prunes add a bit of sweet richness. This dish tastes extravagant but in fact it's economical to make when you can pick up cheap birds from butchers during the shooting season (1 October to 1 February).

POT-ROAST PHEASANT
WITH PRUNES AND LENTILS

Serves 3–4

2 tbsp olive or rapeseed oil

30 g/1 oz/2 tbsp unsalted butter

2 oven-ready pheasants

4 slices of unsmoked streaky bacon

2 leeks, sliced and well rinsed

2 carrots, finely diced

2 celery stalks, finely diced

2 garlic cloves, roughly chopped

150 ml/5 fl oz/⅔ cup dry white wine

2 sprigs of thyme

salt and pepper

12 prunes

6 tbsp brandy

250 g/9 oz/1¼ cups small lentils such as pardina, Castelluccio or Puy, rinsed

3 tbsp double (heavy) cream

1 tbsp grainy mustard

Preheat the oven to 160°C/325°F/Gas mark 3.

Heat the oil and butter in a large cast-iron casserole with a well-fitting lid and brown the pheasants. Use tongs to turn the birds and make sure they get a good colour. You're creating lots of flavour too. Set the pheasants aside.

Add the bacon to the pan and cook for about 5 minutes and then throw in all the vegetables and garlic. Turn down the heat and cook until soft.

Pour in the wine and bring to the boil. Place the pheasants, breast side down, among the vegetables, add the thyme and some salt and pepper, cover and put in the oven. Cook for 1 hour, turning the birds over after 30 minutes.

Meanwhile, put the prunes in a small pan with the brandy and bring to the boil for 2–3 minutes. Set aside and leave the prunes to plump.

Put the lentils in a pan and cover with 5 cm/2 in of cold water. Bring to the boil, then simmer until tender but still whole – anything from 30 minutes to 1 hour. Drain.

Once cooked, take the pheasants out of the pot and cover with foil to keep warm.

Add the lentils, prunes and any brandy, the cream and mustard to the pheasant juices. Taste and season with more salt and pepper as necessary.

Chop the pheasant into legs and breasts and return to the pot. Serve with some dark winter greens.

HOW ABOUT?

… increasing the quantities and using the leftovers to make a wonderful soup. Lengthen with chicken stock, purée a few of the lentils to add some creamy texture and shred in some of the cooked pheasant flesh. Eat within a couple of days or freeze.

… using the same recipe for guinea fowl or 4 partridge.

Possibly the quickest, most satisfying crowd-pleaser of a bean recipe in my repertoire. It appeared in my book *The Real Taste of Spain*, but I couldn't leave it out of a book on pulses.

For the very best results, try to track down the soft cooking chorizo that is available in many delis and specialist Spanish shops; it breaks down into the sauce beautifully. The jars of cooked Spanish *judiones* are spectacularly good too, their creamy texture really explains why they were named butter beans.

The finished dish benefits from sitting for a few hours, or even overnight if you have the time, so that the beans really soak up all the flavours.

CHORIZO WITH RED PEPPER AND BUTTER BEANS

Serves 4

2 tbsp olive oil

2 onions, diced

1 red pepper, deseeded and sliced

2 garlic cloves, diced

250 g/9 oz chorizo, hot or mild, sliced

500 g/1 lb 2 oz home-cooked or 2 x 400 g/14 oz cans of butter beans
    (large lima beans)

400 g/14 oz canned chopped tomatoes

salt and pepper

2 tbsp roughly chopped fresh parsley

extra-virgin olive oil

Heat the olive oil in a large pan and cook the onions and the pepper until they soften, then add the garlic and chorizo. Once the chorizo fat has rendered down and the pan is swirling with its crimson juices, tip in the beans, stirring to coat them in the oil.

Add the tomatoes and cook for 10 minutes. Set aside to rest, and then reheat, if possible.

Sprinkle with the parsley and a drizzle of olive oil before serving.

HOW ABOUT?

... substituting chickpeas or other beans for the butter beans.

... frying fillets of firm white fish, just until golden, and laying them on top of the bean and tomato mixture to finish cooking. Cover with a well-fitting lid and simmer for a couple of minutes, allowing the fish to steam to perfection.

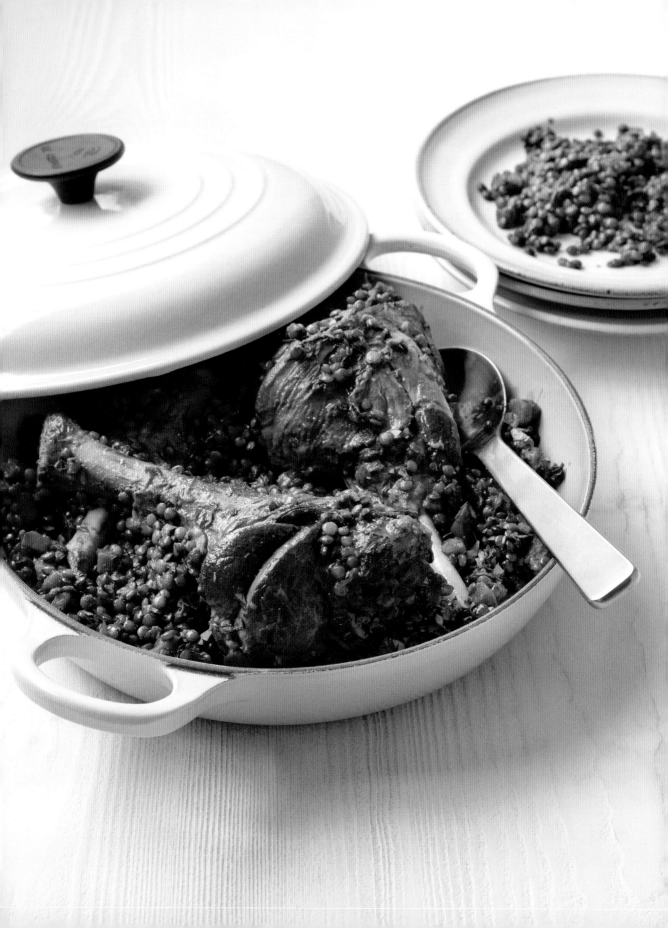

The mystery ingredient in this recipe is the anchovy, which gives a deeply satisfying savoury note. You may baulk at the idea, but think of it as a seasoning rather than a flavour, just like the fish sauce in a Thai curry.

The lentils make this a superb one-pot dish with no last-minute fuss. I like to serve it with steamed green beans tossed in melted butter with chopped parsley and capers, but a simple green salad would work well too.

BRAISED LAMB SHANKS WITH LENTILS

Serves 4

3 tbsp olive oil

4 lamb shanks

2 onions, roughly chopped

2 carrots, finely diced

50 g/1¾ oz can of anchovies in oil, drained and chopped

4 garlic cloves, finely sliced

pinch of chilli flakes

1 sprig of rosemary

300 ml/10 fl oz/1¼ cups red wine

about 1 litre/1¾ pints/4 cups vegetable or meat stock

250 g/9 oz/1¼ cups small firm lentils such as Puy, Castelluccio, *pardina* or beluga, rinsed

salt and pepper

5 tbsp balsamic vinegar

handful of fresh parsley, roughly chopped

Preheat the oven to 160°C/325°F/Gas mark 3.

Heat 1 tablespoon of the oil in a large cast-iron or heavy-duty casserole and sear the lamb shanks, a couple at a time, until they are browned all over. Set aside and spoon off most of the fat from the pan.

Add the remaining oil to the same pan and cook the onions and carrots until soft and just beginning to caramelize.

Throw in the anchovies and garlic, give them a stir, and then toss in the chilli and rosemary. Return the lamb shanks to the pan and pour in the wine and enough stock to cover most of the meat.

Cover with a tight-fitting lid and place in the oven for about 2 hours, turning the lamb shanks after about an hour.

When the shanks are fairly tender, remove them from the pan and set aside. Bring the juices to the boil over a medium-high heat and reduce by about a third. Tip in the lentils (they should be well covered by the liquid) and replace the lamb shanks.

Cover with the lid and put back in the oven for another hour, until the lamb is meltingly tender and the lentils are plumped up with all the fabulous juices.

Taste and season; the anchovies will have added salt, but you may want a bit more peppery heat. The sweet-and-sour balsamic vinegar will really liven things up – add it a little at a time to balance the flavours. Stir in the parsley and serve.

HOW ABOUT?

... using cooked beans such as haricots or flageolets instead of the lentils. Just add the beans for the last 30 minutes of cooking to absorb all the flavours.

.. getting ahead: cook the shanks for the first 2 hours up to a day in advance. Bring the juices to the boil, add the lentils and lamb and place in the oven for the final hour.

... serving with salsa verde (see p.242).

Meltingly tender lamb and tiny green flageolet beans are a French classic. Slow cooking at its best, filling your kitchen with tantalizingly good smells. The lamb takes about 7 hours to reach perfection and the beans will need soaking ahead (unless of course you are cheating with canned). The result is a dish that requires very little attention, with none of the last-minute Sunday lunch angst over gravy, roast spuds and all the trimmings.

Many recipes call for the flageolets to cook with the lamb, but since the cooking time for the beans can vary so much, I prefer to cook them separately and then combine for the last hour to soak up all the glorious juices. That way there is no chance of beans like bullets or a sludgy mash.

SLOW-ROAST SHOULDER OF LAMB WITH FLAGEOLET BEANS

Serves 4–6

2 tbsp olive oil

1 shoulder of lamb, about 1.8 kg/4 lb

2 onions, diced

4 garlic cloves, crushed

1 tbsp finely chopped rosemary

½ bottle dry white wine

salt and pepper

700 g/1 lb 9 oz home-cooked or 3 x 400 g/14 oz cans of flageolet beans

3 leeks, sliced roughly

250 g/9 oz green beans, topped but not tailed

2 tbsp roughly chopped flat-leaf parsley

dash of balsamic vinegar

Preheat the oven to 160°C/325°F/Gas mark 3.

Heat the oil in a large, deep roasting pan or a large cast-iron cooking pot over a high heat and sear the lamb until brown all over. Add the onions, garlic, rosemary, wine and a little salt and pepper. Cover with a well-fitting lid or cover the whole pan carefully with foil (you want to create a steamy environment for the meat to cook in). Roast the lamb for 3 hours and then turn the oven down to 140°C/275°F/Gas mark 1 and cook for another 4 hours.

About an hour before serving, remove the pan from the oven and skim off any excess fat. Taste the lamb juices and season with salt and pepper. Add the beans and leeks to the pan, replace the lid or foil, and cook for a further hour. There should be plenty of liquid for the vegetables to soak up, but do add a little stock or water if it seems dry.

Remove the pan from the oven, lift out the meat and set aside to rest for a few minutes while you steam or boil the green beans until just tender. Add the fresh beans to the flageolets, season well and add the parsley.

You should now be able to break up the tender lamb with a fork. Spoon the beans onto individual plates, and top with the lamb. Add a dash of balsamic vinegar – you need a bit of acidity – and serve.

HOW ABOUT?

... seasoning the lamb with 1 tablespoon of smoked paprika and stirring some sliced piquillo peppers into the beans.

... adding a can of chopped tomatoes when you add the flageolets and leeks.

... making a zippy sauce with a few tablespoons of the lamb juices, 2 tablespoons of capers, plenty of freshly chopped mint and a good splash of red wine vinegar.

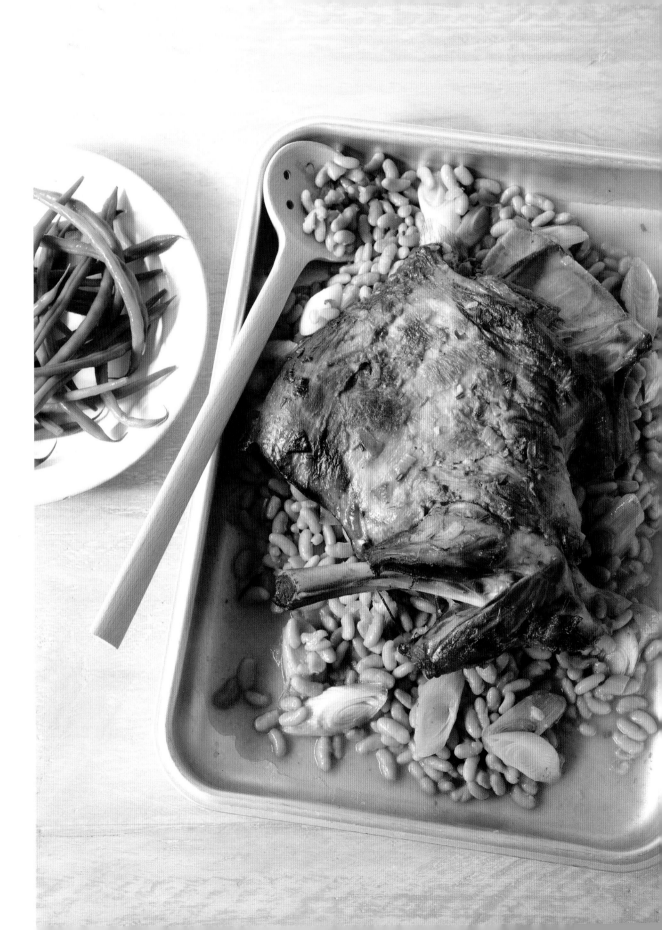

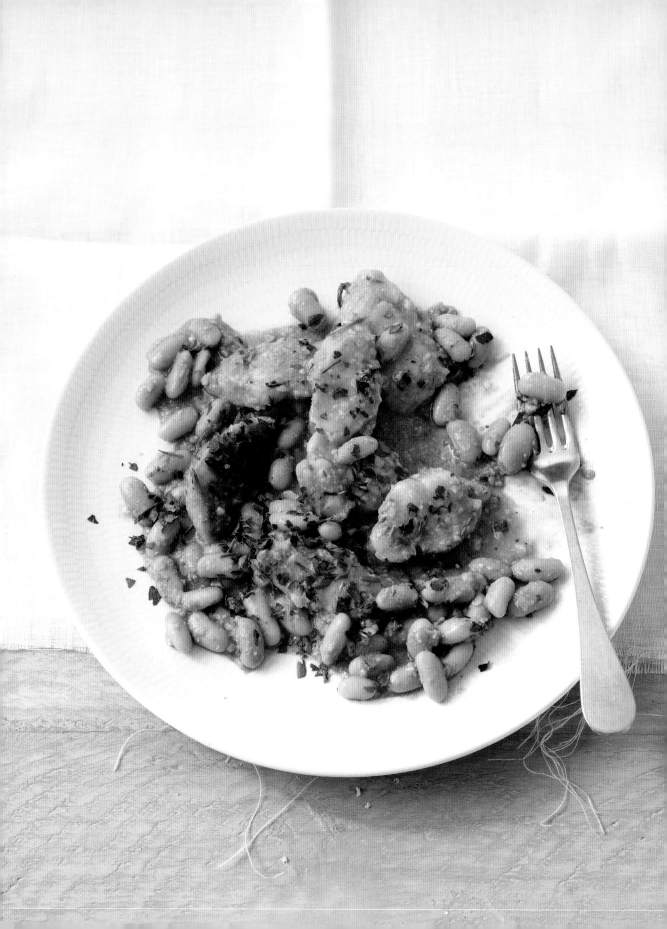

The Spanish are obsessive about their legumes, with more EU protected varieties than any other country in Europe. Each region has its bean, and when you get to Catalonia the *mongete del ganxet*, with its delicate skin and creamy texture, is king of the castle. Locals will be up in arms but, since they consume most of the beans themselves, I'd recommend any good-quality white bean for this dish.

Romesco sauce is another Catalan speciality, made with nuts, garlic, paprika and tomato.

MONKFISH, ROMESCO AND WHITE BEAN CAZUELA

Serves 4

4 pieces of monkfish fillet, about 175 g/6 oz each, well trimmed

salt and pepper

3 tbsp olive oil

romesco sauce (see p.243)

150 ml/5 fl oz/⅔ cup dry white wine

400 ml/14 fl oz/scant 1¾ cups good fish stock

450 g/1 lb home-cooked or 2 x 400 g/14 oz cans of ganxet, haricot (navy) or cannellini beans

juice of ½–1 lemon

large handful of flat-leaf parsley, roughly chopped

extra-virgin olive oil

About 1 hour before cooking, sprinkle the monkfish with a little salt: this will draw out excess moisture and allow the fish to brown rather than sweat in its own juices when you come to cook it.

Heat the oil until really hot in a large wide pan. Add the monkfish and sear until just golden but not cooked through. Set aside.

Add the romesco sauce to the hot oil. Let it bubble for a minute or two, stirring all the time, and then add the wine and about half of the fish stock. Bring to the boil, give it a good stir, add the beans and simmer for about 10 minutes. Add more stock if the beans seem dry, but remember this is not a soup. Stir gently from time to time, you don't want the bottom to catch, but equally you want to keep those precious beans intact.

Meanwhile, slice the monkfish fillets into medallions. They should still be slightly translucent and uncooked in the middle.

Taste the beans and season with more salt, pepper and lemon juice. Remove a large cupful of beans from the pan and purée them with a hand-held blender or the back of a fork to thicken up the sauce a little. Return the pureed beans to the pan, bring them up to a bubble and carefully add the monkfish, sliding the slices in among the beans. Cover the pan and remove from the heat at once.

Leave to rest for about 5 minutes, until the fish has cooked through. Serve with plenty of chopped parsley and a dash of extra-virgin olive oil.

HOW ABOUT?

… adding raw, shell-on prawns and mussels. Cook them for a few minutes with the beans while they are simmering, before you add the fish.

I love the chunky texture of a traditional Cumberland sausage but any good-quality pork sausage will be delicious. Feel free to change the beans too. In fact, once you have this recipe in your repertoire, the possibilities are endless. Swap the cider for wine, add different herbs to suit your sausage, throw in fennel or leeks along with the onion.

This makes a generous quantity as a one-pot supper. If you serve it with baked potatoes, then you will have plenty for six.

CUMBERLAND SAUSAGE WITH BEANS AND CIDER

Serves 4

2 tbsp olive oil

4 slices of smoked streaky bacon, chopped

450–500 g/about 1 lb sausages (or 1 traditional Cumberland sausage, cut into 10-cm/4-inch lengths)

2 red onions, diced roughly

4 garlic cloves, thinly sliced

12 sage leaves, finely chopped

750 g/1 lb 10 oz home-cooked or 3 x 400 g/14 oz cans of haricots (navy beans) or butter beans (large lima beans)

300 ml/10 fl oz/1¼ cups dry cider

300 ml/10 fl oz/1¼ cups chicken or vegetable stock

2 tbsp wholegrain mustard

salt and pepper

5 tbsp double (heavy) cream

large handful of kale or Savoy cabbage, finely sliced

large handful of flat-leaf parsley, roughly chopped

lemon juice or cider vinegar (optional)

Preheat the oven to 180°C/350°F/Gas mark 4.

Heat the oil in a large, heavy-bottomed casserole or ovenproof pan and cook the bacon with half of the sausages, until golden brown. Set the meat aside, brown the remaining sausages and set side.

Add the onions, garlic and sage to the fatty juices, cover with a lid and cook gently for about 10 minutes, until meltingly tender and golden.

Tip in the beans, cider, stock and mustard. Cut the sausages in half (a slightly diagonal cut looks attractive) and add to the casserole. Season and place in the oven for 45 minutes.

Remove from the oven, and if the sauce seems a little thin, use a hand-held blender or a potato masher to purée just a few of the beans. Stir in the cream and kale or cabbage and cook for a further 10 minutes.

Taste and adjust the seasoning. You may need to add a dash of lemon juice or cider vinegar to sharpen things up. Stir in the parsley and serve.

HOW ABOUT?

... using Italian Luganega sausage, red wine, chilli, fennel bulb and cannellini beans (no cream required).

... or Toulouse sausage, white wine, thyme, leeks and flageolets.

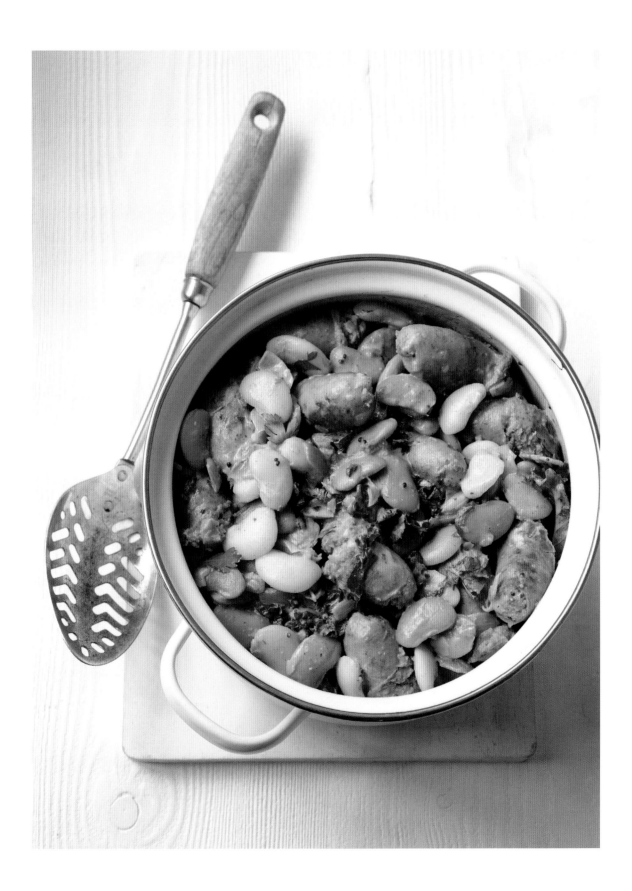

The dish that spawned a multimillion-dollar industry, but where's the real thing? We Brits eat baked beans by the ton, yet many of us have never have tasted, and probably never will taste, a true Boston baked bean. Supermarket aisles are stacked with cans of pretenders: low-salt, no-salt, sugar out, pickle in, spiced up, cheesy, and the one with the anaemic rubber sausage lurking in it. I know, I sound like a bean snob. While I have nothing against straightforward baked beans (there's always a can in my cupboard), it's a terrible shame not to savour the genuine, rib-sticking one-pot wonder.

BOSTON BAKED BEANS

Serves 4–6

750 g/1 lb 10 oz (preferably) home-cooked or
   3 x 400 g/14 oz cans of haricot (navy) beans
1 heaped tsp English mustard powder
   or 1 tbsp English mustard
2 tbsp maple syrup (or light brown sugar)
2 tbsp black treacle

2 tbsp tomato purée
2 small onions, peeled and studded with 4 cloves
350 g/12 oz piece of streaky bacon or pork belly,
   rind removed
salt and pepper
Worcestershire sauce (optional)

Preheat the oven to 140°C/275°F/Gas mark 1.

Drain the beans. If using home-cooked, keep the liquid to use as stock later. If using canned, tip the gloop away and give the beans a rinse. Pour the beans into a large cast-iron pot or casserole.

Mix the mustard, maple syrup, treacle and tomato purée with a couple of spoonfuls of water and tip over the beans. Toss the onions into the pot too.

Nestle the piece of pork among the beans. If it's bacon, and therefore salty, don't add salt to the dish. If it's pork belly, add a good teaspoon of salt. Grind over plenty of black pepper.

If you cooked your own beans, add the nutritious cooking water, to just cover the beans. Otherwise use tap water. Cover the pot with a tight-fitting lid or cover tightly with foil and place in the oven for 3 hours.

Remove the lid and taste the beans. Add more salt and pepper as necessary, and a dash more maple syrup and/or Worcestershire sauce. If the beans seem a little dry, add a splash of water, but the finished dish should be thick and sticky.

Lift out the pork or bacon and chop it into large chunks. Place it fat-side up on top of the beans and then put the pot back into the oven, uncovered, for another 45 minutes to 1 hour.

Serve with crusty bread (I might crave a green salad to follow).

HOW ABOUT?

... keeping up with tradition and sloshing a few tablespoons of rum into the beans for the last hour of cooking.
... leaving out the pork for a veggie version and maybe adding some red peppers instead.
... adding some diced carrot to the pot (about 3 medium carrots) – unorthodox but good.

Chilli con carne, *carne con chili*; minced meat, chunks of meat; no beans, full of beans. Oh, the controversy! It's amazing that a humble dish that reputably evolved on the cowboy campfire of the American South-West (or was it in a Texan jail?) can stir up such strong feelings.

And then there's what to serve it with. In San Antonio, Texas, the self-proclaimed home of the 'bowl of red', it's most likely to come with rice or a tortilla, while the famous 'chili parlors' of Cincinnati serve their chilli with spaghetti, Cheddar and salted crackers. Conclusion: each to their own. And, to all the chilli, *chile*, *chili* pedants out there… just chill out.

CHILLI CON CARNE

Serves 6–8

5 tbsp olive oil

900 g/2 lb chuck (braising) steak,
    cut into 3-cm/about 1-inch cubes

2 onions, diced

6 garlic cloves, crushed

1 tsp cumin seeds, roasted and ground,
    or 1 tsp ground cumin

1 tbsp dried oregano

2–3 tsp chilli powder

1 can or small bottle (about 330 ml) of bitter, or dark beer

400 g/14 oz can of chopped tomatoes

2 tbsp brown sugar

2 tsp Worcestershire sauce

salt

550 g/1¼ lb home-cooked or 2 x 400 g/14 oz cans of red
    kidney, pinto or black beans

large handful of coriander (cilantro), roughly chopped

Heat half the oil a large cast-iron pot or heavy saucepan over a high heat and brown the meat in batches. It needs to be well coloured to give plenty of flavour. Set the meat aside.

Add the remaining oil to the pan, add the onions and cook until soft. Add the garlic, cumin, oregano and chilli, and stir for a minute or two – the chilli will make you gasp. Return the meat to the pan before the garlic catches and burns.

Tip in the beer, tomatoes, sugar, Worcestershire sauce and season with a good pinch of salt. Bring to the boil, then cover and simmer really gently for about 2 hours or until the beef is really tender.

Stir in the beans, simmer for a further 10 minutes and check the seasoning.

Serve with the chopped coriander or, better still, leave the chilli for a day or two for the flavours to mingle, marry and mature.

HOW ABOUT?

… a bowl of salsa (see p.242) or guacamole (see p.243), some grated cheese (I love Wensleydale) and sour cream on the side.

… serving with boiled rice, a baked potato, tortillas or even polenta.

… playing with fire: try using fresh chillies or tracking down some of the Mexican dried chillies available in specialist shops or online.

When it comes to bean dishes, *cassoulet* is perhaps the jewel in the European crown. A classic from the French region of Gascony, and just like any other iconic dish there's the inevitable controversy over the most authentic version.

The town of Castelnaudary, the most widely accepted home of *cassoulet*, has its own brotherhood of impassioned gastronomes, the *Grande Confrérie du Cassoulet*, who strive to maintain the purity of their dish. Up the road in Toulouse, they may add lamb, while a partridge may wing its way into the Carcassonne recipe, but in Castelnaudary it's all about the beans, with a little duck, pork and sausage. Tomatoes are off limits for some, others will swear by a good sprinkling of breadcrumbs to enhance the crust. You'll be sure to have some self-proclaimed *cassoulet* expert in a tizz whatever you do.

The locally produced *lingot*, white coco or Tarbais beans are the beans of choice, but since it's said that over 70,000 tons of cassoulet are consumed each year in France, they're like gold dust and you'll most likely be using a cannellini.

Note: All time-pressed cooks and impatient diners think again. *Cassoulet* takes a couple of days to make and almost another to digest: it's a labour of love to share and savour with friends. *Illustrated on pp.228–229.*

CASSOULET

Serves about 8

4 duck legs, confit or roast (see p.251)

500 g/1 lb 2 oz Toulouse sausage in one long coil, or about 8 x 10 cm/4 inch sausages

2 tbsp duck fat (from the confit or from roasting the legs)

1 onion, diced

5 garlic cloves, finely chopped

4 tomatoes, peeled, deseeded and roughly chopped

1 tbsp fresh thyme leaves

salt and pepper

2 tbsp duck or goose fat or olive oil, to finish

FOR THE BEANS

1 kg/2¼ lb dried white kidney beans (Tarbais, *lingots*, *coco* or cannellini), soaked overnight

1 bouquet garni

1 onion, halved

1 carrot, halved

2 celery stalks, halved

1 leek, trimmed, washed and halved

150 g/5½ oz thick slice of smoked streaky bacon or pancetta, or smoked lardons

1 small ham hock (optional)

100 g/3½ oz pork loin fat, rind on, cut into thick strips

1 litre/1¾ pints/4 cups chicken stock

For the beans: drain and discard the soaking water. If you're particularly anxious about their flatulence-inducing reputation, you can place them in a large pan, cover them in cold water, bring to the boil for a couple of minutes, then drain and discard this water too. If you're feeling French, then don't bother.

Place the beans in a large saucepan with all the remaining bean ingredients. Top up the pan with water to cover the beans by about 5 cm/2 in. Bring to the boil and then simmer for about 1½ hours or until the beans are just tender.

Meanwhile, you can prepare your meats and vegetables. If you are roasting your duck, now's the time to do it. If you are using confit duck legs, remove most of the congealed fat. Whichever type of leg you are using, trim away any excess skin and cut the legs into drumsticks and thighs.

Take a tablespoon of duck fat from the confit or from your roasting pan and heat it in a large frying pan. Brown the sausages; they will continue to cook in the *cassoulet*, so don't worry about cooking them through. If using confit duck, brown that too. Set aside the meat.

Using the same pan, sauté the onion until golden. Add the garlic, tomatoes and thyme, and cook for a further 5 minutes.

Preheat the oven to 220°C/425°F/Gas mark 7.

Drain the beans, reserving their stock. Remove the vegetables, bouquet garni, ham hock (if using) and pork rind. It seems a shame to throw out the vegetables, so you can chop them roughly and put them back into the beans with the lardons. Shred the meat from the ham hock and return to the beans. Discard the pork rind and bouquet garni.

Add the sautéed onion and tomatoes to the beans.

Place about half of the beans in a 4-litre/7-pint ovenproof casserole or traditional *cassole*. Pile in the sausages and duck and then tip the remaining beans on top.

Taste your beans. If you used a ham hock, they will already be lightly seasoned, but most likely they will need some salt; this will guide you when seasoning the stock. Now taste the bean stock and season well with salt and plenty of black pepper. Tip enough of the bean stock over the *cassoulet* to just cover the beans; if you don't have quite enough, then top up with water.

Dot with a little goose or duck fat and place in the hot oven for 30 minutes, then turn the heat down to about 160°C/325°F/Gas mark 3 and cook for another hour. Every half hour, break the crust by pushing it down into the beans and their juices, allowing a new crust to form. The idea is to end up with a thick, browned crust.

Bring the *cassoulet* to the table and break the crust in front of your guests. Serve with a wonderfully robust red wine, a large green salad (sacrilege I know, but I must have some greenery) and a good few hours to eat and digest.

HOW ABOUT?

.. replacing the duck with some well-cooked lamb shanks.

... cheating and buying some of the ready-made duck confit sold in delicatessens and supermarkets.

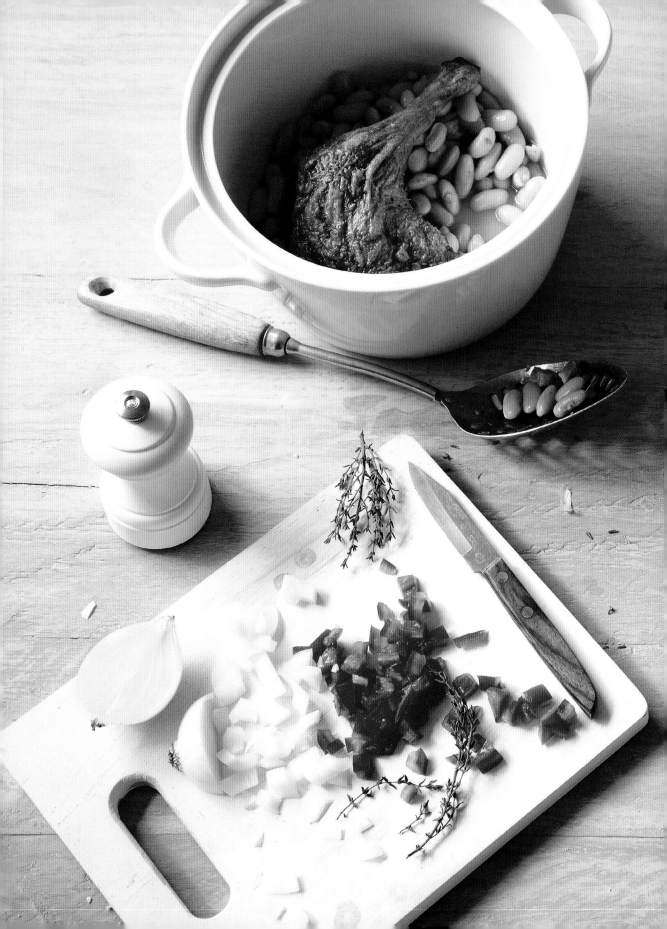

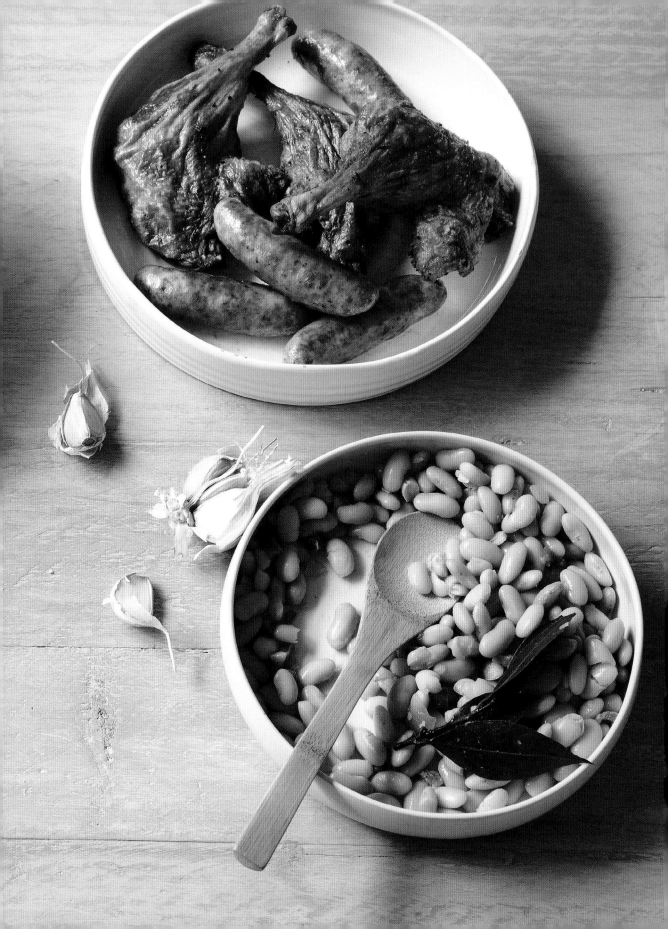

Here's a dish to feed a crowd. You can really get ahead of yourself as the chilli will be even better after a couple of days in the fridge.

The recipe comes from Jennifer Joyce's *Meals in Heels*, a collection of 'do-ahead dishes for the dinner party diva'. Jennifer's food always bursts with gutsy, intense flavours and this is no exception.

SMOKY PORK AND BEAN CHILLI

Serves 6–8

900 g/2 lb pork shoulder, diced into 2 cm/¾ inch cubes

salt and pepper

5 tbsp olive oil

2 large onions, roughly chopped

6 garlic cloves, finely chopped

1 heaped tbsp smoked paprika

1 heaped tbsp ground cumin

1 tsp chipotle paste or Tabasco sauce

800 g/1 lb 12 oz canned plum tomatoes, puréed

4 tbsp cider vinegar

40 g/1½ oz light brown sugar

550 g/1¼ lb home-cooked or 2 x 400 g/14 oz cans of black, pinto or borlotti (cranberry) beans

TO SERVE

red onion, chopped

avocado, chopped

coriander leaves (cilantro), chopped

grated cheese

boiled rice

Season the pork with salt and pepper. Place a large saucepan with a tablespoon of olive oil over a medium heat and cook the pork in batches for a minute or two on each side, until browned all over. Set the meat aside.

Turn down the heat, add the remaining oil with the onions and garlic, season with salt and pepper and cook very gently for about 5 minutes, until soft.

Add the spices and chipotle paste and continue to cook for a couple of minutes.

Now throw in the tomatoes, vinegar, sugar and pork, cover with a lid and cook gently for about 1 hour or until the pork is tender.

Add the beans and warm through.

Serve in bowls, topped with the red onion, avocado and coriander and some grated cheese and boiled rice alongside.

HOW ABOUT?

... serving the chilli with tortillas, sour cream and guacamole and letting everyone assemble their own 'burrito' (see p.196).

... cooking this in the oven at about 160°C/325°F/Gas mark 3.

This chilli is the sort of thing we used to whip up in my student days, although here I am using rich, sweet lamb instead of beef. True chilli enthusiasts will question its credentials but they should give it a try. Easy, tasty, great to prepare ahead and a very economical way to feed a crowd.

SIMPLE LAMB CHILLI

Serves 6–8

3 tbsp olive oil
2 onions, finely diced
2 carrots, finely diced
3 garlic cloves, crushed
600 g/1 lb 5 oz minced lamb
2 tsp chilli flakes
2 tsp cumin seeds, roasted and ground
2 tsp dried oregano
2 x 400 g/14 oz cans of chopped tomatoes
2 tbsp tomato purée
2 x 400 g/14 oz cans of red kidney beans
salt and pepper
dash of Worcestershire sauce
large handful of fresh coriander (cilantro), roughly chopped
juice of 1 lime

Heat the oil in a large saucepan and fry the onions and carrots until the onion has softened and begun to colour.

Add the garlic, stir until fragrant, then add the lamb. Stir for a minute or two and then add the chilli, cumin, oregano, tomatoes and tomato purée. Simmer gently for about 20 minutes.

Add the beans and season with salt, pepper and Worcestershire sauce. Simmer gently for a further 30 minutes; the tomatoes' acidity will prevent the beans from breaking down. Check the seasoning and zip up the dish with the lime juice.

HOW ABOUT?

... serving with sour cream or yogurt.
... serving with tortillas instead of the more usual rice.
... making a double quantity:
it freezes brilliantly.

Feijoada is considered the national dish of Brazil, a famously hearty pot of slow-cooked beans, pork and sometimes beef too. It's difficult, well-nigh impossible, to track down the right smoked sausage or the authentic *carne seca* (salt-cured beef) outside Brazil, but don't get hung up on it. After all, the *feijoada* developed out of the need to feed a crowd on beans and whatever bits of pig's ear, tail, trotter or other meat scraps were available – it was the food of the slaves.

At the mention of a book on beans, my Brazilian friend Leti immediately cooked up a feast of *feijoada* with white rice, greens, slithers of fresh orange, tomato vinaigrette and even the offer of a fried egg on top! Many recipes call for a huge variety of different salted and smoked meats, but Leti's version is really simple and tastes phenomenally good.

You can, of course, throw in a ham hock, a slab of bacon or some salted ribs (be sure to soak overnight) along with the beans if you want to vary or increase the meat. Canned beans just won't do here.

BRAZILIAN PORK AND BLACK BEANS
FEIJOADA

Serves 8–10
2 tbsp olive oil
800 g/1 lb 12 oz pork loin, cut into large chunks
salt and pepper
500 g/1 lb 2 oz smoked sausage such as Portuguese *linguiça*, or smoked chorizo,
    cut into chunks
2 onions, finely diced
4 garlic cloves, finely chopped
2 tsp ground cumin
2 tsp paprika
1 bay leaf
1 kg/2¼ lb black beans, soaked overnight

In a large pot, big enough for all your beans, heat the oil and brown the chunks of pork loin. Season with a little salt and pepper and set aside.

Now add the smoked sausage, onions and garlic to the pot and fry until everything is covered in glistening red oil. Add the cumin, paprika, a bay leaf and a good grind of black pepper.

Stir in the beans to coat them in the oil, and then add enough cold water to cover by at least 5 cm/2 in. Bring to the boil and then turn down to a low simmer, cover and cook for about 45 minutes.

Add the browned pork, make sure that the beans are still covered in liquid, cover and continue to simmer until the stock begins to thicken and the beans are cooked through but still intact (anything up to another hour). Give the pan a shake or stir once in a while to make sure that nothing is catching on the bottom.

If you want a thicker sauce, you can ladle out a couple of spoonfuls of beans and mash them to a paste with the back of a fork or using a hand-held blender, and then stir them back into the pot.

Taste and season. As Leti says, this should be quite a salty dish, which is balanced by all the accompaniments (see below).

FOR THE *FEIJOADA COMPLETA*

Serve with boiled white rice.

Make a tomato vinaigrette (below).

Chop up a couple of oranges into segments (think hockey match half-time rather than dainty dinner party).

Cook up some hearty greens such as spring greens (in Brazil it would be *couve mineira*), slice them finely and then sauté them in oil and garlic.

Serve with some hot chilli sauce.

For the seriously hungry, add a fried egg.

For the truly authentic, track down some coarse manioc or cassava flour and fry it up with some diced onion for the traditional accompaniment, *farofa*.

Fry some plantain slices to serve alongside.

Get hold of some cachaça and limes and stir up some caipirinhas.

TOMATO VINAIGRETTE

3 large tomatoes, diced
1 onion, diced (I use red as it is more digestible, but locals don't seem to worry)
large handful of parsley, roughly chopped
100 ml/3½ fl oz/7 tbsp white wine vinegar
3 tbsp extra-virgin olive oil
salt and pepper

Mix everything together. Yes, it's a lot of vinegar, but you need plenty of acidity to bring the beans to life.

HOW ABOUT?

... ladling off a bit of the stock just before everything is ready. Serve in little shot glasses, to get everyone's mouths watering.

... using a pressure cooker, as Leti does, to speed everything up.

... a bit of gastronomic sacrilege! Prepare it with white beans and you're approaching the traditional Portuguese *feijoada*. Throw in some chorizo and black pudding with your white beans and it's virtually a northern Spanish *fabada*. Just think beans, salted pork, smoky pork and perhaps a touch of salted beef and it'll be delicious in any case.

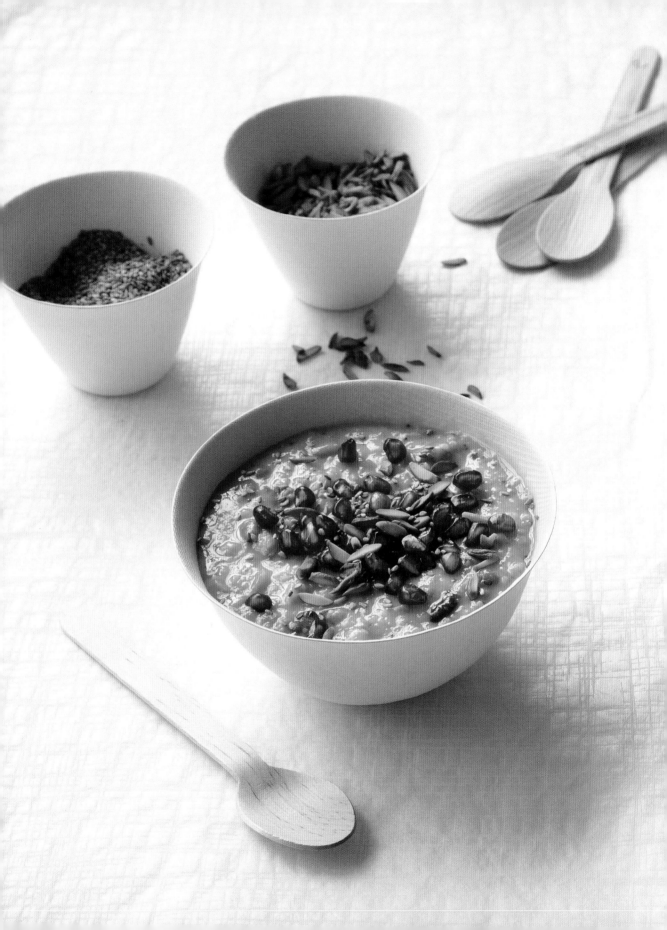

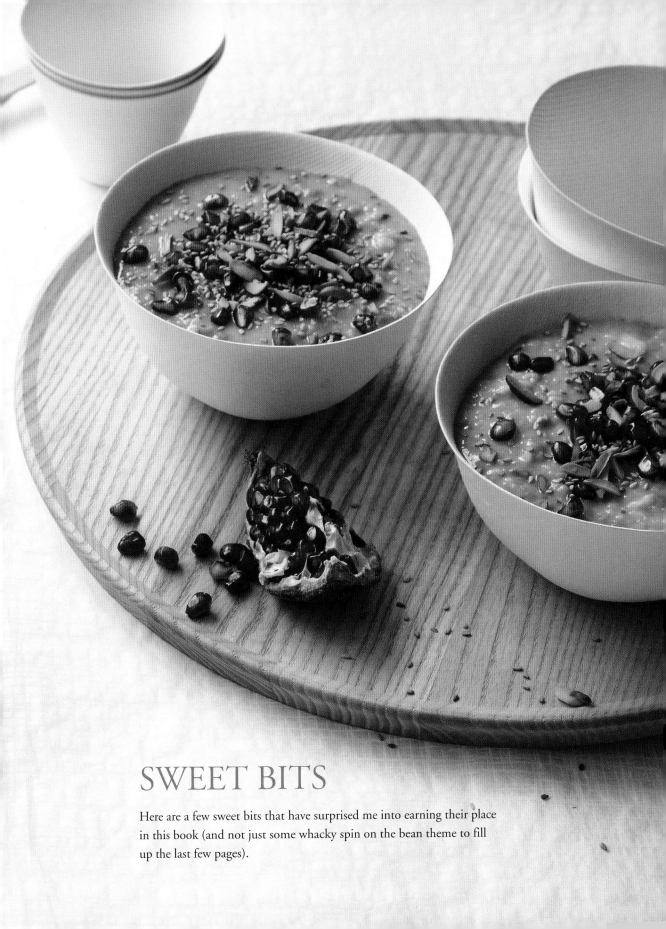

SWEET BITS

Here are a few sweet bits that have surprised me into earning their place
in this book (and not just some whacky spin on the bean theme to fill
up the last few pages).

A legendary dessert that I first stumbled upon in a legendary book, *The Independent Cook* by Jeremy Round. The pudding is an unlikely combination of pulses, wheat, rice and dried fruit that Noah is said to have scraped together from the last provisions left on the Ark as the flood waters subsided. And there's the beauty of the dish – it's a chance to clear out your storecupboard, too.

Ashure is prepared in Turkey, and much of the Middle East, during the Islamic holy month of Muharram. It is loved by Muslims, Christians and Jews alike and is traditionally shared with neighbours as a symbol of peace and generosity. So, all in all, a feel-good dessert. It's not worth making a small quantity. You'll need to begin soaking a day in advance. *Illustrated on pp.234–235.*

NOAH'S PUDDING
ASHURE

Serves 8–10

200 g/7 oz wheat berries (see p.133), soaked overnight

50 g/1¾ oz/¼ cup dried chickpeas, soaked overnight

115 g/4 oz dried haricot (navy), cannellini or butter beans (large lima beans) – a mixture is ideal – soaked overnight

50 g/1¾ oz/¼ cup sultanas, currants or raisins – or a mixture

12 dried apricots, roughly chopped

6 dried figs, stems removed and roughly chopped

50 g/1¾ oz/¼ cup short-grain pudding rice

100 g/3½ oz walnuts, blanched almonds, skinned hazelnuts (ideally a few of each), roughly chopped

280 g/10 oz/1½ cups caster (superfine) sugar

zest of ½ lemon or orange, in very fine strips

2–4 tbsp rosewater

FOR THE TOP

seeds from 1 pomegranate

3 tbsp roughly chopped pistachios, almonds or toasted pine nuts

1 tbsp toasted sesame seeds

Put the wheat berries in a large pot with 2.5 litres/4½ pints/2½ quarts of cold water, bring to the boil and then simmer for about an hour, or until the grains have burst and become quite soft (some wheat berries take longer).

Meanwhile, cook the chickpeas and beans in separate pots until tender (see p.29) and drain. (Perfectionists would have you skin them, but that's up to you.)

Soak all the dried fruit in warm water to cover.

Once the wheat is cooked, remove a few spoonfuls with some of the cooking liquid and purée with a hand-held blender. Add the purée and the rice to the wheat berries and boil for about 15 minutes, stirring from time to time. Add more water if the pudding seems too thick and sticky.

Throw in the beans, chickpeas, fruit and nuts. Stir in three-quarters of the sugar and strips of zest and simmer for about 20 minutes.

Add a little water or milk if the pudding seems very thick (it will set as it cools) and remove from the heat. Add the rosewater and the remaining sugar (or some honey if you prefer) to taste. Leave to cool. Sprinkle with nuts and seeds and serve.

HOW ABOUT?

... a quicker version: substitute pearl barley for the wheat berries and use canned chickpeas and beans in place of home-cooked.

... a creamier version: use half milk, half water to cook the wheat berries and serve with whipped cream.

... a more aromatic version: add 1 teaspoon of ground cinnamon or allspice or 4 crushed cardamom pods along with the rice.

... a fruitier version: top with quarters of fresh fig, slices of apricot and nectarine.

Adzuki beans are incredibly popular throughout East Asia. They are cooked in some savoury dishes, such as the Japanese sticky rice and red bean dish, *sekihan*, that's served at special occasions, but mostly they are eaten as a sweet paste. Red bean paste turns up in all manner of confectionery, pastries and desserts. It's the chocolate of East Asia. I've tried it in a few traditional incarnations, such as Chinese mooncakes and delicate Japanese rice cakes – I'd say they're an acquired taste! But bring on this ice cream, with its Filipino heritage, and I'm smitten.

ADZUKI BEAN ICE CREAM WITH CRYSTALLIZED GINGER

Serves 4

FOR THE RED BEAN PASTE
200 g/7 oz/1 cup adzuki beans
175 g/6 oz/generous ¾ cup caster (superfine) sugar
good pinch of salt
about 50 g/1¾ oz crystallized ginger, cut into wafer-thin
　　slices, to serve

FOR THE ICE CREAM
570 ml/1 pint/scant 2½ cups full-fat milk
300 ml/10 fl oz/1¼ cups double (heavy) cream
225 g/8 oz/generous 1 cup caster (superfine) sugar
8 egg yolks (yes, it's time for a meringue frenzy)
few drops of vanilla extract

To make the red bean paste: put the beans in a pan of cold water and bring to the boil, turn off the heat and leave for 5 minutes and then drain. (Purists repeat this process, but I found no noticeable difference when I did a taste test.)

Start again and this time simmer the beans until tender, around 40 minutes to 1 hour. The beans should still be whole but will squash to a creamy paste between your fingers. At this stage, the beans should still just be submerged in water.

Add the sugar and salt (some recipes call for equal quantities of beans and sugar, so if you have a *really* sweet tooth, go ahead) and stir the beans as they simmer. Mash with the back of a spoon and cook until the sugary water has almost disappeared. Drag a spoon across the bottom of the pan; it should leave a clear track.

Now you can blitz the beans in a blender to make them smooth or leave them textured, as I prefer; both are traditional. Spoon the paste into a bowl to cool.

To make the ice cream: put the milk, cream and sugar in a pan and slowly bring to the boil. Don't leave the pan, or it will suddenly froth up.

Meanwhile, beat the egg yolks and vanilla together in a large bowl. Pour the scalding-hot milk mixture over the yolks, whisking all the time, and then strain the mixture back into the pan. Stir over a low heat until the mixture thickens enough to coat the back of a spoon and then tip back into the bowl.

Whisk in about 250 g/9 oz of the red bean paste and leave to cool. Pour the cooled mixture into an ice-cream maker to churn. Freeze until ready to serve.

Serve with slithers of crystallized ginger.

HOW ABOUT?

... cheating! No ice-cream maker? Buy a tub of good-quality vanilla ice cream, leave it to soften just a little and then whizz it up with the red bean paste in a food processor. Refreeze until ready to use.

... using the leftover red bean paste to sandwich between tiny Scotch (American-style) pancakes – the Japanese do something similar.

... upping the game: make one quantity of adzuki bean ice cream and then make another batch, replacing the vanilla and red bean paste with 3 teaspoons of *matcha*. This fine green tea powder from Japan gives a fabulous flavour and an amazing green colour. Just whisk the powder into the custard before it cools and churn as before. Serve the two ice creams together – a showstopper.

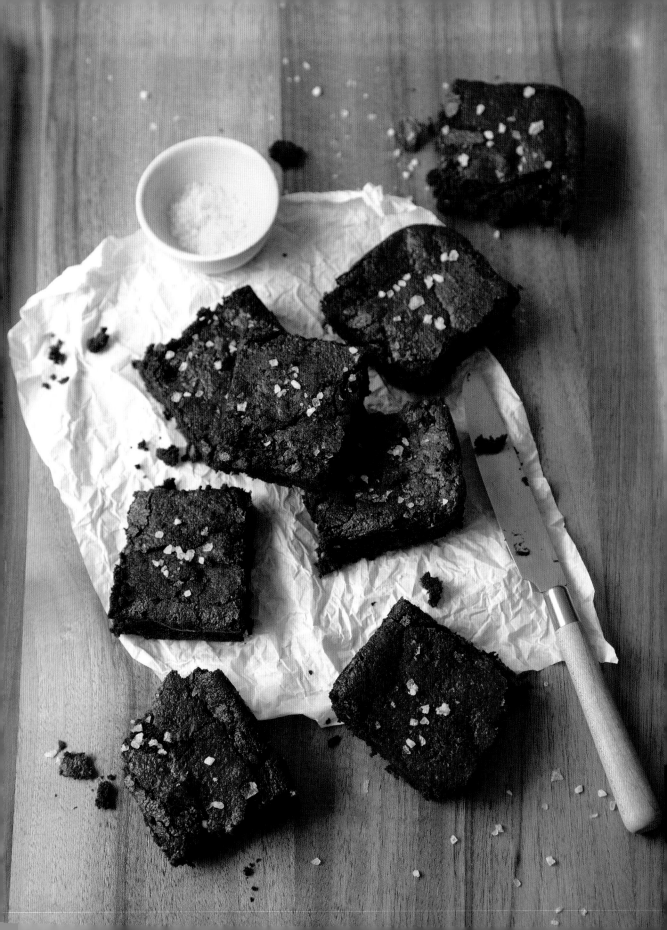

West Coast Americans got into a frenzy of excitement about beany brownies a couple of years ago and of course I had to find out why. To be honest, the idea of a 'healthy', butter-free, low-fat brownie seemed like a sad aberration, why not eat an apple instead? But a fabulously juicy brownie that just happens to contain beans instead of flour, making it more delicious, more nutritious and available to all the coeliacs out there, well, now you're talking.

BLACK BEAN BROWNIES

Makes 12–16 brownies

200 g/7 oz dark chocolate, broken into small pieces

140 g/5 oz/generous ½ cup unsalted butter, cut into small cubes

1 tbsp unsweetened cocoa powder

2 tsp vanilla extract

1 x 400 g/14 oz can of black beans or 250 g/9 oz home-cooked black beans

3 eggs

85 g/3 oz roughly chopped walnuts, pecans, pistachios or almonds

200 g/7 oz/1 cup caster (superfine) sugar

1 tsp sea salt for sprinkling

Preheat the oven to 180°C/350°F/Gas mark 4. Butter a 24-cm/9½-in square baking tin or line with baking parchment.

Melt the chocolate and butter together in a large bowl placed over a pan of simmering water or in the microwave on low. Leave to cool a little, then add the cocoa and vanilla.

Meanwhile, blend the beans with the one of the eggs in a food processor or using a hand-held blender. The mixture should be as smooth as possible, otherwise the brownies will have a mealy texture. Gradually stir the bean mixture and the nuts into the chocolate.

Beat the remaining eggs with the sugar until light and creamy, and then fold into the brownie mixture.

Pour into the tin, sprinkle with salt and bake for about 25–30 minutes, until just set but still a little wobbly.

Place the tin on a wire rack and leave to cool completely before attempting to cut up into small squares. (If the brownies seem very gooey, placing them in the fridge for half an hour will make them easier to slice.) In the unlikely event of leftovers, you can keep the brownies in an airtight container for up to 5 days.

HOW ABOUT?

... adding chunks of white chocolate and dried fruit such as sour cherries or cranberries.

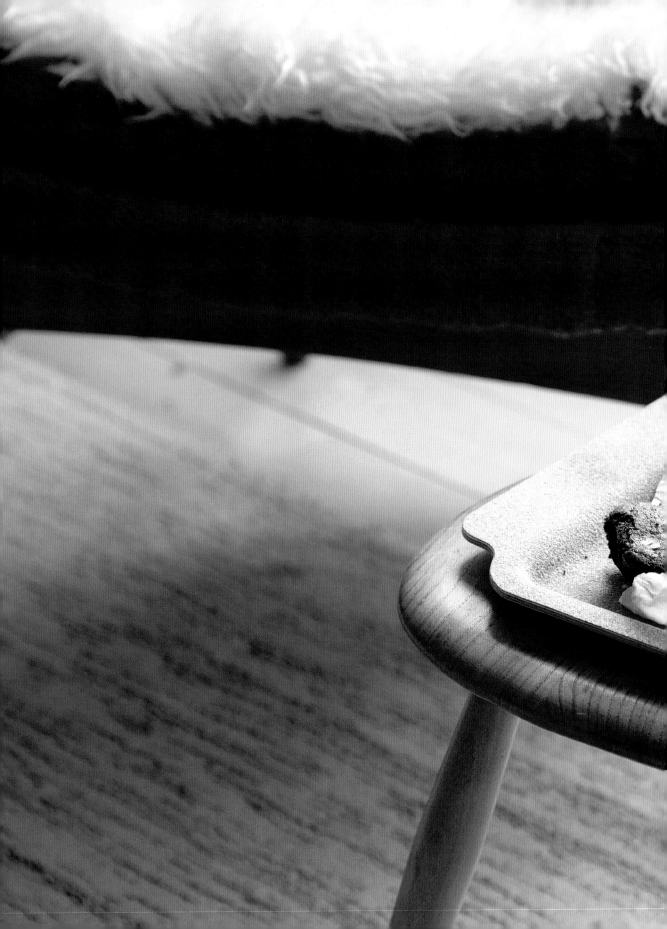

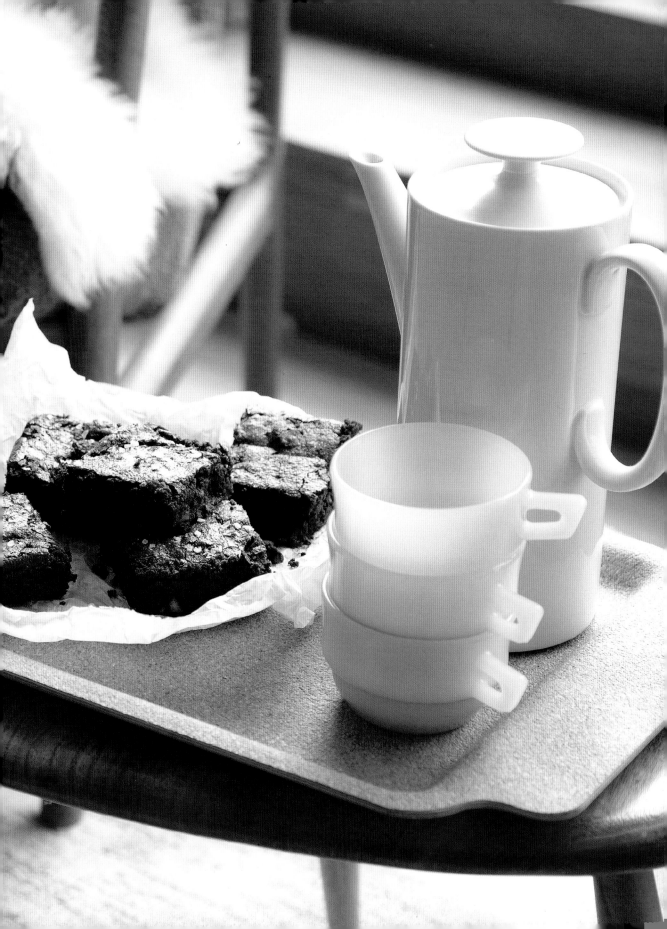

SAUCES, SALSAS AND SEASONINGS

MAYONNAISE

I never make less than a 2-egg quantity of mayonnaise, it's just too fiddly. Any leftover will be delicious for up to 5 days if stored in the fridge.

I love the slightly nutty flavour of rapeseed oil – do buy cold-pressed, it tastes so much better – but you could use any light vegetable oil.

Makes 300 ml/10 fl oz/1¼ cups
2 egg yolks
1 tsp Dijon mustard
300 ml/10 fl oz/1¼ cups rapeseed oil, or a mixture of
    light olive oil and rapeseed oil
juice of ½ lemon
salt and pepper

Mix the yolks and mustard together in a large bowl. Now whisk in the oil extremely slowly, literally drip by drip to begin with, and then as the mixture begins to thicken you can continue in a thin, steady stream.

Once you have added about half of the oil and the mayo has become stiff and wobbly, beat in the lemon juice.

Gradually pour in the remaining oil, whisking all the time. Season with salt and pepper to taste and add a touch more lemon juice if required.

Aioli

Fabulous with all things fishy. Catalans won't approve; their *allioli* contains no egg yolk – the large dose of garlic is enough to emulsify the oil – but I favour the Provençal approach. Using a light olive oil and a few tablespoons of a more characterful extra-virgin olive oil will give the aioli its true Mediterranean flavour.

Use the mayonnaise recipe above, incorporating 2–3 very well-crushed garlic cloves right at the beginning along with the mustard.

Citrus mayonnaise

For a super-lemony mayo, add the lemon zest as well as the juice. Seville orange or lime juices and zests are delicious too.

Herb mayonnaise

Not everyone loves garlic; sometimes a herbed mayonnaise is a great option. Use the mayonnaise recipe above, adding a couple of tablespoons of chopped herbs. Try:
• chervil and dill
• tarragon, parsley and chives
• basil, zest and juice of ½ lime (instead of the lemon)
    You could up the ante with a teaspoon or so of grated fresh ginger, horseradish or wasabi.

SALSA VERDE

Piquant and fresh, Italian salsa verde is the perfect way to zip up beans and lentils. It also makes a great partner for richer meats and fish such as lamb and salmon.

Makes about 200 ml/7 fl oz/generous ¾ cup
large handful of fresh parsley, roughly chopped
2½ tbsp capers
6 anchovy fillets, chopped
2 garlic cloves, finely chopped
1 tsp Dijon mustard
2 tbsp red wine vinegar or 1 tbsp lemon juice
6–8 tbsp extra-virgin olive oil
salt and pepper

Place all the ingredients together in a food processor and pulse until you have a rough pesto consistency. Go easy on the salt as the capers and anchovies can be very salty.

HOW ABOUT?

... adding extra greenery: try chives, basil, mint, oregano or tarragon.
... substituting cornichons and green olives for the anchovies and capers.

ROMESCO

This Catalan dried pepper and nut sauce is fabulous with a white bean salad, great with roasted vegetables and sublime with fish. Romesco will keep for up to 4 days, covered in a layer of oil, in the fridge.

You could use dried ñoras peppers from a specialist Spanish supplier, Mexican ancho chillies (a different but very delicious flavour), or opt for the easier-to-find dried paprika.

Makes about 400 ml/14 fl oz/1¾ cups

6 dried ñoras peppers or ancho chillies, destemmed,
    or 1 tbsp sweet (not smoked) paprika
1–2 hot dried chillies
2 tomatoes
½ bulb of garlic, divided into cloves
50 g/1¾ oz/scant ½ cup blanched almonds
50 g/1¾ oz /scant ½ cup hazelnuts, without skins
150 ml/5 fl oz/⅔ cup extra-virgin olive oil
1 slice of rustic white bread (optional)
4–6 tbsp red wine vinegar
large pinch of salt

Preheat the oven to 180°C/350°F/Gas mark 4.

Cover the ñoras peppers or ancho chillies and the hot chillies in boiling water and leave to soak.

Place the tomatoes and garlic cloves (skin on) on a baking sheet and roast until just beginning to soften, about 20 minutes. Set aside to cool.

On a separate baking sheet, toast the almonds and hazelnuts. They will take between 5 and 10 minutes to turn golden. Set the timer or you will forget – burnt nuts are an expensive mistake.

Drain and chop the dried peppers; don't worry too much about the seeds, you can discard some of them if you like.

Heat the oil in a frying pan and cook the peppers in the oil for a couple of minutes (if using paprika, you will just be frying the hot chilli). Remove from the pan and place in a food processor or blender.

Fry the bread in the same oil; the idea is to soak up the chilli-flavoured oil and toast the bread at the same time. Break up the bread and throw this into the blender too. You can leave out the bread for a thinner sauce.

Add the nuts, the paprika (if using), the tomatoes and the garlic flesh (just squeeze it like a purée from the cloves) to the blender with the peppers and bread. Pour in half of the vinegar, a little salt and half of the oil. Blitz the mixture until it is fairly smooth and then add the remaining oil.

Taste and adjust the salt, vinegar and oil; you may even want a little extra paprika or chilli to zip it up.

GUACAMOLE

This lusciously creamy combination is a must with almost every Mexican and Latino bean combination. Leave it rough and chunky.

Your avocados must be really ripe, so buy them a few days in advance and put them in a paper bag or wrap in newspaper if you need to speed up ripening. Adding a banana or an apple to the bag will help the ripening too. No ripe avocados? Make a tomato salsa instead.

Serves 4

½ red onion, very finely diced
1–2 chillies, diced very finely
juice of 1–2 limes
2–3 ripe avocados (depending on size)
3 tomatoes, diced
handful of coriander (cilantro) leaves, roughly chopped
salt and pepper

Place half of the onion and chilli in a bowl and tip over the juice of 1 lime.

Now peel and roughly chop the avocados, add them to the bowl and mash roughly with the back of a fork. Stir in the tomatoes, most of the coriander and some salt and pepper.

Taste and balance the guacamole with more onion, chilli, lime juice, salt and pepper as required.

PESTO

What a difference between shop-bought and homemade. Even the 'freshly made' pesto from the deli doesn't begin to compare. Pesto tastes extraordinarily good within hours of making and then quickly loses its magic.

Makes about 200 ml/7 fl oz/generous ¾ cup
large bunch of basil leaves
2 garlic cloves, peeled
pinch of sea salt
3 tbsp finely chopped Parmesan cheese
2 tbsp pine nuts
100 ml/3½ fl oz/7 tbsp extra-virgin olive oil

Blend all the ingredients together. Purists will use a pestle and mortar, I just pulse mine in a small food processor and leave it quite rough and textured.

TOMATO SALSAS

These make fabulous accompaniments to beans; the sweet, sour, spicy blend is just what a pulse screams out for. You could quite simply take 250 g/9 oz drained beans (canned or home-cooked), add one of the salsas below and an extra slosh of extra-virgin olive oil and you have a salad to go.

Mexican style

Great with black beans, pinto beans, red kidney beans and basically anything from the Latino, Mexican and Caribbean world.

Serves 4
6 medium tomatoes or 12–15 cherry tomatoes,
    roughly chopped
½ red onion, finely diced
1 red or green chilli, finely diced (optional)
juice of ½–1 lime
small bunch of coriander (cilantro), finely chopped
2–3 tbsp extra-virgin olive oil
½ tsp salt
pinch of sugar (optional)

Mix everything together except the sugar. Taste and season with more chilli, lime juice and salt if necessary. You may not need sugar if the tomatoes are very sweet.

HOW ABOUT?

... using any green tomatoes that don't ripen: they give a lovely tart flavour to the salsa.

Italian style

Best with borlotti, cannellini, butter beans, haricots, chickpeas, firm lentils.

Serves 4
6 medium tomatoes or 12–15 cherry tomatoes,
    roughly chopped
½ red onion, finely diced
2 tbsp capers, rinsed and chopped
1 red or green chilli, finely diced (optional)
small bunch of parsley, finely chopped
1–2 tbsp balsamic vinegar
4 tbsp extra-virgin olive oil
½ tsp salt

Tumble everything together in a bowl, holding back on the salt, as your capers may be very salty. Taste and adjust the seasoning if necessary.

French style

Delicious with haricots, flageolets, borlotti (be sure to call them *haricots coco roses*, it sounds so elegant), chickpeas and Puy lentils.

Serves 4
6 medium tomatoes or 12–15 cherry tomatoes,
    roughly chopped
1–2 shallots, finely diced
small bunch of parsley, leaves finely chopped
small bunch of tarragon, leaves finely chopped
a few chives, finely chopped
1–2 tbsp red wine vinegar
1 tbsp Dijon mustard
4 tbsp extra-virgin olive oil

½ tsp salt

plenty of freshly ground black pepper

1 tsp honey or sugar (optional)

Put the tomatoes, shallots and herbs into a bowl. Place all the remaining ingredients in a jar with a tightly fitting lid and give it a good shake. Taste and adjust the seasoning. Tip over the tomatoes and stir carefully.

RED ONION MARMALADE

Particularly delicious with lentils; add a bit of goat's cheese and you have a meal. Stored in sterilized jars, this will keep for weeks unrefrigerated. However, when I make it I tend to fill a large Kilner jar, keep it in the fridge and it's always gone within the week.

Makes about 300 ml/10 fl oz/1¼ cups

3 tbsp olive oil

6 red onions, sliced

salt and pepper

150 ml/5 fl oz/⅔ cup red wine

4 tbsp balsamic vinegar

2 tbsp muscovado or light brown sugar

Warm the oil in a large, heavy pan with a lid. Add the onions with a good pinch of salt and plenty of pepper. Cover and cook over a medium heat for about 30 minutes. Remove the lid after the first 10 minutes and remember to stir once in a while so that the onions don't catch and burn.

Add wine, vinegar and sugar, turn up the heat and simmer for 20–30 minutes, until the liquid has almost disappeared. Taste and season with more salt and pepper if required.

HARISSA

Call me a wimp, but those tubes of traditional harissa are just too hot for me. I want to taste the aromatic spicing as well as feel the heat. By adding some inauthentic roasted peppers to the paste, the whole thing is lengthened and heat is taken down a notch or two. Stir it into soups, dollop into a bowl of chickpeas with yesterday's leftover lamb and a pile of fresh coriander, or add to dips and purées for a bit of fire.

Makes about 200 ml/7 fl oz/generous ¾ cup

1 tsp cumin seeds

1 tsp coriander seeds

1 tsp caraway seeds

2 red peppers, roasted, peeled and seeded (see p.249)

about 12 dried red chillies, or to taste

2 garlic cloves, crushed

4 tbsp extra-virgin olive oil

juice of ½ lemon

salt

Heat a dry frying pan over a medium heat, add the cumin, coriander and caraway seeds and toast until they are fantastically aromatic. Pound them in a pestle and mortar or whizz in a spice grinder until finely ground.

Blitz the peppers together with the ground spices, chillies, garlic, oil and lemon juice in a blender or food processor and season with salt to taste. The paste should still put hairs on your chest, otherwise it really isn't harissa. Store, covered, in the fridge for up to 1 week.

TARATOR

This Middle Eastern tahini (a paste made from ground sesame seeds) and lemon sauce is the classic accompaniment to felafel (see p.50) and takes just a minute to make. It goes well with anything to do with chickpeas.

Serves 4–6

5 tbsp tahini

juice of 1–2 lemons

2–3 tbsp water

2 garlic cloves, crushed

2 tbsp finely chopped flat-leaf parsley

salt

Put the tahini in a bowl and gradually mix in the lemon juice and water a tablespoon at a time, alternating between the two to get the right balance of flavour at the same time as creating a thick creamy consistency. Add the garlic, parsley and salt to taste.

ZA'ATAR

Za'atar isn't just the Arabic name for the wild thyme that grows in the Middle East, but also for the extraordinarily delicious mix of dried thyme, sesame seeds and sumac, a sour, red ground spice, which you can get from specialist spice suppliers, Middle Eastern stores and some supermarkets. Try this sprinkled on flatbreads with a dash of olive oil, with a poached egg, with roast vegetables, or best of all with hummus.

Makes a small pot (about 8 tbsp)

4 tbsp sesame seeds

2 tbsp dried thyme

2 tbsp sumac

about 1 tsp salt

Heat a dry frying pan over a medium heat, add the sesame seeds and roast until they begin to pop and smell toasty.

Pour the hot seeds into a pestle and mortar. Add the thyme and the sumac and pound together for a moment while everything is warm. Add salt to taste and leave to cool completely. Best eaten within a couple of days but can be stored in a jar for up to a month.

RAITA AND TZATZIKI

These yogurt-based dips or sauces are close cousins; raita from the Indian subcontinent and tzatziki from the eastern Mediterranean. Recipes vary, but both usually contain cucumber. Beware, north European/greenhouse cucumbers are much more watery than the local varieties, so do take the time to remove the seeds or the yogurt will be very runny. Some cooks like to strain their yogurt too, but I find if I use a thick, full-fat Greek-style yogurt, there's no need.

Raita

Makes a wonderful cooling partner for a spicy curry and a refreshing accompaniment to fried food.

Serves 4

200 g/7 oz/generous ¾ cup Greek yogurt, or plain yogurt
   for a lighter option

½ small cucumber, peeled, seeds removed and diced

handful of fresh coriander (cilantro), chopped

salt and pepper

OPTIONAL EXTRAS

3 fresh green chillies, finely sliced

1 tsp cumin seeds, roasted

2 tomatoes, deseeded and diced

Combine the yogurt, cucumber and coriander and season with salt and pepper to taste.

And if you want to add a little pizzazz to the raita, then throw in some chilli, cumin and tomatoes.

HOW ABOUT?

... adding 3–4 tbsp freshly grated coconut or unsweetened desiccated coconut, along with some toasted mustard seeds and grated fresh ginger. Fabulous with bhajia (see p.56).

Tzatziki

Adds a little luxurious creaminess to the *meze* table and is especially good with felafel (see p.50) or Syrian-style lentils (see p.36).

Serves 4

200 g/7 oz/generous ¾ cup Greek yogurt, or plain yogurt
   for a lighter option

½ small cucumber, peeled, seeds removed, and diced

2 garlic cloves, chopped

handful of fresh mint, chopped

handful of fresh dill, chopped

salt and pepper

Combine the yogurt, cucumber, garlic and herbs. Season with salt and pepper to taste.

FRESH MANGO PICKLE

Traditional sweet mango chutney has its place, but I often crave the fresh, sour flavours of this fabulous pickle from Kerala, southern India. The acidity cuts through the richness of fried foods such as pakora and dosa just brilliantly.

You can buy 'raw' mangoes in Asian shops; these small green mangoes are ideal but I've found that an unripe supermarket mango works just fine too.

Serves 4

2 tbsp vegetable oil
2 tsp black mustard seeds
1 tsp urad dal, skinned and split, or red lentils at a push
10 curry leaves
5 tbsp diced shallots
2 green chillies, finely diced – seeds left in or scraped out,
    depending on how hot you like it
large pinch of ground turmeric
salt
2 unripe mangoes, or about 4 raw mangoes, cut into needles
3 tbsp lemon or lime juice
1–2 tbsp white wine vinegar (optional)

Heat the oil in a large frying pan. Throw in the mustard seeds and as soon as they begin to hop around, add the urad dal and curry leaves. Fry until the little split beans begin to colour; they give a wonderful crunch to the pickle.

Add the shallots and chillies, cook for a couple of minutes, and then sprinkle in the turmeric and a pinch of salt.

Stir in the mango. If you're using raw mangoes, you should cook the pickle for a few minutes to soften the fruit a bit. If your mango is a slightly softer, larger type, then just warming the flesh through will be enough.

Add the citrus juice and a touch more salt to taste. And, if you didn't manage to find raw mangoes, a dash of vinegar will sharpen up the pickle too.

TAMARIND PASTE

The sweet, sour, almost caramel flavour of tamarind is adored in much of southern India, Asia and Mexico. Many of us are well acquainted with the flavour without even knowing it: tamarind plays a starring role in Worcestershire sauce and is said to be one of Coca Cola's secret ingredients. The sour paste, when teamed with sweet palm sugar or jaggery (concentrated, unrefined sugar cane juice), is magic in a fabulous yin and yang way.

You often see the pale brown pods of tamarind seeds piled up in Asian stores. The brittle pod encases the sticky flesh surrounding little pebble-like seeds (you'll need a filling if you bite on one). You just need to soak this flesh (seeds and all) in a little hot water for about 10 minutes, and then, using the back of a fork, squash the paste through a sieve, leaving behind the fibre and seeds. Follow the same procedure with the blocks of tamarind pulp you find in Asian stores; these will keep in the fridge for months once opened. The DIY paste is so much tastier – and cheaper – than the concentrate or ready-made stuff.

You can use the paste stirred into soda water for a lip-puckeringly refreshing summer drink, as well as in all the amazing southern Asian soups, dals and curries.

GARAM MASALA

Every north Indian family will have its own blend of *garam*, 'warming', spices. Warming refers to spices that are believed to create heat in the body, rather than chilli heat. OK, you can buy garam masala ready ground and mixed, but since it stales rather quickly, there's nothing like grinding your own blend. That's as long as your spices haven't been lurking in the back of your cupboard for a decade. Buy spices whole and try to use within the year.

1 tbsp cardamom seeds – or the seeds from 2 tbsp
    cardamom pods
1 cinnamon stick, broken up as much as possible
1 tsp black peppercorns
1 tsp whole cloves
1 tsp cumin seeds
1 tsp fennel seeds
¼ of a nutmeg – crack it with a good bash of the rolling pin
1 bay leaf

Place everything in a spice grinder and grind until you have a fine powder. If you're using a pestle and mortar, you will certainly have a workout and you will need to sieve the spices before storing. Keep in an airtight jar in a cool, dark cupboard for up to 2 months.

BASICS

BREADCRUMBS

We should all have a ready supply of breadcrumbs for crisp toppings, crusts and to use in recipes such as bean burgers (see p.66). Forget about those pricey pots of goldfish food from the supermarket; making your own breadcrumbs costs next to nothing.

When we teach bread classes at the Bertinet Kitchen cookery school, we recommend that people keep their bread in a fabric bag, as they do in many parts of Europe. If you put your bread in a clammy bread bin, it will go mouldy rather than dry. Bread goes through different stages: day 1 – fresh and soft; day 2 – great for toasting; day 3 – ideal for crostini, bruschetta, etc.; day 4 – if there's anything left over – you make breadcrumbs. A sourdough loaf's lifespan is even longer and the breadcrumbs are fabulous.

Break or slice the stale bread into smallish pieces. If the bread is not completely dry, pop it into a warm oven to dry out and become brittle, then whizz it in a food processor until really fine and store in a jar or airtight container.

You can make fresh breadcrumbs for stuffings and fillings by blitzing 2- or 3-day-old bread in the food processor. Keep the crumbs in a bag in the freezer.

ADDING CHILLI HEAT
Chillies and other peppers

A little chilli heat or peppery warmth can really lift a bowl of beans, but go carefully, as we all have very different levels of heat tolerance. When cooking for the family, I often serve my six-year-old and then add a dash of Tabasco or other chilli sauce to the pot for the rest of us.

If you're using a fresh green or red chilli, you need to remember that the capsaicin (the compound that creates the burning sensation), and therefore the heat levels, vary dramatically between different varieties and individual crops. So taste a chilli before throwing it into the pot with wild abandon. Have a little milk or yogurt or a spoonful of sugar at the ready in case you need to calm your tongue. The tip is the mildest part of the chilli so start there, tasting a minuscule piece. If your mouth is burning, you will probably want to slice open the chilli and scrape out the pithy membrane and seeds. Try to handle only the outer skin of the chilli to avoid burning your fingertips too. If the tip has no bite at all, then taste a tiny piece of the pithy membrane (the hottest part of the chilli) to be sure that you want to unleash its heat into the dish.

Dried chillies, chilli flakes, cayenne pepper and hot paprika can all add a bit of fire and are usually added during the cooking so that their heat permeates the entire dish.

Turkish Urfa chilli flakes and Aleppo chilli flakes from Syria are a recent discovery for me and I'm addicted. They are fairly mild, with a slightly oily, chewy texture and a sweet raisiny taste. They're great to add to salads or towards the end of the cooking time.

Spanish paprika can be hot, bitter-sweet or mild and – surprising to some – it's not all smoked. Look at the tin carefully before buying. A little smoky heat works incredibly well with pork and seafood dishes.

Two other Spanish peppers to look out for are the pickled *guindillas* and roasted *piquillos*. Both come in jars or cans, or you can sometimes buy them loose from the deli. The long green *guindillas* can be quite fiery and sharp. They're traditionally served alongside your beans, great to bite into for an exhilarating heat rush between mouthfuls. *Piquillo* peppers look more like miniature capsicums and are ideal for stuffing or chopping up into salads. Their flavour is bitter-sweet and slightly smoked.

The Mexicans use dozens of different peppers. My favourite, and rather conveniently one of the most widely available, is the chipotle, a smoked and dried jalapeño pepper. You can sometimes buy whole dried chipotle peppers: you will need to soak them in warm water for about 20 minutes before chopping up to add to your dish. Alternatively you may be able to track down small cans of chipotles in adobo (tomato and onion sauce), chipotle ketchup or chipotle purées and pastes. All will have different degrees of heat and smoke, so do taste before using.

POACHING THE PERFECT EGG

Now, it is up to you how you poach your eggs; every chef, food writer and home cook seems to have a different approach and a strong opinion to go with it. So, if you have a foolproof method, just stick to it.

I poach mine individually in a pan of salted water. I crack an egg into a small cup, add a drop of vinegar to the boiling water, whisk the water to create a whirlpool effect, slip in the egg, turn down the heat and barely simmer for 2–3 minutes (or just 1 minute for a quail's egg). At this point, you can scoop the egg out with a slotted spoon and set aside for a few minutes on some kitchen paper while you cook any remaining eggs. If serving in a hot soup, the egg will soon warm through; alternatively you can dunk all your eggs back in the pan of hot water just before serving.

If you're feeding a crowd, poached eggs can be kept in a bowl of water in the fridge and then plunged en masse into boiling water just before serving. Just be sure to slightly undercook the eggs first time around.

BOILED EGGS

All too often salads are topped with desperately unappetizing hard-boiled eggs, with powdery grey-tinged yolks and a waft of the school chemistry lab. Here is the simple key to a bright, barely set yolk every time. A medium egg will take just 7 minutes: lower into boiling water, time from the moment the water comes back to the boil and then, once the time is up, place in a bowl of cold water. Follow the same procedure for quails' eggs but boil for just 3 minutes.

ROASTED PEPPERS

The natural sweet flavour and creamy texture of roast peppers is unbeatable. If you're after sweetness, then remember to go for red, orange or yellow peppers. Green peppers are unripe and so, even roasted, their bitter tang will come through (it's just the ticket for certain dishes).

I definitely prefer to roast rather than grill my peppers: the process takes a bit longer but it allows the flesh to soften and sweeten up beautifully. Try to prepare your peppers when you have the oven on for another job; they will keep for at least 3 days in the fridge.

Preheat the oven to 200°C/400°F/Gas mark 6.

Throw the peppers into a roasting pan and put about a tablespoon of olive oil into your hand. Turn the peppers in your hands to give them a light oiling. Roast the peppers for about 30 minutes, turning them once, until the skin is thoroughly blistered and starting to blacken. I can't be faffing about with plastic bags, so I just pile up the peppers in their roasting pan and cover with an upturned bowl or saucepan as they cool (the steam helps the skins to loosen for easy peeling).

Once cool, cut the peppers in half, reserving all those ambrosial juices, remove the seeds and peel off the skins.

SEMI-DRIED TOMATOES

This is a highly extravagant, but extraordinarily delicious, thing to do with tomatoes. Having said that, sun-blush, sun-kissed, or whatever they like to call them, tomatoes from the deli counter are astoundingly pricey too. Make these during the summer tomato glut (I have 91-year-old Royston to thank for my annual tomato mountain) or when they're going cheap. Cherry tomatoes are perfect and quicker to dry out, but any ripe and tasty tomato is very good.

Preheat the oven to 120°C/250°F/Gas mark ½.

Cut your tomatoes in half (or quarters if using larger ones) and give them a little squeeze to remove a bit of juice (if you're preparing a large quantity, you might end up with enough for a miniature Bloody Mary as a treat).

Lay the tomatoes on a baking sheet, cut side up. Don't crowd them, otherwise they will sweat rather than roast. Sprinkle with equal quantities of salt and sugar and a good grinding of black pepper. Place in the oven for 2 hours, longer for really large tomatoes, or until they are fairly dry but still soft. Remove from the baking sheet at once otherwise the caramelized sugar will stick like glue. Use immediately or place in a sterilized jar, cover with olive oil and store in the fridge for a couple of weeks.

HOW ABOUT?

... sprinkling some fresh herbs such as thyme or rosemary over the tomatoes before they go into the oven.
... adding a dribble of balsamic vinegar instead of the sugar.
... devouring on toast right away with some cheat's creamy beans (see p.40).

HAM HOCKS

Pork and pulses are natural partners and nothing could be more useful, or economical, than cooking a few ham hocks. The cooking water will provide fabulous stock for soups, purées and risottos, and the meat (which will keep in the fridge for 5 days) can end up in salads, sandwiches or soups, and can even provide Sunday lunch.

Hocks (the pig's ankle, just above the trotter) are sold smoked or unsmoked – I prefer the latter. Either way, it is always best to soak them for a few hours just in case they are excessively salty. Butchers sell cooked or raw hocks; it's best to ask for a 'gammon' hock if you want to cook it, as 'ham' usually refers to cooked meat.

2 or 3 gammon hocks, soaked in cold water for 4 hours
1 carrot, halved
1 onion, halved
1 celery stalk, halved
1 leek, halved
12 peppercorns
1 bouquet garni

Put the hocks and all the remaining ingredients into a large saucepan and cover with cold water. Bring to the boil over a medium heat, then turn the heat right down and simmer for 2–4 hours (hocks vary in size enormously), skimming off the frothy scum from time to time, until the meat is really tender and falls from the bone.

Once cool, store the ham in the fridge; it will keep better whole. Keep the cooking water in the fridge too.

CRISPED JAMÓN

These crispy shards are fabulous on top of canapés, salads and soups, or on grilled fish. *Jamón serrano* and prosciutto, the Spanish and Italian cured hams, have an amazingly complex depth of sweet and salty flavours, and either work fine here. I generally go for *jamón* – but don't use the exquisite (and expensive) *jamón ibérico*: it's virtually sacrilege to do anything but savour it in its raw state.

You can keep the crisped ham in an airtight container for a couple of days (it should be really brittle, so just re-crisp in a hot oven if it has softened).

Preheat the oven to 180°C/350°F/Gas mark 4.

Lay the ham slices in a single layer on a baking sheet covered with greaseproof paper or a non-stick baking sheet. Check the ham after about 5 minutes; it will begin to buckle in places and it's sometimes good to turn it over if it is cooking unevenly. Put it back in the oven and check at 2-minute intervals – this would be a very costly cremation. Once the ham feels crisp, remove from the baking sheet and cool on a wire rack. Store in an airtight container.

POACHED CHICKEN BREASTS

Juicy poached chicken is great in any number of salads, such as chicken, edamame, melon and blueberry (see p.131). A few slices of the tender breast can be added to vegetarian salads to keep those stubborn carnivores happy too.

Place the chicken breasts in a pan, add enough cold water to cover them and pop in some stock powder or ½ stock cube (if I have a few parsley stalks and ½ onion I'll throw those in too). Bring the liquid up to a simmer and bubble gently for 8–12 minutes, depending on the size of your breasts (the chicken's, of course). Check one of the breasts: it should feel quite firm to the touch, but it will continue to cook in the liquid. Remove the pan from the heat and leave the breasts in the poaching liquid for about 15 minutes.

Remove from the stock, check that the chicken is fully cooked, and eat right away or chill until you're ready to use.

DUCK LEGS: CONFIT OR ROAST

There's no doubt about it, confit of duck is absolutely delicious but preparing it at home is quite an undertaking. There's nothing particularly tricky about the method, it's the sheer quantity of goose or duck fat involved: it will probably cost as much as the duck legs themselves. Although you can reuse the fat for about three more batches of confit, it's just another thing to find space for. However, you may love the idea of a jar of preserved duck legs lurking in the larder to dive into at a later date.

So, here I give you two options. Cassoulet purists will stick with the traditional confit – which does give the most melt-in-the-mouth flesh imaginable – while most of us will happily roast the duck, with wonderful results. Either way you need to begin with the salt cure 12 hours before you cook the duck. Depending on the size of your duck legs – and your pans – you can prepare up to 8–10 duck legs at the same time.

For the salt cure
2 tbsp coarse sea salt
½ tbsp black peppercorns, crushed
1 tsp juniper berries, crushed
2 sprigs of thyme, leaves removed from stalks
2 bay leaves, roughly chopped or ripped

Place the duck in a large bowl, lidded container or plastic bag and sprinkle over the salt, spices and herbs. Turn the legs to coat them well. Leave in the fridge for 12–24 hours.

To confit (or preserve) the duck:
Preheat the oven to 110°C/225°F/Gas mark ¼.

Take 1.5 kg/about 3¼ lb duck or goose fat, available in tins or jars from shops and supermarkets. Melt the fat in a deep ovenproof pan into which you can just fit the duck legs. Wipe all the salt and spices off the legs and place them in the pan, making sure they are completely submerged in fat.

Place in the oven for 2½ hours. The meat should fall away from the bone when you spear it with a fork. The legs are now ready to be browned for the cassoulet or preserved in their fat for up to a couple of months.

If you are planning to preserve the duck – and that is after all what a confit is all about –then you will require a large sterilized jar or pot. Remove the legs from the pan and set aside. Ladle the fat from the pan into the jar, scooping it off the top and taking care to leave the cooking juices behind. Allow the fat to cool a little before adding the duck, using tongs and not fingers, and ensuring that the meat is completely covered in the fat. Give the pot a good tap to expel any air, leave to cool completely, cover and chill.

Always brown the duck in a pan before serving to crisp up the skin.

To roast the duck:
Preheat the oven to 180°C/350°F/Gas mark 4.

Wipe away the salt and aromatics from the duck legs. Place the legs in a roasting pan with a tablespoon of duck fat or olive oil, just so that they don't stick, and roast for about 1½ hours, until tender and browned.

HOW ABOUT?

… trying the duck, either way, with the Wine-braised lentils (see p.152), Seville orange lentils (see p.152) or Braised haricots with fennel and orange (see p.158).

CHECK YOUR PULSE: THE IDENTIFICATION PARADE

Pulses are the edible seeds of plants from the *Leguminosae* family, such as beans, peas and lentils. These seeds all grow in pods (the fruit of the plant) and in some cases the pods are eaten too. Many pulses or legumes are commonly eaten fresh, such as peas and broad beans, some – such as the Italian borlotti – are left on the plant to semi-dry, but most are fully dried.

The selection of pulses on offer in supermarkets has grown considerably in recent years, health food shops often have a huge choice of shiny beans just waiting to be scooped up, and in some Asian and other ethnic shops the variety can be overwhelming.

There are simply thousands of varieties of pulse, or legume, grown around the world. Heirloom varieties are increasingly popular among gardeners but rarely available to buy. It did make me giggle as I perused the seed catalogues: in Britain we have distinctly unglamorous bean names such as 'Lazy Housewife' and 'District Nurse', while the North Americans are growing the evocative-sounding 'Black Calypso' and 'Red Nightfall' beans. I'll leave the allotment growers to their endless discussions over the differences between a black cow pea and a purple hull. People do seem to get hot under the collar about the ignorance of calling an adzuki a red cow pea, or the great conundrum of whether the mung bean should in fact be referred to as a pea. I had to detangle entire internet forums to come up with the somewhat simplified guide that follows.

This identification parade has been divided into the following categories: chickpeas, lentils, peas, broad beans, other Old World beans, soya beans, New World beans, groundnuts. These are the legumes that you are most likely to come across. Some may require a bit of tracking down but most are widely available.

CHICKPEA, GARBANZO BEAN (*CICER ARIETINUM*)

Chickpeas are a native of the arid Middle East and have been cultivated for about 9,000 years. They are a staple food in a band of countries stretching from North Africa through the Levant to East India. Chickpeas were embraced by the ancient Greeks and Romans and later the Spanish (after they were introduced by the Moors) and now chickpeas are cooked all around the Mediterranean. The Iberians took them to the New World, but they've never begun to compete in popularity with the indigenous beans in the Americas, or in the Far East for that matter.

The name 'chickpea' derives from the Latin *cicer*. It's said that the Roman orator Cicero had a large wart on his chin and the legume was named in its rather dubious honour – or was the great man with the wart named after the chickpea?

Chickpeas can be eaten fresh: they taste like a cross between an edamame and a fresh pea. I've only found them once or twice in Britain, but in the Middle East at harvest time they are snapped up for salads. The Californians are developing a taste for them too, so watch this space.

Desi chickpea, brown chickpea, Bengal gram, kala chana, black chickpea
Desi is the most common type of chickpea grown in Asia and is the closest relation of the wild chickpea. The tiny brown desi chickpea has a tough skin, a nutty, earthy flavour and is higher in fibre than its cousin the Kabuli (see opposite).

In India, this is the most widely used of all the legume family, and this is the variety you'll find in many traditional Asian curries. You'll probably find desi chickpeas only in Asian shops, but you can always substitute the readily available Kabuli chickpea.

Chana dal, daria dal

Chana dal are skinned and split Bengal gram used to make wonderfully creamy dals, a staple of vegetarian India. You can use them in any of the dal recipes (p.154), but do remember to soak for 2–3 hours otherwise they take an age to cook.

Nowadays we tend to associate chana dal primarily with the Indian subcontinent, but they have been found in ancient Egyptian tombs with the mummies – a quick snack for the afterlife.

Roasted chana dal are known as daria dal, a popular ingredient in Indian chutneys and snacks.

Chickpea flour, gram flour, besan

This is ground from the skinned and split chickpeas. It's used widely in India for fried snacks such as pakoras, bhajia and poppadams.

In the Mediterranean, the flour is traditionally made into roasted flatbreads called *socca* or *farinata*, as well as deep-fried nibbles. It's a fabulous ingredient for those on gluten-free diets. You will find chickpea flour in health food shops, Middle Eastern and Asian stores.

Kabuli chickpea

This is the type most of us are familiar with; it is grown in Europe and the Middle East. The chickpeas are pale beige with a wonderfully nutty flavour. There are dozens of varieties of Kabuli chickpeas. The huge *garbanzo lechoso*, or *blanco lechoso*, from Spain is one of my favourites, which I seek out from delis or Spanish suppliers for a special treat. The jars of cooked Spanish chickpeas are fabulous, too; they have such a creamy texture and make the best hummus imaginable (if you're not on a budget).

Many children consume chickpeas on a regular basis without being aware of it. Supermarkets sell hummus in many colours and flavours, ready to dip into with carrot sticks or pile into a sandwich. Making your own hummus takes just a few minutes in a food processor, it's delicious, it's cheap, you know what's in it: it makes sense.

Chickpeas need a long soak and may take up to 4 hours of simmering to become tender. The upside is that, unlike beans, they won't collapse to a mush. It's always worth cooking a large batch, which you can use in several different ways or even freeze some.

Tinned chickpeas are a useful standby; tossed into a salad, curried, made into felafel, stirred up with chorizo. I use them more than any other legume.

LENTIL (*LENS CULINARIS*)

We've been eating lentils since neolithic times, and they were probably the first of all the pulses to be cultivated, in the Fertile Crescent of the Middle East. The Latin name for a lentil, *lens*, gives us the word for the lentil-shaped glass in your camera or spectacles.

Lentils play an important role in European and Middle Eastern kitchens, but in southern Asia they are a staple. Nowadays India is by far the greatest producer and consumer of lentils, where they provide cheap and valuable protein for a huge vegetarian population.

There are dozens of varieties of lentil around the world, so we will deal with the most common or readily available. To complicate matters further, many of the dals of southern Asia that are commonly considered lentils, such as *toor dal* or *urad dal*, are in fact split beans.

Lentils are wonderfully convenient: they require no soaking and cook in anything between 20 and 45 minutes. Why would you buy ready-cooked lentils? Dried lentils are a cinch to prepare and you can control their texture and flavour.

The key things to keep in mind are that tiny, whole lentils tend to hold together well, larger flatter lentils begin to soften and break down more quickly, and hulled split lentils will always be soft and mushy once cooked. So choose the lentil to suit your dish.

Tiny, premium lentils

Ideal for salads and other dishes where you want the lentils to remain whole and well defined. These are all pretty interchangeable, although I'm sure some local chefs will be up in arms at such a suggestion.

PUY LENTIL

The king of the castle, a marbled teal-green and slate-hued lentil from the volcanic soils of the Auvergne in France. This is the celebrity lentil with its own Appellation d'Origine Contrôlée, like a fine wine. Puy lentils have a wonderful nutty and almost peppery flavour.

Confession: I have also cheated with the Puy lookalikes, labelled small French lentils, with very acceptable results.

CASTELLUCCIO, OR UMBRIAN, LENTIL

Italians love their lentils. They are traditionally served at New Year, each lentil representing a tiny coin that swells in the stock and promises a prosperous year ahead. The tiny greenish-brown Umbrian lentil, with its sweet earthy flavour, grows on the Castelluccio plains and is sought out by chefs all over Europe. Like the Puy, it has its own protected geographical status.

PARDINA LENTIL

The *lenteja pardina* is the Spanish tiny, hold-its-shape lentil. It doesn't look very glamorous (*pardo* translates as dull brown),

but these are some of my favourite lentils to use. They have a nutty, almost herbaceous, flavour and they have their own protected status too.

BLACK BELUGA LENTIL

The glistening black North American lentil may look like caviar when it's raw, but it does lose a bit of its designer edge once cooked. I wouldn't bust a gut seeking these out over any of the other tiny lentils, but they are a very tasty option and do add a certain glitz to your menu description.

Rustic lentils

The brown or green lentil (depending where you are and who's selling it) is the common-or-garden lentil for soups, stews and mashes. It's bigger and flatter than its diminutive cousins (above). There are no flashy names or high price tags, but don't turn your nose up at the rustic flat lentil, it could be just what you're after. Sometimes you do want a lentil that will soften and break down into a creamy mash for a soup or stew. These softer lentils are perfect in Middle Eastern dishes with fried onions or rice, or in a Spanish porky *cazuela*.

Split lentils: red lentils, Egyptian lentils, masoor dal

These are all very similar. They are hulled (skinned) and split lentils and so they cook more quickly, collapse to a mush and are more easily digested than whole lentils. Split lentils make fabulous soups and dals. With a bag of these in the cupboard, a cheap and nutritious dinner is never far away.

Many other split pulses are used to make the Indian dals, but these are actually split gram (beans or chickpeas) rather than lentils.

PEA (*PISUM SATIVUM*)

Peas are one of the ancient crops from the Fertile Crescent of the Middle East, which have been cultivated for around 9,000 years. They quickly spread across Europe and Asia and became a key source of protein in much of northern Europe. Peas are a winter crop in the Mediterranean basin, thriving in the cooler, damper weather, and so they are brilliantly suited to the northern climate.

'Pease' were consumed in huge quantities in Britain from the Middle Ages right into the 20th century, but these weren't the tender, green garden peas that we all have in the freezer as our default vegetable – they were dried. 'Pease pudding hot, Pease pudding cold, Pease pudding in the pot nine days old.' The old English nursery rhyme is a reminder of how our ancestors ate: pease porridge and a spot of bacon if you were lucky or a bowl of gruel if you weren't.

Of all the pulses, dried peas seem to take the longest to cook. This is why split peas are so much better for soups than any of the whole dried peas. So, although in most cases I'm not a great fan of adding bicarbonate of soda to my pot (see p.15), when I use whole peas I make an exception, otherwise they could be bubbling all day before they soften. A pressure cooker can really speed things up.

Fresh peas

Eating fresh peas did not become fashionable until the late 17th century, when they were seen as rather a novelty, a luxury item consumed in the royal courts. If you can track down very fresh peas in the pod, or better still grow your own, then a fresh pea is an amazingly sweet thing.

Garden peas make wonderful quick soups and purées and their tough pods contribute a lovely flavour to a vegetable stock. Canned garden peas make no sense to me at all: tried once, never again!

Tender-podded peas – which you eat pods and all – are delicious in salads.

Marrowfat peas

The only acceptable pea to use for Britain's traditional mushy peas. These are peas that have been left to plump up, mature and partially dry on the plant. They are then fully dried. When cooking, an alkaline such as bicarbonate of soda is useful to ensure soft, mushy results.

You can buy marrowfats dried, canned, or already processed into mushy peas. I have to admit that I'd always turned my nose up at the canned peas until I came upon a quick trick from the fabulous Nigella. Just whizz up a drained can of peas with a ripe avocado, a clove or two of crushed garlic and a dash of fresh lime juice. An inspired, instant crostini topping.

Carlin peas

Also known rather fabulously as Black Badger Peas, Red Fox Peas or Maple peas, these old Northern English peas have been enjoying a bit of a come back of late. Traditionally served as 'parched peas' with nothing more than salt and vinegar, they are wonderfully nutty in flavour and work well in curries and salads.

Blue and Yellow peas

Not that easy to come by, these peas do take some time to cook but give wonderful results in spiced dishes. You could try sprouting them for a great burst of sweet flavour over the top of a salad.

Rather confusingly, once a blue pea is skinned and split it becomes a split green pea!

Split peas

These are dried peas that have been skinned and split in half.

Green and yellow split peas are interchangeable in any recipe.

Green split peas have more of a 'pea-like' flavour. Yellow are the most traditional in all the old English and northern European classic soups and pottages, but there's nothing to stop you throwing in the green instead. Both make a fabulous backdrop for a hearty winter soup or play starring roles in many of the creamy dals of India.

Split peas are ideal for infants and anyone who finds pulses tricky to digest. There's no need to soak them either, although it will cut down the cooking time. Split peas can be substituted for red lentils but will take longer to cook.

BROAD BEAN, FAVA BEAN (*VICIA FABA*)

The Old World's original bean, the fava, was an Egyptian staple back in the days of the pharoahs, although it was considered fit only for slaves and animals. The fava was the only bean known to Europeans for millennia but it did not always enjoy great popularity. The Greeks believed that any wind experienced as a result of eating the beans was the souls of the dead passing from their resting place in the ground, through the soil, into the bean and finally through your body. Now there's a thought next time you suffer from a little flatulence.

Broad beans were associated with death and burials by the Romans and Celts too. All these morbid connections are perhaps no coincidence, since there is a potentially fatal syndrome connected with eating fava beans. Favism is a rare condition that strikes people with a particular enzyme deficiency, many of whom live in, or can trace their origins back to, the southern Mediterranean or the Middle East.

Today the broad bean is proudly considered the Egyptian national dish in *ful medames* (see p.181). China is the world's largest producer: the beans are served as a vegetable and also used, fermented, in the Sichuan sauce *doubanjiang* (along with soya beans and chilli).

Fresh broad beans

Tiny broad beans are heaven, they'll be the first thing I'll grow on my allotment, when I make the time for one (I've only been dreaming about it for a decade now). It's just so bizarre how older gardeners feel that a broad bean is only worth harvesting once it's a leathery giant.

Eaten raw, pods and all, they are absolutely fabulous, but you'll need to pick them while they're the length of your little finger. Next come the diminutive baby broad beans, popped out of their downy pods; eaten raw with sheep's cheese as they do in Rome, or fried up with some Iberian ham, they are unbeatable. Sprinkle them over a salad with fresh mint and you have the essence of summer.

The juicy, slightly more mature bean (still only the size of your thumb nail) requires only super-quick cooking. Just like the pea, tasty sugars begin to turn to starch within hours of picking. It's a question of using either very fresh or, perfectly acceptable, frozen broad beans. If they are on the large side, and let's hope they're not, you can blanch them (when using frozen that job's been done) and pop them out of their skins to reveal the vibrant green bean inside. Amazing in salads, soups, risottos and side dishes.

Dried fava beans

Dried broad beans or fava beans, known as '*ful*', are consumed in huge quantities across the Eastern Mediterranean, Middle East and the Horn of Africa. Surprisingly, huge quantities of the beans are grown in East Anglia, dried and then shipped to the Arab world. So, rather ironically since they are one of Britain's only homegrown dried pulses, they are not easy to track down in British supermarkets, although Greek, Turkish or Middle Eastern shops will certainly stock them.

WHOLE BEANS

The whole, dried brown beans are typically used in the Egyptian national dish of *ful medames*, but you will find variations on the size and type of fava bean used all around the Levant.

The slightly bitter flavour of broad beans (from the tannins in their skin) can be an acquired taste. You will remove some of the bitterness by tipping away the soaking water and also by changing the water that you cook the beans in after about 20 minutes. Favas do take a long time to soften, so be patient, add a teaspoon of bicarbonate of soda to the cooking water or, better still, use a pressure cooker.

SPLIT FAVAS

Quicker cooking, shelled and split varieties are better suited to making felafel (the Egyptians use fava beans rather than chickpeas) and purées rather similar to hummus. They're fabulous for thickening stews, too.

OLD WORLD BEANS

The beans of the *Vigna* genus, native to the Old World, are some of the principal pulses in the Asian and African diet, yet many of these beans still seem rather exotic to us in the West. You may have to make a trip to an Asian, African or specialist store to track them down, although many supermarkets carry an increasingly wide range of beans, reflecting the cultural mix of the local community.

The advantage of many of these predominantly tiny beans is that they cook quickly and are easy to digest, causing few of the windy problems associated with legumes. So, all in all, a very good place to start if you are trying to include more beans in your diet.

Adzuki, aduki, azuki, red chouri (*Vigna angularis*)

Was it the Japanese, the Koreans or the Chinese who first cultivated these tiny maroon-red beans? It's a hotly contested issue, so let's just call the adzuki an East Asian bean.

The idea of sweet beans may seem strange to most of us in the West, but in the Far East most adzuki are traditionally cooked with sugar and made into the red bean paste that is used in many desserts and sweets, such as mooncakes, dumplings and ice cream.

The adzuki bean is fabulous in savoury dishes too. The cooked beans are sometimes stir-fried in China. In India, where they are often known as red chouri, they end up in dals and curries. The adzuki is also a big player in some parts of Africa: in Somalia, it is mixed with butter and sugar in the staple sweet dish *cambuulo*.

Adzuki beans cook in about 40 minutes from dry and even more quickly if you get around to soaking them. Their nutty flavour is wonderful in salads, stir-fries and curries, and they're also one of my favourite beans to sprout.

Mung bean, green/golden gram, moong dal (*Vigna radiata*)

The chameleon of beans, the mung bean pops up in different guises around the world. We've all been eating mung beans for years, perhaps without even knowing it. Back in my student days, it was only the crisp white **bean sprouts** and a dash of soy sauce that lent those rather dubious stir-fries a touch of the exotic. In China, the mung bean is eaten mostly as a bean sprout but also, in common with most of East Asia, sweetened with sugar and served as a dessert.

Another mung bean incarnation is the cellophane or **glass noodle** made from mung bean starch. These spectacularly light noodles are fabulous in soups and salads, soaking up flavours and adding their wispy body to a dish.

In the Arab world **mung beans** are often prepared with rice and spices or cooked in vegetable casseroles. The beans require no soaking and are usually ready in about 45 minutes, so they make a great storecupboard standby.

In Indian cuisine, the bean becomes completely unrecognizable. **Moong dal** (aka green gram or golden gram) is skinned and split, revealing the golden interior often confused with a lentil. The split beans break down into the most fabulously creamy texture for delicious dals.

Moth bean, mat/matki bean, dew bean, Turkish gram (*Vigna aconitifolia*)

You are not going to find moth beans (pronounced 'moat' ... sound a bit more appetizing?) in your local corner shop unless you live somewhere with a large Indian community. However, as a keen sprouter, I just couldn't leave them out. These rather unassuming-looking little beans burst into crunchy sprouts in about 24 hours and then make the most fabulous stir-fry (see p.188). Moth beans make good substitutes for mung beans and can be cooked from dry in about 20 minutes.

Urad dal, urd, black gram, kali dal (*Vigna mungo*)

You will probably only find tiny urd or urad beans in specialist Indian shops or online. They are highly prized in their homeland, where they are considered to make the very best dals and have religious significance to the Hindus. The tiny black beans are sometimes confused with black lentils, but on close inspection they are quite obviously beans. They are sometimes cooked whole, but more often than not they are skinned and split, revealing their white interiors (unlike the mung bean which is more golden). The dry split beans are often quick-fried, almost like a spice, to add texture and flavour to various pickles.

The flour ground from the split beans is used in all sorts of southern Indian specialities such as pappads, idli and poppadams.

Cow pea, black-eyed pea, lobhia (*Vigna unguiculata*)

Let's start by pointing out that it's not a pea at all; scientifically speaking, it's a bean, but as far as the cook's concerned, does it really matter? Not all cow peas have the distinctive black marking of the black-eyed pea, but it is the most common variety.

The cow pea originated in Africa and is still one of the most important sub-Saharan crops. The plants are incredibly hardy and can withstand extremely hot, dry conditions and grow in poor sandy soils. Cow peas were grown in ancient Greece (they're still a Greek favourite) and Rome and quickly spread throughout Asia, turning up in Indian dals and as fresh yard-long beans in China and the Far East.

Black-eyed peas are hugely popular in the southern United States (and I'm not talking hip-hop now), where they are cooked up with pork and rice for the traditional New Year's dish of Hoppin' John. Many mistakenly assume that they're an American native, but in fact the black-eyed peas made their way over to America, Brazil and the Caribbean with African slaves. Not just the beans, but traditional dishes came too. *Acarajé*, the deep-fried dried shrimp and black-eyed pea cakes sold on the streets of Brazilian Bahia, are closely related to Nigerian *akara*.

These little beans cook in less than an hour, and you can halve the time if you remember to soak them. They are fabulous in salads, rice dishes and stews, with their earthy, almost minerally flavour.

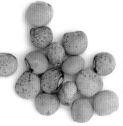

Pigeon pea, gungo pea, Congo pea/bean, gandule bean, toor/tu-var/toovar dal (*Cajanus cajan*)
Another bean posing as a pea. Pigeon peas are probably most familiar in the Caribbean dish of rice and peas. They are also a vital crop in Africa (they arrived in the Americas with the slave trade), where as well as using them dried, they are often eaten fresh: shoots, leaves and all.

Pigeon peas are also immensely popular in India. You are most likely to find them skinned and split as toor dal, used to make the nutritious porridgey soups known as dal. Toor dal can be confused with split yellow peas or chana dal (split chickpeas): while they may have rather different textures, flavours (toor are quite gelatinous and very savoury) and cooking times, you could get away with substituting one for another.

You may also come across oily toor dal, which have been treated with vegetable oil to prolong their shelf life. You need to give them a good rinse before cooking.

SOYA BEAN, SOYBEAN (*GLYCINE MAX*)
This Old World bean is relatively new to the West, but has achieved global dominance in the past 80 years. The Jekyll and Hyde of the bean world, soya is by far and away the most widely produced and consumed pulse on the planet; it is also both the most celebrated and the most controversial. Soy has been a food crop for over 5,000 years; originally considered the food of the poor in ancient China, it is now one of the mainstays of industrial food production throughout the world.

The soya bean is streets ahead of all the other pulses in its oil content (about 20%) and protein content (about 40%). It is, unlike other pulses, considered a 'complete' protein capable of providing all the essential amino acids, and is thus a great alternative protein source to meat, fish and dairy.

Edamame
Edamame are fresh, green, immature soya beans that are usually sold in the pod. Blanched quickly, they make a delicious snack served with a pinch of salt. These are now available in the salad and snack cabinets of many supermarkets. Edamame has become such a by-word for healthy snacks that even a chocolate-coated roasted edamame is apparently an energy-enhancing treat.

Frozen green soya beans
These are podded edamame, which you can find next to the peas and broad beans in the freezer cabinets in some supermarkets. The beans are usually a little bit bigger than the edamame sold in pods.

Frozen soya beans require very little cooking, just a quick steam or boil, but I do find them rather bland and mealy on their own. However, their fabulous lime-green colour will lift all sorts of bean salads and stir-fries, and they are a low-fat, high-protein addition to any healthy meal.

Dried soya beans and today's Western derivatives
In its mature dried form, the soya bean is very difficult to digest. The beans need to be cooked for hours to remove toxins and to render them vaguely tender, and the flavour is excessively 'beany'. There are so many other beans out there, why bother? Some people buy the dried beans to extract their own 'milk'.

In East Asia, cooked soya beans have been converted by various ancient processes into more appetizing and digestible products, such as tofu, tempeh, miso and soy sauce, for thousands of years. But it was not until the 1930s that the West developed a way to unlock the protein and oil content of the soya bean to suit its own needs. Nowadays a vast proportion of the world crop is processed into the soya oil and high-protein soybean meals that make their way into our food supply. Remarkably, the world's soya crop has doubled in the last 15 years.

Today we consume much of our soya unwittingly in processed foods, where it is used as a 'meat extender' in many ready meals. It's cheap, it's low in fat, it's high in protein, it's the food industry's magic ingredient. Soy lecithin is used an emulsifier in margarines, chocolate and many other products. Soy is used as a flour 'improver' in the commercial baking industry. Soy oil is one of the cheapest and most ubiquitous of cooking oils (usually labelled vegetable oil). And that's without mentioning all the low-fat, dairy-free milks, yogurts and dubious cheeses that are made from soya beans. However, probably the most surprising to many of us is that a huge amount of the livestock feed in Europe is soybean meal imported from the Americas. Commercial dairy, pork and chicken farming rely on this high-protein meal for the increasingly large milk yields and fast growth demanded by the food industry.

So, does all that soy in our diets matter? Many, and I'm one of them, would scream 'yes'. Conservationists are increasingly concerned that, with soaring world demand and prices to match, developing economies such as Argentina and Brazil (the second and third largest world producers after the US – in 2010 China came in fifth) will continue to expand their production. Vast swathes of rainforest and grassland will continue to be lost to soya, with a huge impact upon the environment. There are plenty of health concerns, too. Hailed by many as the great weapon against cancer, particularly breast and prostate, some scientists are suggesting that the effects of consuming excessive quantities of soya may be quite the opposite. The previously celebrated high levels of plant oestrogens (phyto-oestrogens) are now being blamed by some for early-onset puberty and infertility issues, too. It's a nutritionist's minefield.

My conclusion is this. Like everything else, it's best to eat soy in moderation. Prepare your own food and then you will know what you are eating. Research suggests that less processed soya products are much better for you, so go for the most natural, organic products available. Follow the lead of the East, with their ancient understanding of the bean, predominantly consuming fresh green (edamame) beans, or fermented soya, in which the levels of phyto-oestrogens are dramatically lower.

Tofu or bean curd

Tofu could be called the cheese of the East. Soy milk, extracted from the cooked beans, is curdled by adding either salty or acid coagulants, and the curd is then pressed into cakes.

Try to buy organic tofu and prepare it yourself rather than buying highly processed tofu products. It is best to drain the firm tofu before use. Recipes often call for you to press it between two plates to squeeze out excess moisture. The tofu is then ready to marinate or to dust in cornflour and fry.

Silken tofu has a much softer, creamier texture than the more readily available firm tofu. In East Asia, it is often prepared as an uncooked savoury dish or as a dessert. It can be useful when preparing dairy-free sauces and puddings.

Tofu can provide an important source of protein for vegetarians and vegans and, in the Far East, has often been thought of as 'famine food' as a result of its incredible nutritional value. However, many of us do not need to increase our protein intake. Instead, we need to find ways of enjoying tofu, rather than suffering it. Tofu on its own is incredibly bland, but given the right treatment can be absolutely delicious (see recipe on p.199).

Tofu becomes much chewier after freezing, which can be an advantage, depending on the recipe.

Tempeh

Tempeh bears little resemblance to the neutral blank canvas that is tofu: it has a distinctive and delicious savoury flavour of its own. Like tofu, tempeh is a bean curd, but it is fermented in an ancient process that originated in Indonesia. You will probably find tempeh in a vacuum pack in your local health store; it won't look like much but I do urge you to give it a go. Fried up and served with a splash of chilli sauce, it might even convert the resolute carnivore (see also the recipe on p.198).

Miso

Miso is a fermented paste that lends an amazingly nutty, salty and savoury depth wherever you use it. The paste is usually made with soya beans, salt, rice or barley and a fungus, or starter culture. It's a staple of the Japanese kitchen but is used in much of East Asia.

Paler, creamy-coloured miso has gone through a quicker fermentation process and is milder and less salty, while darker misos have a more mature, stronger flavour. Miso is the key to that *umami*, savoury, depth of flavour sought out in Japanese cooking. I find it invaluable in vegetarian recipes too, where a quick dash can give an instant third dimension.

Soy sauce

The traditional Chinese and Japanese condiment has become a universal ingredient. It is traditionally made by fermenting a mixture of soya beans, wheat and salt with various types of bacteria and yeast, over several months. There are many inferior soy sauces made by a much speedier process and so I always look for those labelled 'organic' or 'naturally brewed'.

As with miso paste, when dealing with the naturally fermented sauces, the darker the sauce, the more pronounced the flavour.

Tamari, one of my favourite soy sauces, is a traditional Japanese sauce made without wheat.

Ketjap manis, the Indonesian soy, is syrupy, sweetened with sugar and flavoured with spices.

Black beans (fermented)

Chinese fermented and salted soya beans are usually referred to simply as black beans. They have no connection with the Mexican black (turtle) bean.

The pungent little beans are used as a seasoning in sauces and stir-fries, giving an amazing range of bitter, sweet, sour, salty flavour.

You can buy the beans by the bag from Asian stores. Once opened, they will keep for several months in an airtight container. It's an idea to rinse the beans before use as they can be very salty. Black bean paste or sauce is available in many supermarkets too.

NEW WORLD BEANS

The discovery of the Americas by the European powers in the late 15th century brought with it many of the crops and foodstuffs that are the kings of the kitchen today. Just imagine our depleted larder without potatoes, peppers, tomato, corn, chocolate, vanilla and the huge variety of beans.

Western Europe embraced the New World beans far more readily than it had many of the Asian species, partly because they were more suited to the climate. Nowadays many of these beans are seen as part of the European culinary heritage. Try telling a Tuscan that his treasured borlotti is in fact a hybrid Mexican bean, or a Basque that the celebrated Tolosa black is just a turtle bean in disguise. Over the centuries, many of the South and Central American beans have evolved in Europe, in North America (where there are simply hundreds of 'heirloom' beans) and even in Asia into varieties with their own distinctive culinary qualities. Back in their Latin American homeland, there's virtually a bean for every dish.

While I aim to cover the most popular and readily available varieties, please don't hurl your book down in disgust when I leave out your favourite calico pole bean or tasty *alubia del ganxet*. Many speciality beans are grown in tiny quantities and are consumed by locals in their own traditional dish. The Tarbais bean may be the authentic cassoulet bean in south-west France, but are you likely to pick one up in Cardiff? I think not. Beans are readily interchangeable, so go forth and experiment if you meet a newcomer – you could be in for a treat.

Butter bean, lima bean, Madagascar bean (*Phaseolus lunatus*)

The butter bean is a bean apart from all the other Latino beans, not just because of its size and creamy texture but also because of its Andean origins. It is from a quite different bean family from all the kidney and haricot beans, and many would say a more aristocratic bean altogether.

Butter beans are perhaps my number one bean; they're wonderful in salads and work well with mustardy vinaigrettes, they have an affinity with leeks and are fabulous with creamy or more acidic tomato sauces. However, they can be quite a challenge to cook. They require a long overnight soak and then a really slow, gentle simmer, otherwise they seem to shed their skins and collapse more readily than other beans.

The Spanish *judiones* are my favourite variety, and I quite often cheat by using the jars of ready-cooked creamy beans. They are an extravagance, but worth every penny – you can really understand why they are called 'butter' beans.

The dried Greek *gigantes* ('giant' or 'elephant') beans are spectacular, although most supermarkets seem to sell them ready-cooked in a tomato sauce.

Definitions get complicated in North America, where many varieties of lima beans are grown and eaten fresh as well as dried. In the southern US, the term 'butterbean' refers to the smaller, flat green beans instead of the large, slippery, creamy variety we are talking about.

Almost all of the *Phaseolus lunatus* family need cooking, be they fresh or dried, as they contain varying levels of cyanide. Commercial varieties have been selected for their safer, lower levels, but should you start growing your own, it's probably best to cut out any garden grazing. For more details, I recommend the joyfully named tome, *How To Poison Your Spouse the Natural Way* by Jay D. Mann.

The common bean (*Phaseolus vulgaris*)

This is by far the biggest group of New World beans. The varieties evolved from a south-western Mexican legume about 7,000 years ago. By the time the Europeans arrived, these pulses were widespread, and cultivated right across the Americas. The common bean has been developed into beans of all sizes, colours, flavours and textures, including haricots, flageolets and kidney beans.

Haricot bean, navy bean, pea bean (*Phaseolus vulgaris*)

If you've only ever eaten one bean as a Brit, it will be this one! The British consume haricots by the ton in all those cans of good old baked beans.

The tiny round haricot is rather bland, not something I would put into a salad, for example, but it soaks up other flavours such as tomatoes and pork wonderfully well. So the haricot is ideal for slow-cooked dishes such as the traditional Boston baked beans and that king of all bean pots, the cassoulet of south-west France.

There are many varieties of haricot that fit their own local dish perfectly, such as the Tarbais or white coco that star in cassoulet, but they are hard to track down outside the region. White coco, and other varieties such as the Spanish *pochas*, are sometimes cooked semi-fresh, straight from the pod. The French *haricots de Soissons* are the giants of the common bean world and have the most velvety texture imaginable when puréed into soups.

Meanwhile in Tuscany, the Italian bean capital, pale yellow *zolfino* and the pearly-white *sorana* beans attract gastronomic pilgrimages. Other white beans to look out for are the diminutive *arrocina*, or 'rice', beans from Spain, which I have found in my local deli. These creamy little beans have lots of flavour and hold their shape well.

The American Great Northern bean is a larger type of haricot with similar qualities to the smaller varieties. It's too subtle and starchy to play centre stage, but works well in casseroles and stews and is a popular substitute for the navy bean in traditional baked beans. Whilst Great Northerns are readily available in the US, I've yet to find them elsewhere.

Flageolet bean (*Phaseolus vulgaris*)

These little green celebrities of the French bean world are also known as *chevrier verts*, in honour of Monsieur Gabriel Chevrier who first cultivated them in the 1870s on the outskirts of Paris. It's a particular strain of dwarf haricot that retains its fresh green colour due to its ability to retain chlorophyll, even once dried in the pod. And, unlike so many beans that lose their glamour in the pot, the flageolet is a stunner once cooked too.

The tiny flageolet not only looks and sounds elegant, it has a fine skin that makes it easily digestible and especially creamy. It works wonderfully with lamb, pork, cream and tarragon.

Another variety of small green bean that is worth a mention is the Spanish *verdina* bean. Slightly less kidney-shaped than the flageolet and with a lustrous jade-green skin, these are the ultimate bean to prepare with clams, as they do in Asturias. You'll probably not find them outside the local area, but the north coast of Spain is a bean Mecca and well worth a visit.

Cannellini bean (*Phaseolus vulgaris*)

One of the most famous Italian beans is the cannellini. It's a white kidney bean, possibly an Argentinian native, that has made itself at home in central and southern Italy.

You may be lucky enough to find fresh cannellini in their pods, as they are sometimes sold in Italy. They are allowed to mature fully on the plant, so they will need plenty of cooking (about half an hour or so), and you will lose about half their weight in the pods, but they are heaven. Dried beans are the more likely prospect. Cannellini are particularly creamy and slightly nutty-tasting and lend themselves beautifully to vegetable soups and salads doused in extra-virgin olive oil.

As a close relation of the red kidney bean, it's a good precaution to boil these for 10 minutes at the beginning of the cooking to avoid any possibility of food poisoning (see red kidney beans below).

Another highly fêted white kidney bean is the Spanish *faba de Asturias*, the star ingredient in the local pork and bean dish, but its production is limited and price usually exorbitant.

Red kidney bean, rajma dal (*Phaseolus vulgaris*)

The ubiquitous bean of chilli con carne. Yet kidney beans have so much more to offer: they look fantastic, have a firm texture, hold together well and have a slightly sweet, almost meaty flavour. They are fabulous paired with sharp and hot, spicy flavours.

Red kidney beans are particularly popular in Latin American, Caribbean and Indian cooking, where they are often teamed up with rice.

Plenty of people are rather cautious about cooking beans from scratch and it's the red kidney we have to blame. Many of the common beans contain a toxin called phytohaemagglutinin, but it's only the red kidney bean that contains high enough concentrations to cause real problems, which can range from an upset stomach to full-on food poisoning. A good long soak and a change of water before cooking are advisable, but the crucial bit is the boiling. The toxin is deactivated by boiling for 10 minutes, so the long, slow simmer required to soften the beans should always be preceded by the boil. Slow cookers are fine as long as you remember to boil for 10 minutes first, otherwise you will actually be increasing the toxin levels.

Borlotti, coco rose, Roman bean, cranberry bean (*Phaseolus vulgaris*)

If there was ever a bean to make a fashion statement, it would be the borlotti, with its pink Missoni-style jacket. The fresh pods are a stunning sight in summer markets. The magic continues as you open the pods to reveal the beans within, each speckled like an exquisite little wren's egg. The most readily available beans are dried, but do try to track down the fresh beans if you can. These require no soaking, will cook in about 30 minutes, and are fabulous smothered in extra-virgin olive oil. The celebrity of the borlotti world is, without a doubt, the Lamon bean from the Italian Alps.

All the borlotti, *coco rose*, Roman and cranberry beans are closely related and probably evolved from the Colombian cargamonto bean. I happily interchange them and tend to use the most evocative name to suit the menu or the dish.

Once cooked, the beans do lose their rather chichi markings, turning a deep reddish brown, but what they lose in looks they more than make up for in creamy, nutty flavour.

Pinto bean (*Phaseolus vulgaris*)

Literally 'painted bean', named for their rather splotchy mottled skins, these are the most commonly used bean in north-west Mexico and the southern United States. The pinto more often than not ends up as the refried bean or piled into a chilli.

Other very similar but not so widely available beans are rattlesnake, appaloosa and anasazi beans. You'd probably have to be in cowboy country to track any of those down, but who knows? There's a huge resurgence of interest in heirloom beans in the US right now; give it a few years and I'll probably spot them on my local supermarket shelf. In the meantime, I'll raise a few eyebrows by suggesting a borlotti in its place. It may not have quite the same sweet beany flavour, and the skin is a little thicker, but by the time you've got all the Mexican trappings, will anybody notice?

The Basques have their own speckled *pinta alavesa* and the rather similar red *alubia de Gernika* and maroon/black *alubia de Tolosa* bean. Oh I know that I'll be chastized for this by some Basque bean fancier or even the local bean brotherhood (and yes, there is one!), but these beans refry very well and are delicious cooked up with all manner of porky things and served with a touch of chilli heat – just like a pinto.

Black bean, black turtle bean (*Phaseolus vulgaris*)

Dramatic black beans turn to a glorious deep purple once cooked in their most traditional guise – *frijoles de la olla*, or pot beans. Growers can track down evocatively named varieties such as Zorro, Black Valentine and Nighthawk, but most of us will have to make do with the good old black turtle. They are all varieties of the same little Mexican bean, with its dense, meaty texture and sweet, almost mushroomy, flavour.

Black beans are a little firmer than the cooked pinto, so this is my bean of choice when I want to make a zippy salad or fling some beans into a spiced vegetable soup. Black beans are very popular in Latin America, where they are the stars of Brazilian *feijoada* (see p.232), and right across the Caribbean. They have nothing to do with Asian fermented black beans (see p.261).

BAMBARA GROUNDNUT, BAMBARA BEAN (*VIGNA SUBTERRANEA*) AND PEANUT, GROUNDNUT, GOOBER PEA, MONKEY NUT (*ARACHIS HYPOGAEA*)

Peanuts and groundnuts are, scientifically speaking, legumes and not nuts. The bambara groundnut and the peanut are extremely unusual in that their edible seeds grow and ripen underground. There are many similarities between the two and yet they have totally different origins.

The bambara groundnut is an African species and is widely cultivated in much of West Africa as it can withstand incredibly hot, dry growing conditions. These nuts provide vital protein for people living on marginal agricultural land.

The peanut came from South America and was introduced by the Europeans to Africa and to North America. The peanut is more productive and easier to harvest than the groundnut, and it's higher in protein and oil. Rather confusingly, it became known as a groundnut as well.

Nowadays huge quantities of peanuts are grown in Asia, where they are used primarily for oil. In sub-Saharan Africa, groundnut stew (and this time we're talking peanuts) is a staple that provides vital protein, minerals, vitamins and calories to millions every day. Meanwhile, in the US and Europe, the peanut is consumed mostly as a snack or as peanut butter.

AND THE REST…

There are hundreds of legumes out there that I haven't mentioned, primarily because you're unlikely to find them, they're used as animal fodder or we don't really eat the seeds. But just so you know that they weren't forgotten, here are a few of the more important ones:

• All those green beans such as runner beans, haricots verts, winged beans, where the pod rather than the bean is the star – that's another book!

• Alfalfa – you might come across this as a sprouted seed but most cultivated alfalfa is actually used as animal fodder.

• Lupins – yes, those towering rods of cottage garden colour are one hybrid of a plant that provides small edible peas, which are used as animal fodder but also turn up as a bar snack on a saucer with your *cerveza* in southern Spain, Portugal, Turkey and the eastern Mediterranean.

• Hyacinth beans, or lablab beans, are grown across Asia and Africa; they need prolonged boiling due to the cyanide they contain (and have generally been avoided by food retailers as a result of it). You'll find them in southern Indian curries and they're popular in Kenya, too, where they are a must for breastfeeding mothers, apparently increasing lactation.

• Tamarind, native to Africa but grown throughout Asia and also in the Americas, are huge trees that produce brittle pods filled with inedible seeds. However, the sweet and sour pulp that surrounds the seeds is delicious and used as a souring agent (see p.247).

• Tepary beans are a super-hardy, drought-resistant bean native to the American south-west and northern Mexico. Supposedly exceptionally nutritious and sweet, they've yet to make it onto the world stage.

INDEX

ACKNOWLEDGEMENTS

For Libbus, you're super human, I'm so proud of you.

HUGE THANKS

To everyone at Pavilion, especially to Emily Preece-Morrison who embraced my idea from the outset and made this book come true. I have so loved working with you on this project, thank you for your encouragement, support and dealing with an overwrite of epic proportions!

To Maggie Ramsay, for your meticulous editing, patience and being fun with it all too.

To all of you who've made this book look stunning, leaving the hippy hessian right out of the picture. To Georgina Hewitt for the stylish layout design and dealing with all those tiny pulse shots. And then for the simply amazing photos: I am so grateful to stylist Wei Tang, to Maud Eden for cooking the dishes so beautifully, to Natalie Costaras for keeping everything running smoothly and to super-talented photographer Clare Winfield for your fabulous vision. Not only do I love the pictures, but you were such a calm and positive team to work with, I so enjoyed the shoot in sunny Sydenham.

To Hannah Cameron McKenna for all your invaluable recipe testing, you have been remarkably generous with your time, your comments, advice and enthusiasm. To Conor too, you probably consumed more pulses in your first year of married life than in all the rest of them put together.

To every cook, chef, food writer and friend who's kindly shared a recipe: Richard Bertinet, Sarah Britton, Mercé Brunés, Ursula Ferrigno, Clara Grace Paul, Barney McGrath and Leticia Valverdes. And to those who have allowed me to re-publish a recipe: Hugo Arnold and Leylie Hayes from *Avoca Café Cookbook* (Avoca Handweavers, 2000), Rosemary Barron from *Flavours of Greece* (Grub St, 2010), Jude Blereau from *Coming Home to Eat – Wholefood for the Family* (Murdoch Books, 2008), Sally Butcher from *Veggiestan* (Pavilion Books, 2011) and Jennifer Joyce from *Meals in Heels* (Murdoch Books, 2010). And to all the dozens of other writers whose fabulous articles, books and blogs have inspired, answered questions and spawned ideas along the way.

To everyone I work with at Books for Cooks, Divertimenti, Leiths and The Bertinet Kitchen for wise words and great encouragement.

To all my eager Bristol guinea pigs who often sampled half a dozen pulse experiments at a time, sometimes with the predictable after effects.

To my family: Mum, Richard and Libbus, you've been unbelievably supportive.

Lastly, I'm infinitely grateful to my wonderful Peter and little Imi for keeping me sane (and miraculously remaining so yourselves too) through months of experimentation, endless beany buffets, a chaotic kitchen, wobbles, triumphs and deadlines.

ABOUT THE AUTHOR

Jenny Chandler trained at Leith's School of Food and Wine before embarking upon a decade of cooking and travel, spending many years as a chef on a luxury yacht. During this time she lived in Spain, Italy and France and travelled extensively in the Mediterranean, Caribbean, Pacific and Indian Oceans, giving her the opportunity to gather recipes, techniques and experiences from all over the world. Jenny now lives in Bristol with her partner Peter and daughter Imogen, and spends most of her time writing and teaching at her own school, The Plum Cooking Company in Clifton. She teaches regularly in London and Bath and is also the author of *The Food of Northern Spain* and *The Real Taste of Spain* (both published by Pavilion). Follow her blog on: **http://jennychandlerblog.com/**

REVIEWS OF *PULSE*:

"The future is all about pulses. They are delicious, nutritious and frugal and they represent an important, healthy and sustainable approach to cookery and well-being. Jenny Chandler brings her customary level of research, flair and knowledge to bear on this important subject, to create a work that is comprehensive and compelling."
Silvana de Soissons, *The Foodie Bugle*

"Truly beautiful, both visually and in its writing style, there is so much to learn from this treasure of a book, through simple instructions and marvellously clear pictures that make everything look so lovely and fresh. Quite simply, a must-have book."
Valentina Harris

First published in the United Kingdom in 2013 by Pavilion
43 Great Ormond Street
London WC1N 3HZ
www.pavilionbooks.com

Copyright © 2013 Pavilion Books Company Ltd
Text copyright © 2013 Jenny Chandler
Photograph on p.12 © Diana Miller

ISBN: 9781862059863

A CIP catalogue record for this book is available from the British Library

10 9 8 7 6 5 4

Reproduction by Rival Colour Ltd, UK
Printed by 1010 Printing International Ltd, China

Commissioning editor: Emily Preece-Morrison
Design and art direction: Georgina Hewitt
Photographer: Clare Winfield
Home economist: Maud Eden
Stylist: Wei Tang
Shoot assistant: Natalie Costaras
Shoot location: Light Locations
Copy editor: Maggie Ramsay
Indexer: Ruth Ellis

NOTES
1 teaspoon = 5ml; 1 tablespoon = 15ml.
All spoon measurements are level.

Both metric and imperial measures are given for the recipes. Follow either set of measures, not a mixture of both, as they are not interchangeable.

Medium eggs should be used, except where otherwise specified. Note that some recipes contain raw or lightly cooked eggs. The young, elderly, pregnant women and anyone with an immune-deficiency disease should avoid these, because of the slight risk of salmonella.

To sterilize jars for pickles, sauces and jams, put the jars in a preheated oven at 150°C/300°F/Gas mark 2 for 20 minutes.

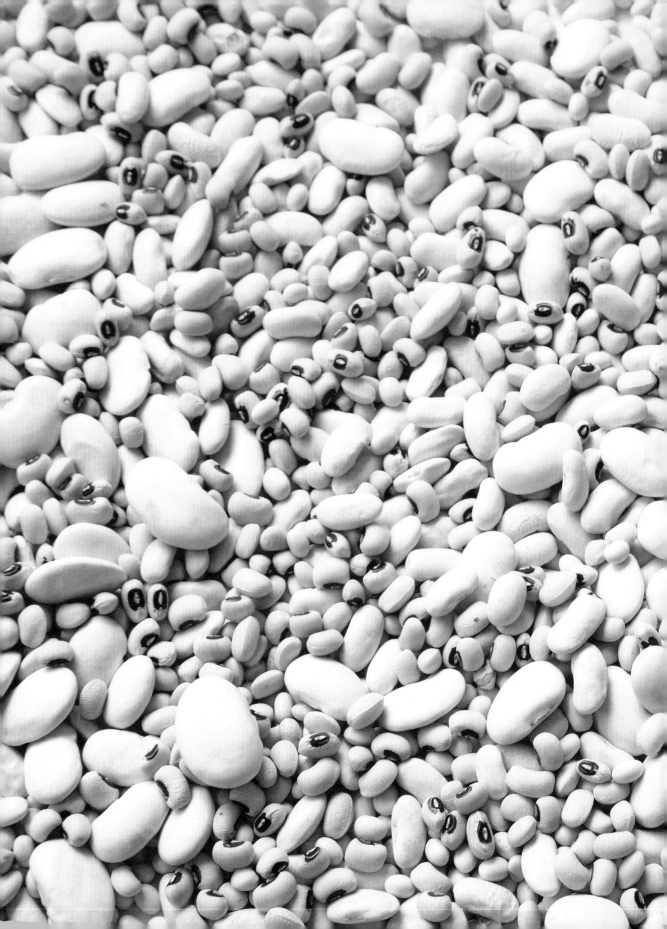